Computerized Cardiopulmonary Exercise Testing

U. J. Winter, K. Wasserman,
N. Treese, H. W. Höpp (Eds.)

Computerized Cardiopulmonary Exercise Testing

Steinkopff Verlag Darmstadt
Springer-Verlag New York

The Editors:
PD Dr. U. J. Winter
Klinik III für
Innere Medizin
Universität Köln
Joseph-Stelzmann-Str. 9
5000 Köln 41

Prof. Dr. H. W. Höpp
Klinik III für
Innere Medizin
Universität Köln
Joseph-Stelzmann-Str. 9
5000 Köln 41

Prof. Dr. K. Wasserman
Harbor UCLA
1000 W. Carson Street
Torrance, CA 90509
USA

Prof. Dr. N. Treese
II. Medizinische Klinik
und Poliklinik
Universität Mainz
Langenbeckstraße 1
6500 Mainz

Die Deutschen Bibliothek — CIP-Einheitsaufnahme

Computerized cardiopulmonary exercise testing / U. J. Winter
... (ed.) — Darmstadt: Steinkopf; New York: Springer, 1991
ISBN 3-7985-0859-3 (Steinkopf)
ISBN 0-387-91404-8 (Springer)
NE: Winter, Ulrich J. [Hrsg.]

Medical Editorial: Sabine Müller — English Editor: James C. Willis — Production: Heinz J. Schäfer
Title-Logo: Graphic Design Pabel-Winkel, Köln

Printed in Germany

Type-setting, printing and bookbinding: Vereinigte Buchdruckereien, Bad Buchau
Printing on acid-free paper

Foreword

The measurement of cardio-circulatory and gas-exchange parameters during physical exercise — the so-called ergospirometry or cardiopulmonary exercise testing (CPX) — as a basis of pathophysiological and clinical research has a long tradition in Cologne. Knipping and his coworkers, especially Hollmann, performed basic research work in healthy subjects. In the area of sports medicine, bicycle or treadmill exercise testing with parallel serial lactate determinations has gained increasing importance for the assessment of cardiac functional capacity. Also, in other medical disciplines, ergospirometry lost its importance. K. Wasserman in Los Angeles is to be credited for having further improved the method to its present standard, a computerized, on-line measuring and practicable cardiopulmonary exercise testing procedure. The prerequisites were technical innovations, such as continuously-measuring gas analyzers and personal computers. Thereby, the knowledge about physiology, pathophysiology, and clinical circumstances of cardiocirculatory and respiratory regulation during exercise were significantly extended. The working groups of W. Hollmann, Cologne, and K. Wasserman, Los Angeles, determined normal values for the gas-exchange parameters and derived values for healthy normals in large populations. Wasserman and coworkers were able to introduce a differential diagnostic concept for patients suffering from various cardiovascular and cardiopulmonary diseases. Many cardiologists, working, for example in myocardial failure or with rate-adaptive pacemakers, belong to those who recommended the modern, computerized ergospirometry. Furthermore, this method is controversely discussed by colleagues working in sports medicine and pulmonary function.

The main topic of the first Cologne CPX Workshop (which was organized by my coworker Priv.-Doz. Dr. U. J. Winter) was the interdisciplinary discussion of clinical and diagnostic values of modern cardiopulmonary exercise testing. This meeting brought together all the experience gained in different medical disciplines. The results of this workshop and these discussions are collected in this book. The active participation of W. Hollmann, pillar of German sports medicine, and of K. Wasserman, the "father" of modern computerized ergospirometry at this meeting was of special benefit for all who attended. I therefore hope for a widespread distribution of this book and a good acceptance by the readers. It is an important source of current information on modern cardiopulmonary exercise testing.

Cologne, FRG — Prof. Dr. H. H. Hilger

Contents

Introduction

Cardiopulmonary exercise testing (CPX) has been proposed to examine the integrity of the heart, lung, and circulation during exercise. This approach is based on the classical view that pulmonary gas exchange, gas transport by the circulatory system, and the cellular gas exchange are functioning together to maintain the "internal milieu" both at rest and during exercise. The analysis of the respiratory gas exchange may provide some insight in possible disorders of this integrated unit. Modern computerized technology has facilitated the analysis of expired gases on breath to breath basis. Therefore interest in this unique tool is growing to readily identify mechanisms of exercise intolerance.

The problem with cardiopulmonary exercise testing today is that this technique originally developed and extensively used in sportsmedicine has now been more and more employed in patients with severely limited excercise capacity. Whereas in sportsmedicine serial lactate determinations have almost resplaced the respiratory gas analysis, cardiologists discover the value of simultaneous assessment of ventilatory and circulatory reserve in their patients.

The first Cologne CPX symposium 1990 was focused on the different views on how to assess cardiopulmonary function. The controversy between sportmedicine using the lactate approach and cardiology employing gas exchange analysis was extensively discussed:

Hollmann gave an unique historical view about the development of ergospirometric devices and experiences with this method since the early beginnings. Fundamental studies from the Deutsche Sporthochschule in Cologne had stimulated the research in this field over a long period of time before switching over to the more metabolic approach using serial lactic acid determination. Heck demonstrated the different concepts and definitions of the anaerobic threshold, based upon serial lactate determinations. Stegemann reported upon a new method with possible application for low exercise capacity. Serial lactate determination as a tool to assess exercise capacity also in patients with cardiopulmonary disorder was appraised by Rost. A critical review of exercise testing in clinical medicine was given by Löllgen, who discussed the possible role of cardiopulmonary exercise testing compared to concurrent methods.

The outstanding contribution of Wasserman and his group from Harbor-UCLA, Torrance in California to the development of respiratory gas analysis during exercise has been appreciated for many years. Their research on the dynamic coupling of external to cellular respiration during exercise has contributed fundamental insight into exercise physiology and presented evidence that the respiratory anaerobic threshold is truly the lactic acidosis threshold. Wasserman discussed his approach to cardiopulmonary exercise testing with the V-Slope Method during an incremental work rate test which allows the non-invasive determination of the anaerobic threshold. It is his methodology which is mostly used by the clinicians today.

While in the United States cardiopulmonary exercise testing has gained wide acceptance, the clinical experience with this technique in our country is still limited to a small number of patients. The first CPX symposium therefore tried to bring together different groups which have alrady gained some clinical experience with respiratory gas exchange analysis during exercise:

Several groups have independently used CPX to assess exercise capacity in rate response pacing. Alt reported on CPX to compare activity controlled and temperature controlled pacing systems. Treese pointed out that this technique allows to optimize pacemaker programming in these patients.

Winter and his group discussed his experience with CPX in patients with coronary heart disease and chronic heart failure. Most interesting was their observation of an oscillatory ventilation pattern in the very severly limited patients. Drexler reviewed clinical studies using cardiopulmonary exercise testing in chronic heart failure. In his own studies a good correlation was found between serial lactate determinations and oxygen uptake at the anaerobic threshold. Kleber reported early results on exercise testing to assess the efficacy of long-term treatment with captopril after myocardial infarction.

The use of cardiopulmonary exercise testing in patients with chronic obstructive pulmonary disease was reported by van Erkelens. The increase of exercise capacity improvement after bronchodilative medication could be demonstrated. Interesting the use of CPX to assess pulmonary function in HIV infected patients as presented by Pothoff.

This first German CPX symposium was thought to encourage further use of cardiopulmonary exercise testing in patients with exercise limitation of various reasons. However, it became also quite clear that a concerted interdisciplinary effort is necessary towards more standardized guidelines for testing and interpretation. A common method is necessary to collect data in larger patient populations and to finally establish the potential diagnostic power and limitations of this interesting technique.

The different papers of this symposium express quite controversial views on how to ideally exercise, however, they demonstrate the increasing importance of exercise as part of the quality of life of many of our patients. We therefore hope that these proceedings will stimulate the interest in cardiopulmonary exercise testing and speed its further application.

Köln, Mainz 1991 — The editors

1. Historical and Methodological Aspects

On the History of Spiroergometry[1])

W. Hollmann, P. Prinz

Institute for Cardiology and Sports Medicine, German Sports University, Cologne

Spiroergometry is a diagnostic procedure for the assessment of the performance capacity of the cardiovascular system, respiration, and metabolism. As far as term and content are concerned, spiroergometry includes two components: spirometry and ergometry. The goal of spirometry is the continuous measurement of respiratory gas metabolism and the continuous registration of respiration (spirography). Here, the measurement of oxygen consumption — which is synonymous with oxygen uptake — is much more important than that of CO_2 expiration. Ergometry constitutes a method for the exact dose of physical work and its precise reproduction at any time. The history of science shows that, initially, spirometry and ergometry were used sporadically and later more systemically in the experimental arrangements of research scientists. H. W. Knipping was the first in the 1920s to unite both elements into a standardized clinical procedure [60, 61]. The following historical overview describes milestones in the joining of ergometry and spirometry.

The first attempts to measure human gas metabolism during quantified physical work were made in 1790 by the versatile French scientist Antoine Laurent Lavoisier and his assistant Armand Seguin [99]. Lavoisier measured his assistant's oxygen consumption under different experimental conditions, e.g. at rest and during physical exercise. Apparently the exercise consisted of weightlifting. It appears that the workload was not preset, but that at the end of the experiment it was calculated as the total height of lift of the weight per unit of time. Two mutually corroborative illustrations of these experiments show that the gas metabolism examinations were based on the attachment method using a face mask. The investigators absorbed the expired carbon dioxide by means of a solution of alkali hydroxydes; the oxygen content of the inhaled air was presumably measured eudiometrically [49], which means that the oxygen was led into a water-soluble compound. The measured oxygen consumption per hour was between 24 liters (sober, at rest, and at 32.5 °C) and 91 liters (exercise during digestion) [99].

Further investigations into the gas metabolism of exercising humans were conducted by the English physician William Prout in 1813. He is particularly known to chemists as the creator of the "Prout Hypothesis" (chemical elements are integral multiples of hydrogen) [17]. During and after walks, Prout collected his own exhaled air in a bag and later analyzed its carbon dioxide content. By varying the walking distance and velocity, he distinguished between moderate and intensive physical exercise. However, Prout obtained no conclusive results [90].

In 1856 a handy method of measuring the amount of inspired air and expired carbon dioxide during exercise was developed by the English physician and hygienist Edward Smith [19]. While wearing a face mask he inhaled ambient air through a

[1]) Supported by the Federal Institute for Sports Science, Cologne

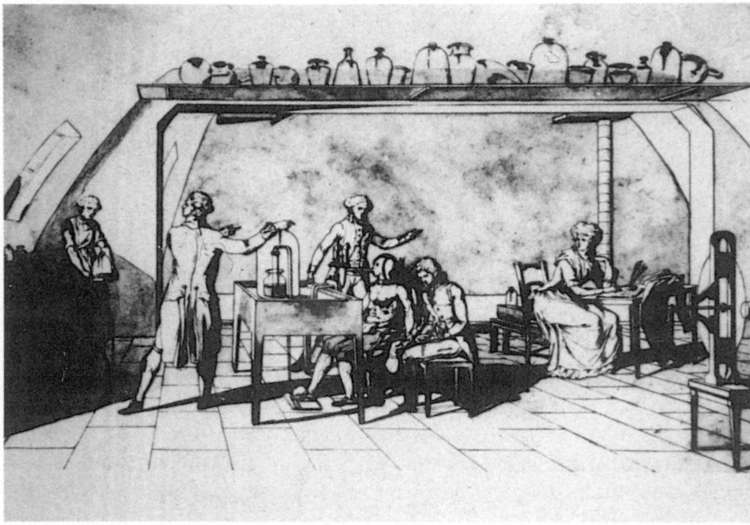

Fig. 1. A working essay of historical significance by Lavoisier and Seguin, written in 1790.

portable spirometer which registered the passing air volume gasometrically. He exhaled into an easily exchangeable box filled with a solution of alkali hydroxides. The increase in weight of this box was an indication of the amount of exhaled carbon dioxide. Because of a sufficiently long rubber tube, he had considerable freedom of movement during the experiment thus he could walk about at a certain speed. His exercise experiments on the treadmill of the Coldbath Fields Prison were particularly spectacular [102]. This was a treadmill which could accomodate several hundred people at the same time. From 1822 on these treadmills were used in several English prisons to punish prisoners assigned to "hard labor". The prisoners sarcastically called this torture "to grind the wind", since most treadmills did not drive machinery, but only a ventilator placed on the roof of the prison [19].

The French engineer Gustave-Adolphe Hirn used an airtight chamber with a built-in treadmill in a series of experiments which he conducted between 1855 and 1857. His motive for these experiments was not a medical but a physical problem. Hirn wanted to measure the human heat equivalent. From a spiroergometric point of view his experiments with machines and humans are remarkable since his gas-metabolic experiments occupy an original and ambiguous place as far as methodology is concerned. They represent the presumably first exercise experiments in a closed system although they were conducted using the attachment method. The subject stood erect in a chamber measuring 2.3 cubic meters and stepped onto a step wheel which measured the distance covered. While doing so, he inhaled through a nose tube from a first gasometer and exhaled through a mouth tube into a second gasometer. Hirn later analyzed the exhaled air for its carbon dioxide, oxygen, and nitrogen contents [31].

In December 1866 the presumably first experiments with a braked crank, the famous Pettenkofer apparatus of the Munich Physiological Institute [88], were conducted in a "genuine" respiration chamber. In this spacious, closed apparatus which permitted a quantitative measurement of carbon dioxide expiration even over longer periods of time [108], Max von Pettenkofer and Carl Voit had a worker turn a

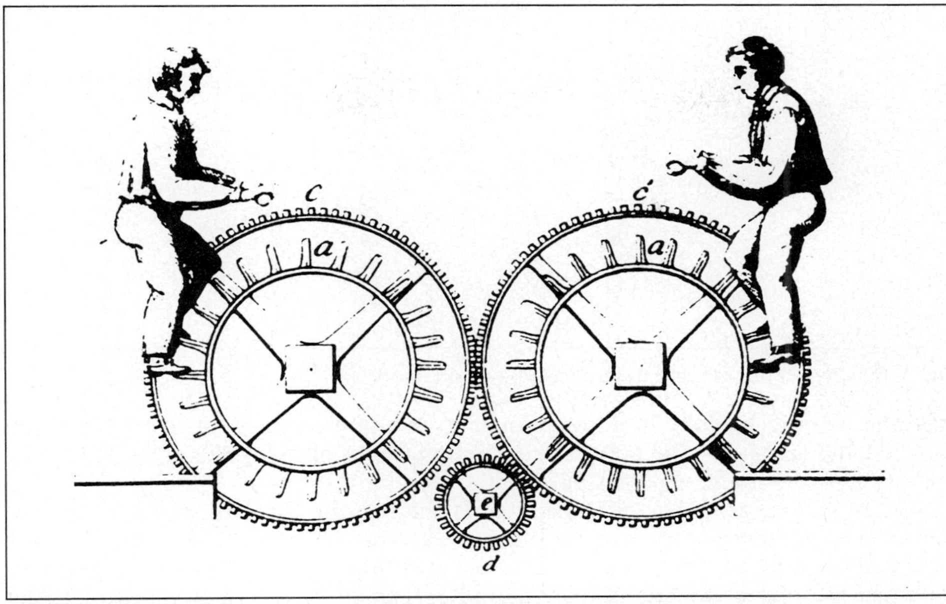

Fig. 2. Treadmill for prisoners sentenced to "hard labor" in England in the 1800s.

flywheel, over which a 25 kg chain was hung. As this chamber was rather unsuitable for detecting short-term changes in gas metabolism, the investigators had their subjects work hard over a period of 9 h. The "breaks were identical with those workers are used to in their normal life" [88].

In 1883 the German physician Carl Speck combined a similarly constructed exercise instrument with an attachment procedure developed by himself in a series of experiments. With his left arm Speck turned an iron spindle, whose friction he could vary by turning a screw. Resistance was changed by weights hung on the crank while the number of revolutions was varied by a string which could be wound. Speck collected the exhaled air in both containers of his double spirometer simultaneously, and he then measured the content by absorbing the carbon dioxide using a solution of barite and potassium hydroxide. For absorbing the oxygen he used pyrogallic acid [103].

Three years later, in 1886, the French researchers M. Hanriot and Charles Richet also presented the results of work experiments with a braked turning wheel. Gas metabolism was measured during exercise and some minutes thereafter [25]. The attachment procedure developed by them was conspicuous for its simplicity: the subject inhaled through a gasometer (I) and exhaled into two gasometers (II, III) connected in series. Between the two latter measuring devices a carbon dioxide absorber was installed. The volume difference between I and III was identical with oxygen consumption, while the difference between II and III corresponded to the amount of expired carbon dioxide [24].

Crank ergometry really got going when the "ergostat" appeared on the scene. This was an invention of the Bohemian physician and Viennese university lecturer Gustav Gaertner [8, 83]. In December 1887 he presented the ergostat to the public. Gaertner had actually designed this mechanically braked apparatus (which meas-

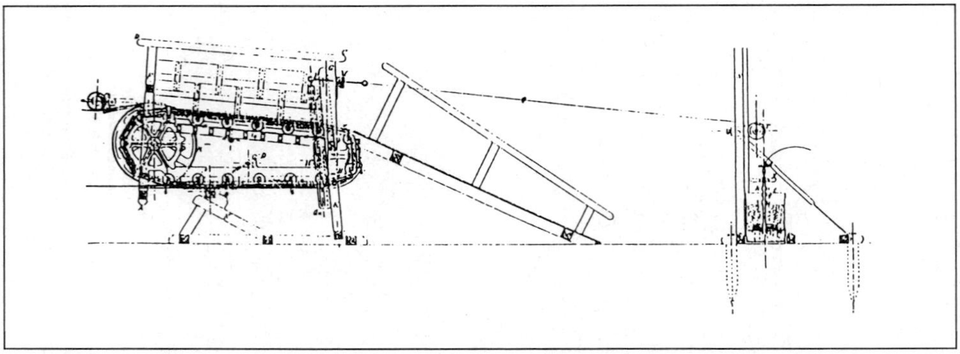

Fig. 3. Moving belt for exercise tests invented by Zuntz in Berlin 1889.

ured the work to be done in kilogrammeters) as a hometrainer for overweight persons. At the same time he considered the possibility of using the ergostat experimentally in systematic work-tests [21].

Nathan Zuntz, professor of physiology at the Intitute for Animal Physiology in Berlin [23], used Gaertner's apparatus. As early as in spring 1888, he and Curt Lehmann conducted the first gas-metabolic experiments with this new exercise instrument [70]. In the following year Georg Katzenstein, directed by Zuntz, conducted the now famous work-tests with Gaertner's ergostat [54]. As far as spirometry is concerned, the Berlin group of research scientists used the Zuntz-Geppert method, which is an attachment procedure during which the total amount of the exhaled air is measured, although only a small aliquot part is collected and its oxygen and carbondioxide content are analyzed quantitatively [82, 108].

During Katzenstein's gas-metabolic studies from the year 1889, a treadmill ergometer was presumably used for the first time in ergometric experiments with humans [54]. Originally Zuntz, Lehmann, and Oscar Hagemann had improved this predecessor of modern treadmills for working experiments with horses [124]. According to Zuntz this "tread work" permitted "a completely satisfying measurement" of leg work [123].

However, in the spring of 1897, a serious alternative appeared: the bicycle ergometer. Its inventor was the Frenchman Elisée Bouny, an assistant to the physiologist Etienne-Jules Marey. Bouny, who was enthusiastic about cycle racing, was not interested in developing a suitable exercise instrument for metabolic experiments. It was rather his goal to measure a cyclist's physical performance as exactly as possible. When Bouny checked the measuring accuracy of Marey's dynamometric pedal by means of a Pony bridle, he struck on the idea to install the mechanic brake directly at the back wheel of a jacked up bicycle frame without a frontwheel. Thus, the first bicycle ergometer was born [16].

Bouny published his invention in April 1897. Only 1 month later the era of gas-metabolic experiments using bicycle ergometers began — however not in Paris, but in a laboratory of the American Wesleyan University in Middletown, Connecticut. This was the location of the famous respiration calorimeter, in which nutritionists working with Wilbur O. Atwater and Francis G. Benedict had their subject exercise on a bicycle ergometer for the first time on May 18, 1897. In the closed apparatus constructed by Atwater and E. B. Rosa, whose respiration part was an imitation of the Pettenkofer apparatus, the subject had to pedal hard for 8 h per day over a total of 4 days. The Americans however, used an ergometric principle which was different from that of the French Bouny. Their stationary bicycle drove a dynamo whose increase in temperature served as a measure of the work performed [5].

While the working group in Middletown developed the dynamo measuring principle further [6] and later developed a bicycle ergometer with an electromagnetic brake [7], most European research scientists of the beginning 20th century preferred mechanical brakes. A corresponding construction by Zuntz [18] and the bicycle-ergospirometric tests conducted by the French Jules Amar in Northern Africa [3] were such.

In 1911 the English physiologist C. G. Douglas introduced a gas bag which was later named after him. In this bag the exhaled air was collected and later analyzed for its content [20]. Today this method is still used in field experiments.

In 1924 Knipping developed an apparatus "for the exact examination of gas metabolism in both clinical and medical practice" [60]. In 1928 he constructed a dynamoergometer. Within a range of 1 to 100 revolutions/min, every desired performance up to 1.5 PS could be selected by changing a field current, load resistance, and the number of revolutions. Even at that time the development of a large flywheel was thought to be important for making constant work possible [61].

In 1929 Knipping combined a spirograph, which was especially designed for physical work, with the aforementioned ergometer and thus created "spiroergometry" [61]. It was finally possible for clinical practice to have patients perform an exactly controlled and at any time precisely reproducible work with simultaneous continuous and non-invasive measurement of respiration and gas metabolism. From then on, time-consuming physiological examination techniques requiring special laboratories with the sample character which was usual until that time were no longer necessary. Thus, spiroergometry was a handy method even for the clinician inexperienced in physiological examinations.

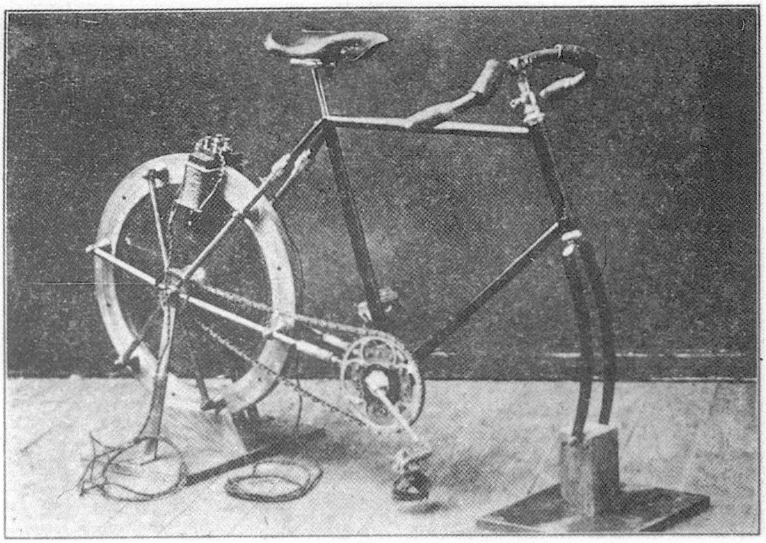

Fig. 4. Bicycle ergometer constructed by Atwater and Benedict in the late 1800s.

As early as in 1924, the English nobel laureate A.V. Hill had found the maximal oxygen uptake as a gross criterion of the cardiopulmonary performance capacity. At the same time he created the terms "O_2 deficit", "steady state", and "O_2 debt" [30]. Knipping and Brauer created the term "vita maxima" for clinical practice. Even today, this term is still used by many clinicians. This term was thought to be the opposite of the then usual "vita minima", i.e. the basal metabolic conditions. Contrary to this, vita maxima was understood as the behavior of the human organism during maximal muscular work. In the beginning a distinction was still made between the maximal performance of the heart and that of the lung, in the former case implying maximal cardiac output, whereas in the latter one maximal ventilation was intended [62].

Subsequently numerous new, mostly pulmonary terms were created, since during that time not cardiac disease but pulmonary diseases (such as pulmonary tuberculosis) were the most important health problems. Among those terms were the maximal breathing capacity [27], ventilatory equivalent [64], respiratory reserve [61], respiratory rest insufficiency, respiratory work insufficiency, and spirographic O_2 deficit [4, 15, 27, 62, 63, 109].

Even at that time, the clear distinction which was made between respiratory rest and exercise insufficiency on the basis of spiroergometric tests was particularly remarkable.

In 1938 Knipping coined the term "exercise insufficiency of heart and circulatory system" [62]. Thus, a distinction was already made between the concept of work insufficiency of the heart contrary to the symptom-free findings during physical rest. Alleröder and Landen [1, 2] developed the so-called heart performance quotient (HLQ = Herz-Leistungsquotient) for the determination of the functional state of work-insufficient patients. In the 1930s Koch [65], a member of Knipping's work group, dealt with aeromedical and sportsmedical problems from the point of view of spiroergometry. In 1937 Borgard, Matthiessen, and Zaeper used spiroergometry

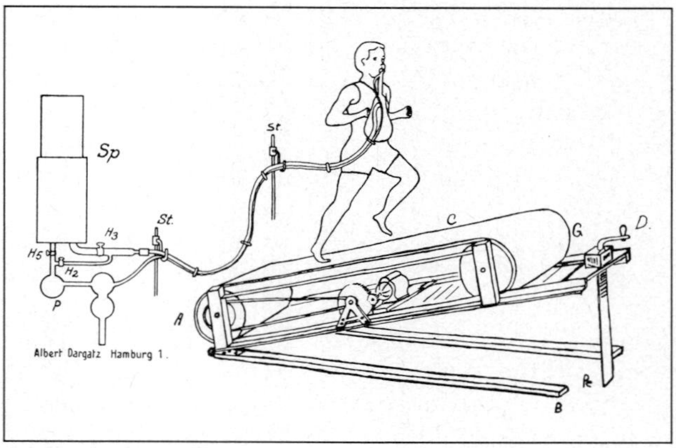

Fig. 5. Line drawing by Knipping 1929, which shows his still practical ideas for constant breathing- and metabolic-registration during exercise testing.

to examine the effect of physical training on respiration and the cardiovascular system [15].

However, it was not before the 1950s that spiroergometry gained general acceptance as a routine method for clinical examinations and as a basic research method. The most important stimulus was the working group around Bolt, Valentin, and Venrath in Knipping's Medical University Clinic in Cologne at the beginning of the 1950s [11, 12, 13, 14, 69, 113, 114]. In 1949 Dargatz et al. in Hamburg were the first to build a spirograph system which fulfilled almost all scientific requirements, even for research purposes up to a maximum O_2 uptake of approx. 3000 ml/min. This apparatus was set up in the Sports University in Cologne to find normal values of the ventilatory and metabolic behavior of healthy, fit men and women at various loads. The men and women examined differed in age and training state. For the first time an accompanying routine registration of the ventilatory equivalent during exercise took place. Today this is an essential criterion of the non-invasive assessment of the metabolic and performance situation [32, 107]. The ergometer used was the eddy-current crank ergometer which was also built by Dargatz. This ergometer was characterized by a large-radius crank and was used with the subject in a standing position, breathing both oxygen and ambient air. Using this ergometer Valentin et al. [115] determined maximal oxygen uptake of persons of different age groups who inhaled O_2. From 1954 on Dargatz built a new closed system with a pump and CO_2 absorption capacity; it was sufficient for maximal O_2 uptake values around 5000 ml/min. By making some technical changes of our own we were at last able to reliably measure O_2 uptake values of more than 6000 ml/min. It was thus possible for us to examine even world-class endurance athletes under maximum exercise stress [33—36].

Until 1954 Knipping's school only worked with crank work performed while standing. This kind of work made it impossible to measure blood pressure during controlled work or to make venous or arterial punctures and blood withdrawals for metabolic blood examinations. That is why in 1954, we borrowed a bicycle ergometer (Zentralwerkstatt, Göttingen; [53, 80, 81] from Prof. Dr. E. A. Müller from the Max-Planck-Institute for Work Physiology in Dortmund. Thus, we introduced bicycle ergometry performed in a sitting position with simultaneous spirographic measurement of gas metabolism into the Medical University Clinic Cologne as an addition to the crank work still favored by Knipping [45]. The first thing we found using this new method was that the so-called "spirographic O_2 deficit" [109] (not identical with "O_2-deficit") was no pathognomonic symptom but could always be observed at a sufficiently high load intensity. At the same time the comparison between bicycle work in sitting position and crank work in standing position showed that in the case of bicycle work, maximal oxygen uptake was higher by 30 % on average, whereas at given submaximal loads the oygen uptake and respiratory minute volume were lower [34—36].

On the bicycle ergometer the usual blood pressure measurement according to Riva-Rocci could not be conducted auscultatorily as the noise of the bicycle chain made blood pressure auscultation impossible. To overcome this handicap, our technical engineer G. Sander constructed the first semi-automatic working apparatus for measurement and for optical as well as acoustic recording of the systolic and diastolic blood pressure during bicycle ergometer work. Using this apparatus the first ergometric blood pressure norm values could be developed [33, 46, 48]. From

1960 on this apparatus was mass-produced, and at the first World Exhibition for Medical Electronics in New York in 1960 it was presented as the first of its kind.

Proceeding from this apparatus, from 1960 on we developed a simple apparatus for blood pressure measurement to be used by non-physicians. The intention was to be able to determine doses of medicine for hypertensive patients more accurately. For example in the case of a two- or three-time measurement of the blood pressure per day, the dosage of the respective medicine was planned to be adapted to the respective measured value. At that time our recommendations were met with fierce resistance from various groups of physicians. In their eyes this was an infringement of an exclusively medical authority.

In the beginning of the 1950s the only reliable parameter for the assessment of the cardiopulmonary performance capacity of patients in the clinic was the measurement of maximal O_2 uptake. However, this method had two disadvantages: the risk of overstressing the patient in the case of an existing organic disease and the possibility of insufficient motivation of the person examined so that the individually highest possible performance was not achieved. For this reason, from the mid-1950s, we looked for methods of assessing performance reliably even using medium or submaximal loads. First we replaced the oxygen respiration, which was used in Knipping's school, by the respiration of normal ambient air. In 1959 our first publication about the existence of an "oxygen threshold for prolonged work" appeared. This oxygen threshold for prolonged work was determined by detecting a "point of optimal efficiency of respiration" (POW = Punkt des optimalen Wirkungsgrades der Atmung) [34]. This had been preceded by the observation of a similar increase of the respiratory minute volume, the respiratory equivalent, and the arterial lactate concentration during bicycle ergometer exercise with load increments at 3-min intervals. Now the cardiopulmonary capacity could be exactly measured using submaximal loads and by determining the respiratory minute volume and/or the arterial lactate concentration [34—40, 42]. From then on we systemically examined healthy and ill men and women from childhood to old age using this submaximal load method [38]. Because of differences in the behavior of the venous lactate concentration as compared with the arterial lactate concentration we, at that time, had to restrict ourselves to arterial punctures and measurements of lactic acid in connection with this [10, 34]. This changed in the 1960s when the enzymatic method of measuring lactic acid was introduced — until then the chemical method according to Barker and Summerson had been applied — and the finding that the composition of the blood taken from the hyperemized earlobe was almost identical with that of arterial blood. From then on the arterial punctures could be abandoned in favor of micro-blood withdrawals from the hyperemized earlobe. These withdrawals could be repeated many times. The registration of the respiratory minute volume was thus gradually replaced by the measurement of the arterial lactate concentration.

In 1964 a similar method was presented by Wasserman et al., who called the oxygen threshold of prolonged work "anaerobic threshold" [117]. This expression has gained international acceptance. Today the measurement of the aerobic-anaerobic threshold is the method most often used in performance diagnostics on an international scale.

In the 1950s and 1960s increasingly more working groups took over spiroergometric examination techniques. In Leipzig it was Böhlau [9], in Freiburg Reindell and Kirchhoff [91], and in Berlin Mellerowicz [78] who expanded spiroergometry. These research scientists used different equipment and methods. The Reindell working group chose pedal work in supine position using Fleisch's metabograph. Böhlau developed the "Polyenergotest", while Mellerowicz worked both with crank and pedal work. Reindell et al. related spiroergometric parameters as for example, the oxygen pulse, to the heart volume, which had been determined radiographically in supine position. In this way they created the equivalent heart volume value or the heart volume performance quotient. Thus, the question as to whether the performance capacity of a heart is sufficient in relation to its volume could be answered [66—68, 92, 93]. The catheterizations conducted during spiroergometry with intracardiac and intrapulmonary pressure measurements revealed the different stadia of exercise insufficiency of the heart [51, 95].

In the early 1960s the ECG-recording during bicycle ergometer work gained acceptance [94]. In view of the rapidly growing importance of coronary heart disease at that time, this method permitted an early diagnosis by recording the ST-depressions during graded ergometer exercise. It was ultimately because of the great number of coronary heart disease that in the following years clinical spiroergometry was increasingly replaced by ergometry in combination with ECG and blood pressure recording and without measurement of gas metabolism and respiratory minute volume. During the last 2 years, a reverse trend characterized by the simultanous recording of all parameters mentioned has taken place in clinical practice.

In the 1960s the technical perfection of closed spirographic systems was followed by the development of open systems. Electronics and computers were introduced into spiroergometry. In 1974 Keiper, in connection with our institute, constructed the first fully electronic and computerized bicycle ergometer ("Dynavit"). This had been preceeded by the development of universal ergometers for crank and pedal work of various kind up to pulse-rate-controlled devices.

In some cases, for special questions and forms of performance measurement, ergometers have been replaced by treadmills. On treadmills higher maximal oxygen uptake values can be achieved [41]; at the same time, in the case of sport-specific examinations (e.g. with runners), more precise statements can be made about the performance state using hemodynamic and metabolic parameters [26, 41—59, 71, 77, 79, 84—87, 89, 96, 98, 101, 104, 106, 110, 112, 116, 118, 119].

In 1976 Mader et al. from our working group described the so-called 4 mmol lactate threshold. This is a statistical mean value, which is 2 mmol higher on average than the aerobic threshold aforementioned. The 4 mmol lactate threshold is the highest load which can be maintained over a period whose length varies from individual to individual without a further increase in lactic acid concentration. This 4 mmol lactate threshold has been a valuable enrichment of spiroergometry (see overview in [26]).

Today, spiroergometry can be found in clinics, hospitals, and institutes all over the world. The performance diagnosis of heart, circulatory system, ventilation, and metabolism has become an important area of clinical medicine. Although the ECG recording during ergometer work, which was added in the beginning of the 1960s, makes the registration of ventilation and metabolism superfluous for cardiological problems, this method remains at interest for several other clinical problems particularly from the point of view of the breath-by-breath analysis, which has been possible since the early 1970s. Thus, a broad range of spiroergometric instruments is available today.

Summary

Spiroergometry — a synonym of ergospirometry — is a diagnostic procedure for the assessment of the function and capacity of the heart, circulation, respiration, and metabolism. The term contains the two components spirometry and ergometry. The first attempts at measuring human gas metabolism while performing a quantified physical work can be traced back to the year 1790. The development of procedures to measure gas metabolism as well as the construction of ergometers in the 19th and 20th centuries is shown. 1929 is the most important year, both for spiroergometry as it is used today and for the start of a routinely performed clinical capacity diagnosis. It was not until the 1950s that the first spiroergometric apparatus was developed to serve all the scientific needs. From a historical point of view, the parameters used and the physiological and pathophysiological findings based on spiroergometry are dealt with. Numerous medical fields have profited from the technique of spiroergometry: cardiology, pulmonology, sports medicine, physiology of functional capacity, biochemistry, clinical pharmacology, surgery, orthopedics, pediatrics, gerontology, etc., besides global fields such as preventive medicine, kinesiotherapy, and rehabilitative medicine.

References

1. Alleröder H, Landen CH (1940) Das Verhalten der Komplementärluft, der Reserveluft und der Sauerstoffaufnahme im Arbeitsversuch. Z exper Med 108: 406
2. Alleröder H, Landen CH (1942) Über den störenden Einfluß äußerer Faktoren im Belastungsversuch bei Herzkranken. Zbl inn Med 63: 273
3. Amar J (1909 Le rendement de la machine humane. Paris: Librairie J B Baillière et Fils
4. Anthony AJ (1937) Funktionsprüfung der Atmung. Barth, Leipzig
5. Atwater WO, Benedict G (1899): Experiments on the metabolism of matter and energy in the human body. US Department of Agriculture, Office of Experiment Stations — Bulletin No 69. Washington: Government Printing Office
6. Atwater WO, Benedict FG (1903) Experiments on the metabolism of matter and energy in the human body. 1900—1902. US Department of Agriculture, Office of Experiment Stations — Bull NO 136. Washington: Government Printing Office
7. Benedict FG, Cady WG (1912) A bicycle ergometer with an electric brake. Carnegie Institution of Washington. Publ No 167. New York: Isaach H Blanchard Company
8. Bett WR (1955) Gustav Gaertner (1855—1937) clinician and inventor. The medical press 234: 308
9. Böhlau V (1955) Prüfung der körperlichen Leistungsfähigkeit bei Gesunden, Kranken und Rekonvaleszenten mit einem vollautomatischen fortlaufend registrierenden Gasstoffwechselgerät. Barth, Leipzig
10. Bolt W, Hollman W, Schild KT, Valentin H, Venrath H (1956) Über den Brenztraubensäure- und Milchsäurespiegel im Blut bei Arbeit. Ärztl Wschr 66: 656
11. Bolt W, Knipping HW, Valentin H, Venrath H (1952) Sport as a therapeutial factor in heart conditions. Sports Medicine, Olympiade Helsinki
12. Bolt W, Knipping HW, Valentin H, Venrath H (1953) Respiratorische Ruhe- und Arbeitsinsuffizienz. Die Gruppierung der verschiedenen Formen und die Abgrenzung von der kardialen Insuffizienz unter besonderer Berücksichtigung der Lungentuberkulose. Beitr klin Tbk 108: 394
13. Bolt W, Valentin H, Venrath H (1950): Herzleistungsbreite der kardialen Linksinsuffizienz Z Kreislaufforschung 39: 718
14. Bolt W, Valentin H, Venrath H, Wullen L (1952) Die Herzfunktion in der Klinik der Hochdruckerkrankungen unter besonderer Berücksichtigung der intrakardialen Druckmessung. Dtsch med Wschr 77: 297

15. Borgard W, Matthiessen G, Zaeper G (1937) Einwirkungen des Trainings auf Atmung und Kreislauf. Klin Wschr 15: 385
16. Bouny E (1897) Études expérimentales. Revue mensuelle du Touring-Club de France. Avril 140
17. Breathnach CS (1985) Prout Biographical sketches — 48. Irish Med J 78: 26
18. Caspari W, Zuntz N (1911) Stoffwechsel. In: Tigerstedt R (Hrsg) Handbuch der physiologischen Methodik, erster Band. Hirzel, Leipzig
19. Chapman CB (1967) Edward Smith (1818—1874) Physiologist, human ecologist, reformer. J History Med All Sci 22: 1
20. Douglas CG, Priestley JG (1924) Human physiology. A practical course. Oxford: Clarendon Press
21. Gaertner G (1887) Über die therapeutische Verwendung der Muskelarbeit und einen neuen Apparat zu ihrer Dosierung. Wiener medizinische Blätter 10: 1554, 1582. Allgemeine Wiener medizinische Zeitung 32: 607, 621
22. Grimaux E (1888) Lavoisier. 1743—1794. D'après sa correspondance, ses manuscrits, ses papiers de famille et d'autres documents inédits. Paris: Félix Alcan
23. Gunga HC (1989) Leben und Werk des Berliner Physiologen Nathan Zuntz (1847—1920). Husum: Matthiesen Verlag
24. Hanriot M, Richet C (1887) Nouveau procédé de dosage de l'acide carbinique expiré et de l'oxygene absorbé dans les actes respiratoires. Comptes rendus hebdomadaires des séances de l'Académie des sciences 104: 435
25. Hanriot M, Richet C (1893) Des échanges respiratoires chez l'homme. In: Richet C (Hrsg) Physiology (Travaux de laboratoire de Richet). Paris Bd 1: 470
26. Heck H (1987) Laktat in der Leistungsdiagnostik. Habilitationsschrift, Deutsche Sporthochschule Köln
27. Hermannsen J (1933) Untersuchungen über die maximale Ventilationsgröße (Atemgrenzwert). Z ges exper Med 90: 180
28. Hermannsen J (1938) Die ergometrische Methode als Funktionsprüfung für Herz und Lunge. Beitr Klin Tbk 92: 395
29. Hermannsen J, van Uytvank P (1933) Einige Untersuchungen über die Kreislauf- und Lungenleistungen bei schwerer Arbeit. Z ges exper Med 88: 279
30. Hill AV (1925) Muscular activity. Baltimore: Williams and Wilkins
31. Hirn GA (1858) Recherches sur l'équivalent méchanique de la chaleur, présentées à la Société de physique de Berlin. Colmar: Bureau de la Revue d'Alsace
32. Hollmann W (1954) Herzleistungsquotient und Wirkungsgrad sowie die Lungenvolumina bei Sportlern unter 35 Jahren. Dissertation, Uni Köln
33. Hollmann W (1959) Der Arbeits- und Trainingseinfluß auf Kreislauf und Atmung. Darmstadt: Dr. Steinkopff
34. Hollmann W (1959) The relationship between pH, lactic acid, potassium in the arterial and venous blood, the ventilation, PoW and pulse frequency during increasing spiroergometric work in endurance-trained and untrained persons. Chicago: Pan-American Congress for Sports Medicine
35. Hollmann W (1961) Zur Frage der Dauerleistungsfähigkeit. Fortschr Med 79: 439
36. Hollmann W (1963) Höchst- und Dauerleistungsfähigkeit des Sportlers. München: Barth
37. Hollmann W (1964) Changes in the capacity for maximal and continuous effort in relation to age. In: Sport and Physical Medicine. Springfield/III: CC Thomas
38. Hollmann W (1965) Körperliches Training als Prävention von Herz-Kreislaufkrankheiten. Stuttgart: Hippokrates
39. Hollmann W, Barg W, Weyer G, Heck H (1970) Der Alterseinfluß auf spiroergometrische Meßgrößen im submaximalen Arbeitsbereich. Med Welt 28: 1280
40. Hollmann W, Bouchard C (1970) Untersuchungen über die Beziehungen zwischen chronologischem und biologischem Alter zu spiroergometrischen Meßgrößen, Herzvolumen, anthropometrischen Daten und Skelettmuskelkraft bei 8- bis 18jährigen Jungen. Z Kreislaufforschg 59: 160
41. Hollmann W, Heck H, Schmücker B, Stolte A, Liesen H, Fotescu D, Mathur DN, Joura K (1971) Vergleichende spiroergometrische Untersuchungen über den Effekt und die Aussagekraft von Laufband- und Fahrradergometerbelastungen. Sportarzt u Sportmed 6: 123

42. Hollmann W, Kastner K (1969) The behaviour of arterial blood gases, arterial substrates, pH and hematocrit in different ergometric work. In: Medicine and Sport Vol 3: 81. Basel New York: Karger
43. Hollmann W, Liesen H (1973) Über die Bewertbarkeit des Laktats in der spiroergometrischen Leistungsdiagnostik. Sportarzt u Sportmed 8: 175
44. Hollmann W, Schlüssel H, Spechtmeyer H (1965) Einige Enzymspiegel bei dosierter dynamischer und statischer Arbeit unter Atmung verschiedener O_2-Gemische. Sportarzt 5: 166
45. Hollmann W, Valentin H (180) 50 Jahre Spiroergometrie. Münch med Wschr 122: 163
46. Hollmann W, Valentin H, Venrath H (1959) Vergleichende Arbeitsuntersuchungen männlicher und weiblicher Personen unter fortlaufender Registrierung von Ventilation, Stoffwechsel, Pulsfrequenz und Blutdruck. Münch med Wschr 39: 1680
47. Hollmann W, Venrath H, Bouchard C, Werne D (1964) Vergleichende Untersuchungen über den Einfluß von einbeinig und beidbeinig verrichteter Fahrradergometerbelastung auf Stoffwechsel und Kreislauf. Sportarzt 6: 169
48. Hollmann W, Venrath H, Valentin H, Spellerberg B (1959) Über den arteriellen Blutdruck bei Menschen während dosierter körperlicher Arbeit. Z Kreislaufforschg 48: 162
49. Holmes FL (1985) Lavoisier and die chemistry of life. An exploration of scientific creativity. Madison/Wisconsin: The University of Wisconsin Press. Reihe: Wisconsin publications in the history of science and medicine, No 4. General editors: Coleman W, Lindberg DC, Numbers RL
50. Jeschke D, Heitkamp HC, Locher R, Schneider D, Simon M, Zintel B (1983) Aerobe Kapazität und anaerobe Schwelle bei unterschiedlichen Belastungsmethoden auf dem Fahrradergometer. In: Mellerowicz H, Franz IW (Hrsg) Standardisierung, Kalibrierung und Methodik in der Ergometrie. Erlangen: Perimed
51. Kaltenbach M, Roskamm H (1980) Vom Belastungs-EKG zru Koronarangiographie. Berlin Heidelberg New York: Springer
52. Karlsson J, Saltin B (1970) Laktate, ATP and CP in working muscles during exhaustive exercise in man. J Appl Physiol 29 (5): 598
53. Karrasch K, Müller EA (1951) Das Verhalten der Pulsfrequenz in der Erholungsperiode nach körperlicher Arbeit. Arbeitsphysiol 14: 369
54. Katzenstein G (1891) Über die Einwirkung der Muskeltätigkeit auf den Stoffverbrauch des Menschen. Archiv für die gesammte Physiologie des Menschen und der Thiere 49: 330
55. Keul J, Doll E, Keppler D (1969) Muskelstoffwechsel. München: Barth
56. Keul J, Kindermann W, Simon G (1978) Die aerobe und anaerobe Kapazität als Grundlage für die Leistungsdiagnostik. Leistungssport 8 (1): 22
57. Keul J, Simon G, Berg A, Dickhuth HH; Doerttler I, Kübel R (1979) Bestimmung der individuellen anaeroben Schwelle zur Leistungsbewertung und Trainingsgestaltung. Dtsch Z Sportmed 30 (7): 212
58. Kindermann W, Keul J (1977) Anaerobe Energiebereitstellung im Hochleistungssport. Schorndorf: Hofmann
59. Kindermann W, Simon G, Keul J (1979) The significance of the aerobic-anaerobic transition for the determination of work load intensities during endurance training. Eur J Appl Physiol 42: 25
60. Knipping HW (1924) Ein einfacher Apparat zur exakten Gasstoffwechseluntersuchung in der Klinik und ärztlichen Praxis. Münch med Wschr 71: 553
61. Knipping HW (1929) Die Untersuchung der Ökonomie von Muskelarbeit von Gesunden und Kranken. Z ges exper Med 66: 517
62. Knipping HW (1938) Ergebnisse der Ergographie in der Klinik. Die Arbeitsinsuffizienz von Herz und Kreislauf. Klin Wschr 17: 1457
63. Knipping HW, Hollmann W (1960) Beurteilung der menschlichen Leistungsfähigkeit. In: Heiss F (Hrsg) Praktische Sportmedizin. Stuttgart: Enke
64. Knipping HW, Moncrieff H (1932) The ventilatory equivalent for oxygen. Quart J Med 1: 17
65. Koch A (1939) Über Arbeit bei Sauerstoffmangel. Luft med 3: 97
66. König K, Reindell H, Musshoff K, Roskamm H, Kessler M (1961) Das Herzvolumen und körperliche Leistungsfähigkeit bei 20- bis 60jährigen gesunden Männern. Zweite Mitt. Arch Kreisl-Forsch 35: 37
67. König K, Reindell H, Roskamm H (1962) Das Herzvolumen und die Leistungsfähigkeit bei 60- bis 75jährigen gesunden Männern. Dritte Mitt Arch Kreisl-Forsch 39: 143

68. König K, Reindell H, Roskamm H (1962) Kriterien der individuellen Leistungsgrenze im spiroergometrischen Belastungsversuch. Dtsch med Wschr 87: 1304
69. Landen HC (1955) Die funktionelle Beurteilung des Lungen- und Herzkranken. Darmstadt: Dr. Steinkopff
70. Lehmann C, Mueller F, Munk I, Senator H, Zuntz N (1893) Untersuchungen an zwei hungernden Menschen. Arch path Anatomie u Physiologie und für Klinische Medizin 131/Suppl 1
71. Lehmann M, Dickhuth HH, Wybitul K, Berg A, Huber G, Keul J (1983) Unterschiede der aeroben Ausbelastung, der freien Plasmakatecholamine und energieliefernder Substrate während Fahrrad-, Laufband- und Gehbandergometrie. Dtsch Z Sportmed 34 (6): 188
72. Lehmann M, Schmid P, Keul J (1985) Plasma catecholamine and blood lactate cumulation during incremental exhausted exercise. Int J Sports Med 6 (2): 78
73. Liesen H, Mader A, Heck H, Hollmann W (1977) Die Ausdauerleistungsfähigkeit bei verschiedenen Sportarten unter besonderer Berücksichtigung des Metabolismus:zur Ermittlung der optimalen Belastungsintensität im Training. Leistungssport (Beiheft) 9: 63
74. Löllgen H (1978) Zur Bedeutung der Tretgeschwindigkeit in der klinischen Ergometrie. Habilitationsschrift, Uni Mainz
75. Mader A (1984) Eine Theorie zur Berechnung der Dynamik und des Steady state von Phosphorylierungszustand und Stoffwechselaktivität der Muskelzelle als Folge des Energiebedarfs. Köln: Habilitationsschrift Deutsche Sporthochschule
76. Mader A, Liesen H, Heck H, Philippi H, Rost R, Schürch P, Hollmann W (1976) Zur Beurteilung der sportartspezifischen Ausdauerleistungsfähgkeit im Labor. Sportarzt u Sportmed 27 (4): 80 (5) 109
77. Margaria R, Carretelli P, Mangili F, (1964) Balance and kinetics of anaerobic energy release during strenuous exercise in man. J Appl Physiol 19 (4) 623
78. Mellerowicz H (1975) Ergometrie. Grundriß der medizinischen Leistungsmessung. München: Urban & Schwarzenberg
79. Mellerowicz H, Franz IW (Hrsg) (1983) Standardisierung, Kalibrierung und Methodik in der Ergometrie. Erlangen: Perimed
80. Müller EA (1955) Regulation der Pulsfrequenz in der Erholungsphase nach ermüdender Muskelarbeit. Int Z angew Physiol 16: 35
81. Müller EA (1958) Die Beziehung zwischen Pulsfrequenz und Muskelarbeit als Test der Herzfunktion. In: Klepzig H (Hrsg) Die Funktionsdiagnostik des Herzens. Fünftes Freiburger Symposium. Berlin: Springer
82. Müller F (1920) Quantitative Bestimmung des Gasstoffwechsels mittels des Zuntz-Geppert'schen Apparates. In: Abderhalden E (Hrsg): Handbuch der biologischen Arbeitsmethoden. Abt VI Angewandte chemische und physikalische Methoden, Teil 10, Heft 1. Berlin Wien: Urban & Schwarzenberg
83. Pagel J (Hrsg) (1901) Biographisches Lexikon hervorragender Ärzte des 19. Jahrhunderts. Berlin Wien: Urban & Schwarzenberg
84. Pansold B, Roth W, Zinner J, Hashrt E, Gabriel B (1982) Die Laktat-Leistungskurve — ein Grundprinzip sportmedizinischer Leistungsdiagnostik. Med u Sport 22 (4): 107
85. Pearce DH, Milhorn HT (1977) Dynamic and steady state respiratory responses to bicycle exercise. J Appl Physiol 42 (6): 959
86. Pendergast DR, Cerretellik P, Rennie DW (1979) Aerobic and glycolytic metabolism in arm exercise. J Appl Physiol 47: 754
87. Pessenhofer H, Schwaberger G, Schmid P (1981) Zur Bestimmung des individuellen aerob-anaeroben Übergangs. Dtsch Z Sportmed 32 (1): 15
88. Pettenkofer M, von Voit C (1866) Untersuchungen über den Stoffverbrauch des normalen Menschen. Zeitschrift für Biologie 2: 459
89. Poortmans JR, Delescaille-van den Bossche J, Leclercq R (1978) Lactate uptake by inactive forearm during progressive exercise. J Appl Physiol 45 (6): 835
90. Prout W (1813) On the quantity of carbonic acid gas emitted from the lungs during respiration, at different times, and under different circumstances. Annals of Philosophy 2/5: 328
91. Reindell H, Kirchhoff HW (1956) Über kombinierte Funktionsprüfungen des Kreislaufes und der Atmung. Erste Mitt.: Untersuchungen an Personen mit durchschnittlicher Leistungsbreite und Hochleistungssportlern. Dtsch med Wschr 81: 592
92. Reindell H, Kirchhoff HW, Musshoff K, Klepzig H (1956) Das Sauerstoffäquivalent, ein Maßstab für die Beurteilung von Herz und Kreislauf. Verh dtsch Ges Kreislauf-Forsch 22: 108

93. Reindell H, König K, Roskamm H (1967) Funktionsdiagnostik des gesunden und kranken Herzens. Stuttgart, Thieme
94. Rosenkranz KA, Drews A (1964) Über eine modifizierte Ableitungsmethode zur Registrierung von Brustwandelektrokardiogrammen während dosierter körperlicher Belastung. Z Kreisl.-Forsch 53: 615
95. Roskamm H (1971) Funktionsprüfung von Herz und Kreislauf. Basel: Sandoz
96. Roskamm H, Reindell H, Müller M (196) Herzgröße und ergometrisch getestete Ausdauerleistungsfähigkeit bei Hochleistungssportlern aus 9 deutschen Nationalmannschaften. Z Kreisl.-Forsch 55: 2
97. Rost R, Holmann W (1982) Belastungsuntersuchungen in der Praxis. Stuttgart: Thieme
98. Rusko H, Luthanen P, Rahkila P, Viitasalo J, Rehunen S, Härkönen M (1986) Muscle Metabolism, blood lactate and oxygen uptake in steady state exercise at aerobic and anaerobic thresholds. Eur J Appl Physiol 55: 181
99. Seguin A, Lavoisier AL (1789, 1862) Premier mémoire sur la respiration des animaux. Histoire de l'Académie des sciences (1789) Neuausgabe in: Dumas, JBA (éd) (1862) Oeuvres de Lavoisier. Mémoires de Chimie et de Physique. Paris: Imprimerie Impériale S 688
100. Simon G, Berg A, Dickhuth HH, Simon-Alt A, Keul J (1981) Bestimmung der anaeroben Schwelle in Abhängigkeit vom Alter und von der Leistungsfähigkeit. Dtsch Z Sportmed 32 (1): 7
101. Sjödin B, Jacobs I, Karlsson I (1981) Onset of blood lactate accumulation and enzyme activities in m vastus lateralis in man. Int J Sports Med 2 (3): 166
102. Smith E (1859) Experimental inquiries into the chemical and other phenomena of respiration and their modifications by various physical agencies. Philosophical Transactions of the Royal Society of London 149: 681
103. Speck C (1892) Physiologie des menschlichen Atmens nach eigenen Untersuchungen. Leipzig: FCW Vogel
104. Stanley WC, Gertz EW, Wisneski JA, Morris DL, Nesse RA, Brooks GA (1985) Systemic lactate kinetics during graded exercise in man. Am J Physiol 249 (Endocrinol Metab 12): 595
105. Stegemann J (1963) Zum Mechanismus der Pulsfrequenzeinstellung durch den Stoffwechsel. Pflügers Arch ges Physiol 276: 481
106. Stegmann H, Kindermann W, Schnabel A (1981) Lactate kinetics and individual anaerobic threshold. Int J Sports Med 2 (3): 160
107. Tietz N (1954) Herzleistungsquotient und Arbeitsökonomie sowie Lungenvolumina bei Sportlern von 35 bis 70 Jahren. Köln: Uni Dissertation
108. Tigerstedt R (1911) Respirationsapparate. Handbuch der physiologischen Methodik, erster Band. Leipzig: Hirzel
109. Uhlenbruck P (1930) Über die Wirksamkeit der Sauerstoffatmung. Z ges exper Med 74: 1
110. Ulmer HV (1975) Zur Methodik, Standardisierung und Auswertung von Tests für die Prüfung der körperlichen Leistungsfähigkeit. Bd 1, Schriftenreihe Medizin des Bundesinstituts für Sportwissenschaft, Köln-Löwenich, Deutscher Ärzteverlag
111. Valentin H, Hollmann W, Venrath H (1960) Über die Möglichkeiten der Prüfstanduntersuchungen von Lungen, Herz und Kreislauf während Arbeitsbelastungen. Med Welt 31: 1573
112. Valentin H, Holzhauser KP (1976) Funktionsprüfungen von Herz und Kreislauf. Köln: Deutscher Ärzteverlag
113. Valentin H, Venrath H (1952) Die Spiroergometrie nach Brauer und Knipping. Ein objektiver und quantitativer Test für die Beurteilung der Leistungsfähigkeit des Herzens und der Lungen. Acta Med Scand 211: 90
114. Valentin H, Venrath H (1952) Die Differenzierung der respiratorischen Arbeitsinsuffizienz von der kardialen Insuffizienz unter besonderer Berücksichtigung der Links- und Rechtsinsuffizienz des Herzens. Beitr Klin Tbk 107: 35
115. Valentin H, Venrath H, v Mallinckrodt H, Gürakar M (1955) Die maximale Sauerstoffaufnahme in den verschiedenen Altersklassen. Eine praktisch wichtige Herz-Kreislauf-Funktionsprüfung im Vita-Maxima-Bereich. Z Altersforschg 9: 291
116. Wasserman K, Beaver WL, Whipp BJ (1986) Mechanisms and patterns of blood lactate increase during exercise in man. Med Sci Sports Exercise 18 (3): 344
117. Wasserman K; McIlroy MB (1964) Detecting the threshold of anaerobic metabolism in cardiac patients during exercise. Amer J Cardiol 14: 844

118. Wasserman K, Whipp BJ, Koyal SN, Beaver WL (1973) Anaerobic threshold and respiratory gas exchange during exercise. J Appl Physiol 35 82): 236
119. Whipp B, Wasserman K (1972) Oxygen uptake kinetics for various intensities of constant load work. J Appl Physiol 33 (3): 351
120. Zaeper G (1937) Bestimmung der Kreislaufleistung als Maß für die Beurteilung der sportlichen Leistungsfähigkeit. Klin Wschr 49: 1705
121. Zaeper G, Haebisch H, Cranford A, Wolf W (1939) Zur Charakterisierung bestimmter Formen kardialer Arbeitsinsuffizienz durch Arbeitsatmung. Klin Wschr 18: 270
122. Zorn O (1950) Funktionsprüfungen von Atmung und Kreislauf mittels der Spiroergometrie nach Brauer und Knipping. Beitr Silikose-Forschg 7: 21
123. Zuntz N (1899) Zwei Apparate zur Dosierung und Messung menschlicher Arbeit (Bremsergometer). Verh Berliner Physiologische Gesellschaft, Archiv für Physiologie (Physiologische Abteilung des Archivs für Anatomie und Physiologie) Jahrgang 1899, 372
124. Zuntz N, Lehmann C (unter Mitwirkung von Hagemann O) (1889) Untersuchungen über den Stoffwechsel des Pferdes bei Ruhe und Arbeit. Landwirtschaftliche Jahrbücher 18: 1

Author's address:

Prof. Dr. W. Hollmann
Institut für Kreislaufforschung und Sportmedizin
Deutsche Sporthochschule
Carl-Diehm-Weg
5000 Köln 41

Dynamic coupling of External to Cellular Respiration During Exercise*

K. Wasserman, A. Koike, K. Sietsema, and R. Casaburi, Harbor-UCLA Medical Center, Torrance, California, USA

Analysis of the pattern of coupling of external to cellular respiration provides considerable insight into circulatory and ventilatory control. Except for the first 15 to 20 s of exercise (Phase I), the circulation does not over-perfuse the tissues nor does the ventilatory control mechanism cause hyperventilation of the pulmonary blood. During Phase I, however, the pattern of response is more complex. At the onset of very low work rate exercise, the increases in heart rate and stroke volume are normally so rapid, that the cardiac output transiently exceeds the metabolic requirement. As a result, $\dot{V}O_2$ and heart rate decrease as work is sustained [15]. At higher work rates, heart rate continues to increase after Phase I, but $\dot{V}O_2$ exceeds the heart rate increase causing an increase in O_2-pulse ($\dot{V}O_2$/heart rate) which is usually complete by one minute [15]. With prolonged exercise, O_2-pulse decreases slightly presumably due to increased skin blood flow secondary to thermoregulation [4, 17].

The increase in ventilation lags behind the increasing metabolic rate, except for the first 15 s when a slight respiratory alkalosis is usually evident (pH increase approximately 0.01) [16]. After the first 15 s a slight respiratory acidosis (approx 2 mm Hg) occurs [16]. For heavier work rates metabolic acidosis becomes evident after a time delay of about 30 s.

These findings suggest that central command or anticipatory homeostasis [11, 13] is the primary control mechanism producing the changes in cardiac output and ventilation immediately following the start of exercise. But this mechanism soon gives way to dominating metabolic control mechanisms which increase blood (and oxygen) flow to the metabolically active muscles and stimulate alveolar ventilation to minimize the hydrogen ion and PCO_2 increase in arterial blood. During recovery, arterial pH returns to rest within 2 min when the acidosis is due to respiratory acidosis alone. The rate of recovery of pH is slower at work rates associated with a lactic acidosis since recovery of arterial pH and PCO_2 are linked to the rate of lactate catabolism [16, 18].

The circulatory transport of oxygen normally increases at a rate which is only slightly above the rate of oxygen consumption (O_2 transport increases about 1.2 L/min. per 1 L of oxygen consumed [19] during exercise. With this narrow difference between the rates of O_2 supply and utilization, the ratio of blood supply/metabolic rate must be quite uniform within the exercising muscles, implying rather precise local vascular control.

Recognizing the essential role of gas exchange in performing work, and the economy of function of the cardiovascular and ventilatory control mechanisms, it would be expected that diseases of the cardiovascular or ventilatory systems distort the pattern of the gas exchange responses. In this presentation, the focus is on recent studies which demonstrate the coupling of external to cellular respiration and chan-

* Supported by Public Health Service Grant HL 11907

ges which occur with disease. In particular, we: 1) address the relationship between $\dot{V}O_2$ and work rate, 2) provide evidence that the lactic acidosis threshold is the anaerobic threshold, 3) describe the cardiovascular implications of altered $\dot{V}O_2$ and $\dot{V}CO_2$ kinetics in response to constant work rate exercise 4) relate O_2-uptake kinetics to lactate production, and 5) introduce the concept of a "training factor" in the control of ventilation during exercise.

The Oxygen Cost of Work

To estimate the oxygen cost of work over the entire work rate range, we have used a calibrated cycle-ergometer. Work rate is controlled and oxygen uptake is continuously measured. Figure 1 shows the $\dot{V}O_2$ for a series of work rates performed for 8 min for a normal subject. At high work rates, $\dot{V}O_2$ continues to rise rather than reaching an asymptote. Therefore the true oxygen cost of these work rates cannot be accurately measured. Similar studies showing lack of steadystate at submaximal work rates have been previously reported [12, 14, 20], which challenge the pervasive concept in exercise physiology and sports medicine that $\dot{V}O_2$ increases linearly with work rate to $\dot{V}O_2$ max and that it is unaffected by lactate metabolism.

Fig. 2 shows the $\dot{V}O_2$ at 2, 4, 6, and 8 min and the lactate concentration at the end of exercise plotted as a function of work rate for the study shown in Fig. 1. It is seen that the $\dot{V}O_2$ values are superimposable at these four exercise durations for work rates below which lactate starts its steep climb. Above that level, (the lactate threshold [1]), $\dot{V}O_2$ is higher at any work rate as related to the time of the measurement. This suggests that lactic acidosis and O_2 cost of work are interrelated. However from the slope of the $\dot{V}O_2$ — work rate relationship, it is easy to see how a superficial analysis in which only one $\dot{V}O_2$ value is measured at each work rate, it might be concluded that $\dot{V}O_2$, as a function of work rate, has the same slope above the lactic acidosis threshold as it has below.

Hansen et al [8] studied the rate of increase in $\dot{V}O_2$ during a progressively increasing work rate (ramp forcing) test. When work rate was increased at different rates,

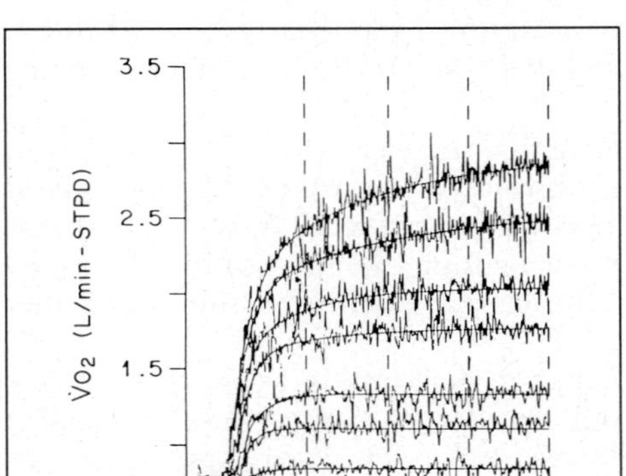

Fig. 1. Oxygen uptake versus time for 7 work rates in a normal subject. Each curve is the average of 3—10 studies. (Modified from Casaburi et al. [7]

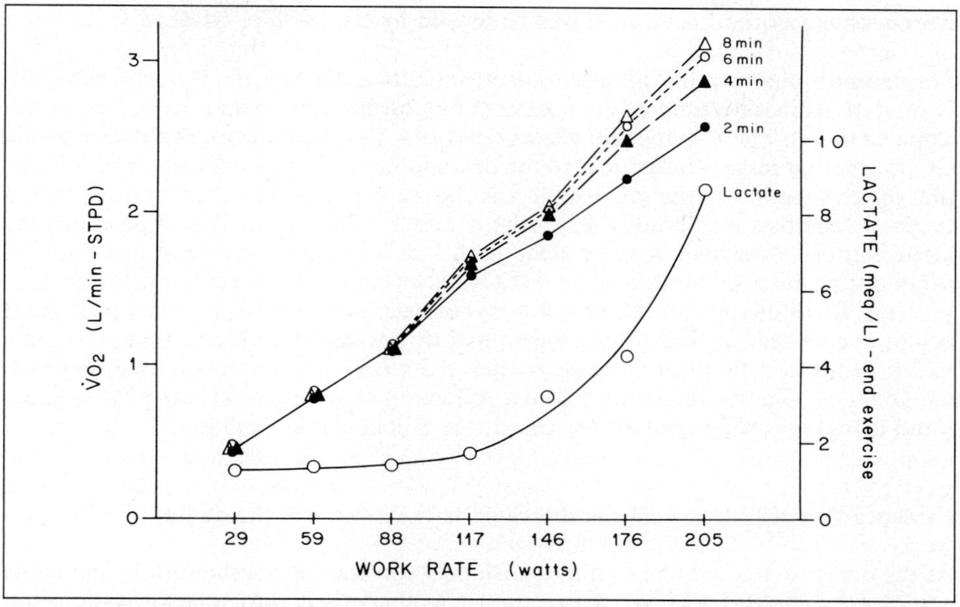

Fig. 2. Data from Fig. 1 taken at 2, 4, 6 and 8 min to show the relationship between $\dot{V}O_2$ and work rate as related to time of the measurement, and the lactate measurements at the end of 8 minutes of the work rate indicated. This study shows that the $\dot{V}O_2$-work rate relationship, consistent at low work rates, steepens for work rates above lactic acidosis threshold.

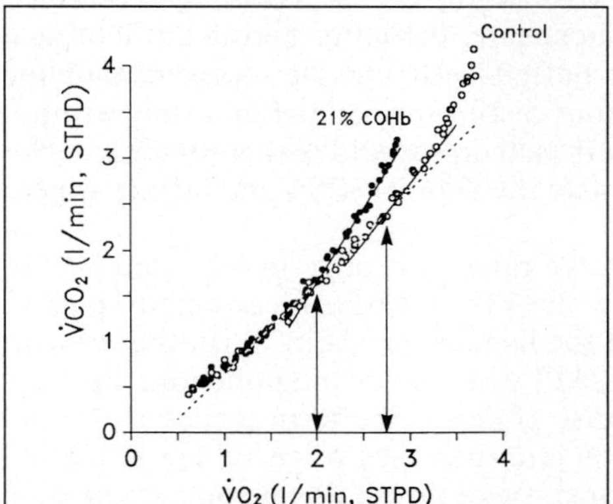

Fig. 3. Plot of $\dot{V}CO_2$ versus $\dot{V}O_2$ taken from Fig. 3, to demonstrate the V-slope method for determining the anaerobic threshold (AT). Not only is AT reduced, but the slope calculated for the data between AT and the respiratory compensation point is steeper in the 21% carboxyhemoglobin (COHb) study. (Taken from data reported in ref. 10)

$\dot{V}O_2$ increased with the same slope regardless of work rate increase until the lactic acidosis threshold (LAT)*. Above the LAT, the $\dot{V}O_2$-work rate relationship was shallower, the faster the work rate increase.

* Lactic acidosis threshold is the $\dot{V}O_2$ above which lactic acidosis develops as evidenced by CO_2 generated from the buffering of lactic acid or the decrease in arterial standard HCO_3^-. It is synonymous to the anaerobic threshold (AT) as described in section 3.

Measurement of the Lactic Acidosis Threshold by the V-Slope Method

For determining the point of onset of lactic acidosis, the rate of CO_2 output ($\dot{V}CO_2$) is plotted against the rate of O_2 uptake ($\dot{V}O_2$) for an incremental exercise test (V-slope analysis). The V-slope plot allows determination of the work rate above which CO_2 output increases consequent to the development of lactic acidosis. The V-slope plot for two studies in the same subject is shown in Fig. 3. The control study shows the lactic acidosis threshold (LAT) to be at about 2.75 L/min. The slope above the lactic acidosis threshold is more steep than 1 and defines the rate of aerobic CO_2 production plus CO_2 produced by HCO_3^--buffering of lactic acid relative to $\dot{V}O_2$ increase. In a study with increased carboxyhemoglobin (COHb) [10], the break-point occurs at a lower $\dot{V}O_2$ than during the air breathing control study and LAT is reduced to 2.0 L/min. Furthermore, the slope above the LAT break-point is steeper in the CoHb study, than in the control study, reflecting an accelerated rate of CO_2 generated from the buffering of an increased rate of lactic acid formation.

Evidence that the lactic acidosis threshold is the anaerobic threshold

At the onset, we would like to distinguish between lactate threshold (LT) and lactic acidosis threshold (LAT). We define the LT as the $\dot{V}O_2$ at which lactate concentration in arterial blood starts its steep increase during a progressively increasing work rate test. We assess this, using the log-log transformation of lactate versus $\dot{V}O_2$, as described by Beaver et al. [1]. However, as also described by Beaver et al. [3], the first lactate increase detected in arterial blood (approximately 0.5 mEq/liter) is buffered by non-bicarbonate buffers (Fig. 4). Possibly, the rate of lactate increase matches the increased hydrolysis of creatine phosphate, the latter taking up hydrogen ions. Alternatively (or in addition), protein buffers with a pK at approximately the cell pH may take up the hydrogen ion without disturbing cell pH and thus without decreasing blood bicarbonate. Thus the bicarbonate threshold is slightly higher than the lactate threshold [3]. Above the bicarbonate threshold, HCO_3^- and lactate appear to change stochiometrically.

The gas exchange method, based on relative rates of change in $\dot{V}O_2$ and $\dot{V}CO_2$, must define the lactic acidosis threshold (i.e. the $\dot{V}O_2$ at which bicarbonate starts to fall consequent to lactate increase) and not the lactate threshold. With that caveat, we use the term lactic acidosis threshold (LAT) when describing phenomena associated with the metabolic acidosis of exercise, and use the term lactate threshold (LT) to describe the $\dot{V}O_2$ at which blood lactate increases when its log is plotted against log $\dot{V}O_2$. The plot consistently demonstrates a threshold response coinciding with the $\dot{V}O_2$ at which the lactate/pyruvate ratio increases. From the following experiments, evidence is provided that the (LAT) is the anaerobic threshold (AT).

Figure 5, taken from the study of Koike et al [10], shows a plot of $\dot{V}O_2$ as related to work rate for a single subject breathing room-air or air with a small amount of added carbon monoxide to increase the carboxyhemoglobin (COHb) to the 10% (a level typical for a heavy cigarette smoker) and 18% levels. The arrows show the lactic acidosis thresholds defined by the V-slope method for the three studies. These studies demonstrate that, above the LAT, $\dot{V}O_2$ is reduced at any workrate in proportion to the increase in COHb level. In contrast, below the LAT, the $\dot{V}O_2$ is the same regardless of the level of COHb. The reduction in $\dot{V}O_2$ above the LAT implies

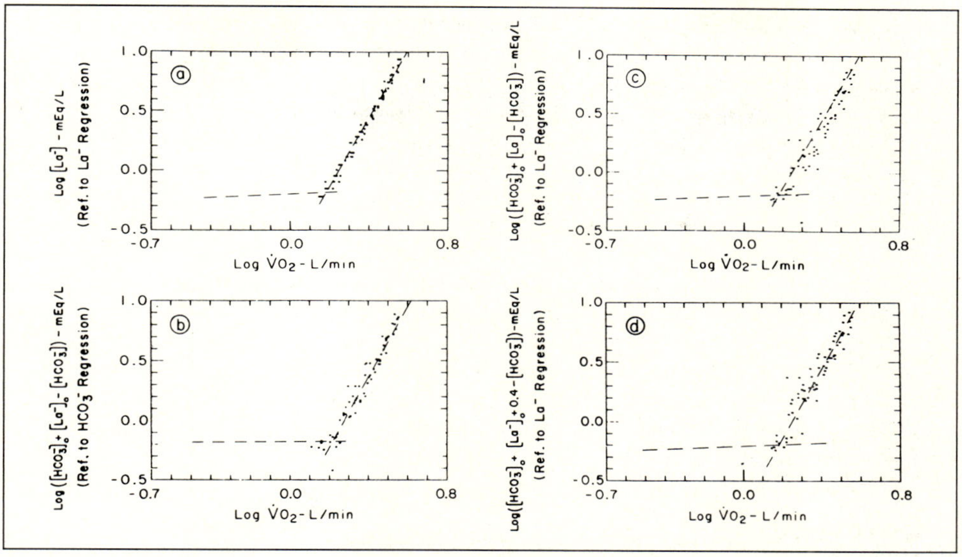

Fig. 4. Results of incremental excercise testing in healthy subjects. Log-log transformation of lactate (panel a) and bicarbonate (panel b) versus $\dot{V}O_2$. In this plot, the bicarbonate concentrations were normalized to the lactate concentrations and expressed as the difference from rest, so that the data for the two measurements could be superimposed (panel C). These studies indicate that the bicarbonate threshold is slightly higher than the lactate threshold, but the displacement is parallel (panel C). By addition of 0.4 mEq/L to the lactate data, these data superimpose on the lactate regression (panel d). (From Beaver et al. (2) with permission)

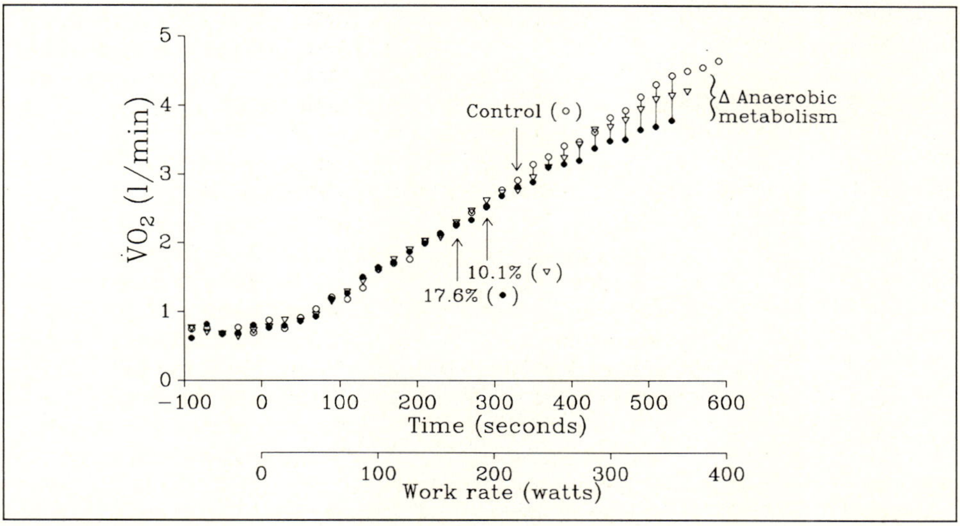

Fig. 5. $\dot{V}O_2$, time, and work rate for progressively increasing work rate test during air breathing without and with a small increase of carbon monoxide to increase the carboxyhemoglobin (COHb) to 10.1 and 17.6 percent, in a normal subject. Arrows show the time and $\dot{V}O_2$ of the lactic acidosis threshold in each of the 3 tests. (From the studies Koike et al. [10], with permission)

that the rate of regeneration of ATP from aerobic metabolism is sensitively affected by O_2 flow to the mitochondria. The reduction in aerobically produced high energy phosphate must be compensated for by increased anaerobic metabolism. Indeed, blood lactate is increased at these work rates. The change in slope of $\dot{V}O_2$ above the LAT demonstrates the sensitivity of this region of the work rate spectrum to O_2-flow and supports the concept that the LAT defines the $\dot{V}O_2$ above which anaerobic mechanisms supplement aerobic mechanisms in the generation of energy for exercise, i.e. a threshold $\dot{V}O_2$ for onset of anaerobic metabolism (anaerobic threshold).

We believe that the most reliable gas exchange method to determine the anaerobic threshold (AT) is one which detects the CO_2 generated as bicarbonate buffers lactic acid. This is the basis of the V-slope method [2]. The results of this method agree with the change in ventilatory equivalent for O_2 without change in ventilatory equivalent for CO_2, and the increase in end-tidal PO_2 without change in end-tidal PCO_2 when these measurements can be accurately interpreted [8]. But since the V-slope method is relatively intensitive, it is more applicable than other ventilatory and gas exchange measurements of the AT.

Oxygen Uptake and CO_2 Output Kinetics: Functional Implications

Oxygen uptake and CO_2 output at the lungs are a function of oxygen consumption and CO_2 production in the cells as modified by the coupling behavior of the circulation between the cells and the lungs (Fig. 6). In the case of CO_2 output, during the cardiac output increase transition, CO_2 stores can increase because of the high solubility of CO_2 in tissues. At work rates above AT, large increases in CO_2 are generated from HCO_3^- buffering of lactic acid during the period of lactate increase. If the metabolic cost of work is very small relative to the fitness of the individual, the magnitude of central command might cause an overshoot in the cardiac output and heart rate will decrease after Phase I [15]. On the other hand, if the oxygen flow exactly matches the oxygen requirement, oxygen uptake kinetics at the lung will be similar to that in the muscle. If oxygen uptake were inadequate for the requirement, oxygen uptake kinetics in the muscle will be slowed by the inadequate O_2 supply. This slowed pattern of oxygen uptake increase in the muscle will be reflected in slow $\dot{V}O_2$ kinetics and speeded CO_2 output kinetics consequent to simultaneous lactic acid generation.

Figure 7 shows the $\dot{V}O_2$ and $\dot{V}CO_2$ kinetics for a normal individual. In order to reduce random noise, six successive tests were performed, with suitable rest periods between each, to average the random noise and enhance the physiological responses. For a moderate work rate (left panel), oxygen uptake and CO_2 output increase abruptly at the start of exercise with little change in the gas exchange ratio through the first 15 s (Phase I). This must be due to the increase in pulmonary blood flow with blood residing in the venous system when exercise began. After capillary blood from the exercising muscles reaches the lungs, the gas exchange ratio decreases, reflecting the rapid increase in oxygen uptake but relatively slow CO_2 output increase because of the retention of some CO_2 produced from aerobic metabolism in the tissues because of its high solubility. Then both $\dot{V}O_2$ and $\dot{V}CO_2$ increase toward the steady-state, with $\dot{V}CO_2$ lagging slightly.

At higher work rates (Fig. 7, right panel), the magnitude of Phase I is only slightly greater, the primary increase in $\dot{V}O_2$ and $\dot{V}CO_2$ being reflected during Phase II. Thus

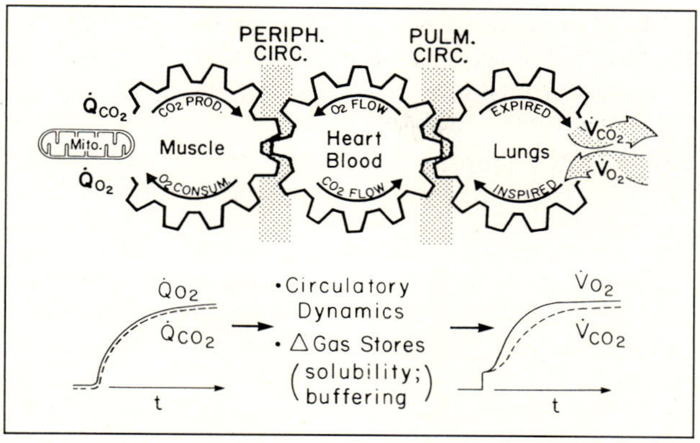

Fig. 6. Schematic illustration of the circulatory coupling of external to cellular respiration. Oxygen uptake at the lungs is determined by oxygen consumption at the cells as modified by the circulatory adjustment to the metabolic requirement. CO_2 output is modified, in addition, by its high solubility in tissues as cellular PCO_2 increases (primarily at the start of exercise), and the CO_2 generated by HCO_3^- as it buffers lactic acid at heavy work rates.

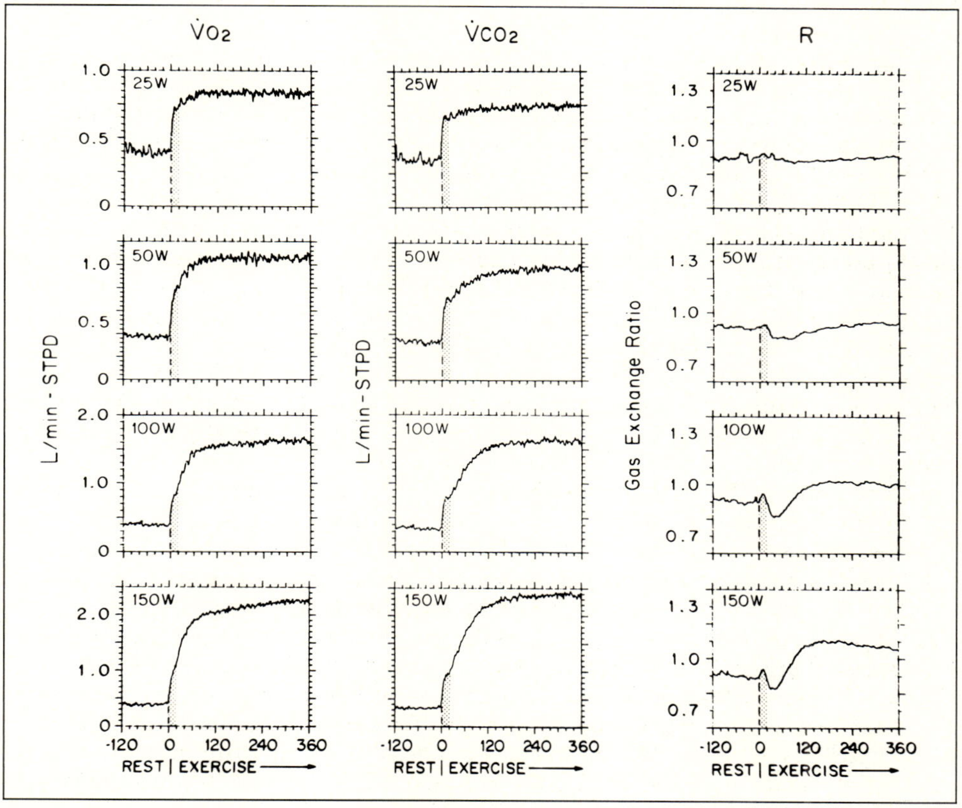

Fig. 7. $\dot{V}O_2$, $\dot{V}CO_2$, and gas exchange ratio (R) for 50 watts and 150 watts work in a normal subject. To reduce random noise, the subject performed each work rate on different days, 6 times. The data were then time averaged to enhance the physiological responses.

the mean response kinetics are relatively slow at the higher work rates, in part because Phase I becomes a smaller fraction of the total response. Thus the magnitude of the immediate (phase I) cardiovascular response to exercise affects the size of the early increase in $\dot{V}O_2$ and $\dot{V}CO_2$.

The dependence of Phase I $\dot{V}O_2$ on the magnitude of increase in pulmonary blood flow at the start of exercise is demonstrated in Fig. 8. In this study, $\dot{V}O_2$ was measured, breath-by-breath, in a patient with congenital heart block and an adjustable

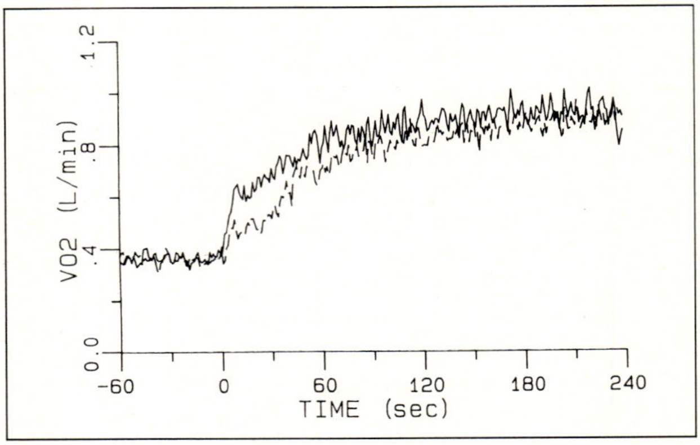

Fig. 8. $\dot{V}O_2$ in response to exercise in a patient with heart block. Exercise started at 0 time and the work rate was 40 watts. The patient's resting heart rate was 40 beats per min. In the study represented by the solid curve, the heart rate was turned up to 80 beats per min at the start of exercise. In the curve indicated by the dashed line, the change in the heart rate was feigned and the heart rate was kept at 40 beats per min. (From Casaburi et al. [6]).

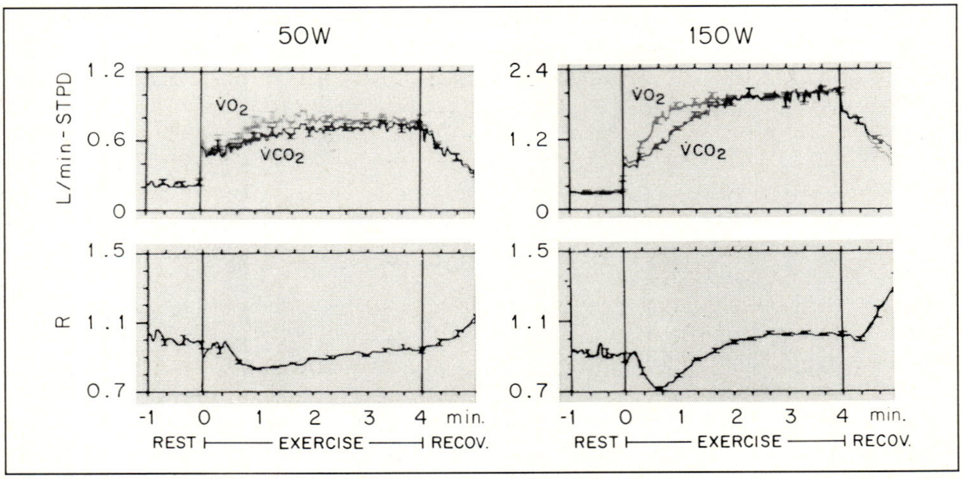

Fig. 9. Oxygen uptake ($\dot{V}O_2$), CO_2 output ($\dot{V}CO)_2$ and R for 25 watts, 50 watts, 100 watts, and 150 watts. The curves are the average responses for a group of ten normal subjects. (Modified from Sietsema et al [15] with permission).

cardiac pacemaker. At zero time, the subject started cycle ergometer work at 40W. Four repetitions were done to reduce the influence of random noise. In the experiment described by the solid curve, heart rate at the start of exercise was increased from a blocked rate of 40 beats/min to 80 beats/min. The broken line shows the $\dot{V}O_2$ change for the same work rate when the subject's heart rate was held constant at 40 beats/min. $\dot{V}O_2$ during Phase I was only half as large when the heart rate was not increased at the start of exercise. This suggests that the cardiac output increase was only about one-half of that which took place when the heart rate was abruptly increased. $\dot{V}O_2$ rises to the same asymptote in both studies.

Figure 9 shows the kinetics of $\dot{V}O_2$, $\dot{V}CO_2$ and the gas exchange ratio (R) for work rates at 25, 50, 100, and 150 watts for a group of normal subjects (modified from studies reported in reference [15]). These data are the average of the responses of 10 normal male subjects between 20 and 42 years of age. These studies demonstrate that phase I is evident at all work rates but it becomes a smaller fraction of the total response for $\dot{V}O_2$ and $\dot{V}CO_2$ as work rate increases. They also demonstrate the drift in $\dot{V}O_2$ at the higher work rates, i.e. above the anaerobic threshold, as illustrated in Fig. 1. Furthermore, for lower work rates, $\dot{V}CO_2$ kinetics after phase I are slower than VO_2 kinetics. This is reflected in a decreasing gas exchange ratio during phase II. For 150 watts (above the AT) $\dot{V}CO_2$ kinetics are faster than $\dot{V}O_2$, resulting in an overshoot in gas exchange ratio; it subsequently decreases, approaching a lower value reflecting the respiratory quotient of the metabolic substrate.

The mean response time for oxygen uptake is related to the cardiovascular fitness of the subjects (Fig. 10). This study shows that for the lowest work rate, the mean response time is approximately the same for all subjects and, in fact, cannot be accurately measured because of the rapidity and size of the cardiodynamic (phase I) response to exercise. But, for the higher work rates, a clear relationship is established with respect to fitness. The higher the work rate is above the subject's AT, the longer is the time constant [7]. This point is made most clearly when relating the mean response time for oxygen uptake to lactate at the end of exercise.

Koike et al. [9] studied the effect of increasing carboxyhemoglobin concentration on the time constant for oxygen uptake kinetics as shown in Fig. 11. They demonstrated that the time constant correlated with the increase in lactate caused by the exercise (Fig. 11), thus $\dot{V}O_2$ kinetics and lactate production appear to be interrelated.

Noting the $\dot{V}O_2$ drift for work rates above the anaerobic threshold, Whipp and Wasserman [20] and later, Roston et al. [14] proposed that the difference in $\dot{V}O_2$ between 6 and 3 min of exercise ($\Delta\dot{V}O_2$ 6—3) was correlated with the magnitude of the lactate increase after 6 min of constant work rate exercise. In contrast to the time constant, which is dominated by data during the first minute of exercise, the $\Delta\dot{V}O_2$ 6—3 describes the kinetics of the slow component. Below the AT, $\Delta\dot{V}O_2$ 6—3 is approximately zero [14].

Figure 12 shows the normal relationship between $\Delta\dot{V}O_2$ 6—3 and blood lactate from the studies of Koike et al. [9]. For a $\Delta\dot{V}O_2$ of about 150 ml per min, lactate is increased to approximately 4 mEq per liter. The correlation of $\Delta\dot{V}O_2$ 6—3 to lactate in this study was quite similar to that of Roston et al. [14].

Figure 13 illustrates a study in a patient with heart failure performing exercise at 70 watts. $\Delta\dot{V}O_2$ 6—3 is determined by the best fit curve from the breath-by-breath $\dot{V}O_2$ data. The value for $\dot{V}O_2$ at 6 min and 3 min of exercise is established from the computerized least square fit of the data. Since $\Delta\dot{V}O_2$ 6—3 is approximately zero for work rates below the anaerobic threshold, a positive value in this study (124 ml/

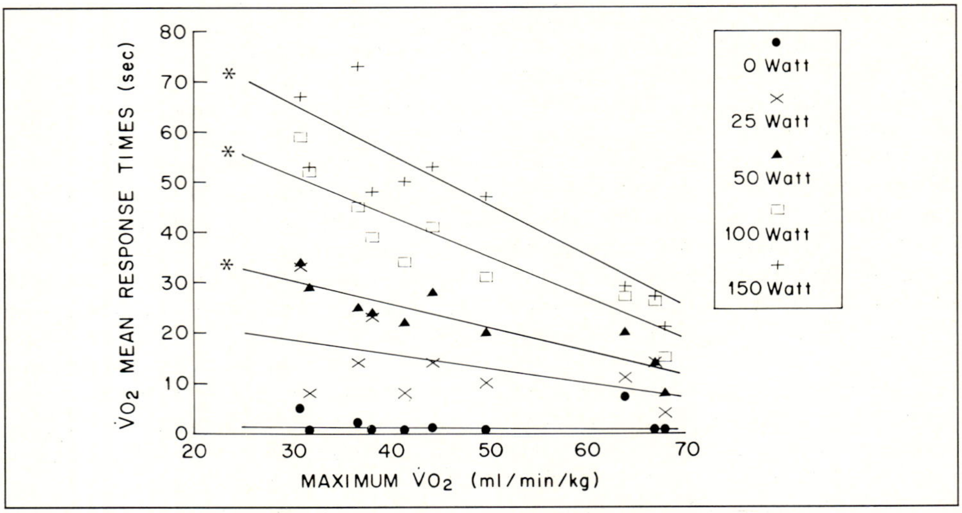

Fig. 10. Time constant for $\dot{V}O_2$ for five different (unloaded cycling, 25, 50, 100 and 150 watts) constant work rates as related to fitness for ten normal male subjects. If the work rate is very low, there is no discrimination of the kinetics since the circulatory coupling more than adequately supplies the oxygen required by the working muscle. However, in the less fit individuals, circulatory coupling of external to cellular respiration begins to limit oxygen utilization and the oxygen kinetics are slowed as related to fitness at the high work rates. (Modified from Sietsema et al. [15])

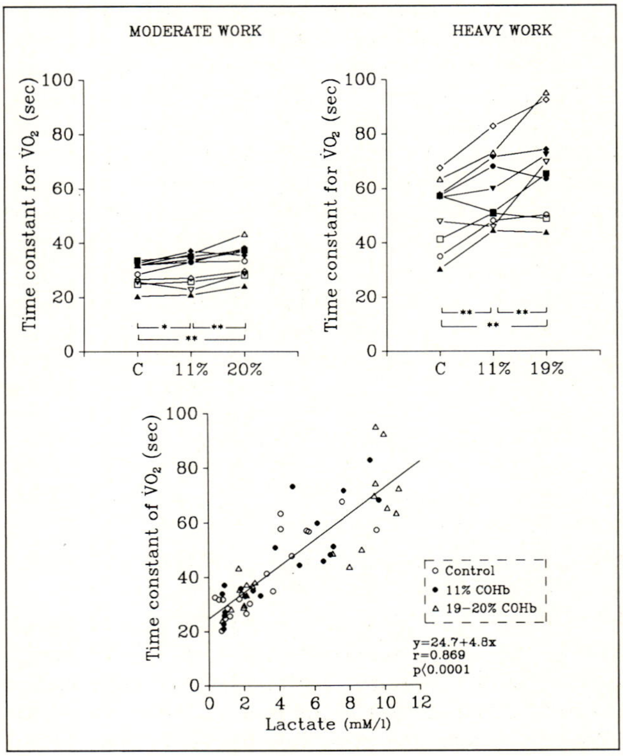

Fig. 11. Time constant of $\dot{V}O_2$ for a constant work rate of moderate and heavy intensity at three different levels of carboxyhemoglobin concentration (COHb) (upper panel) and the time constant plotted as a function of lactate concentration (lower panel) in ten normal subjects. From Koike et al. [9], with permission.

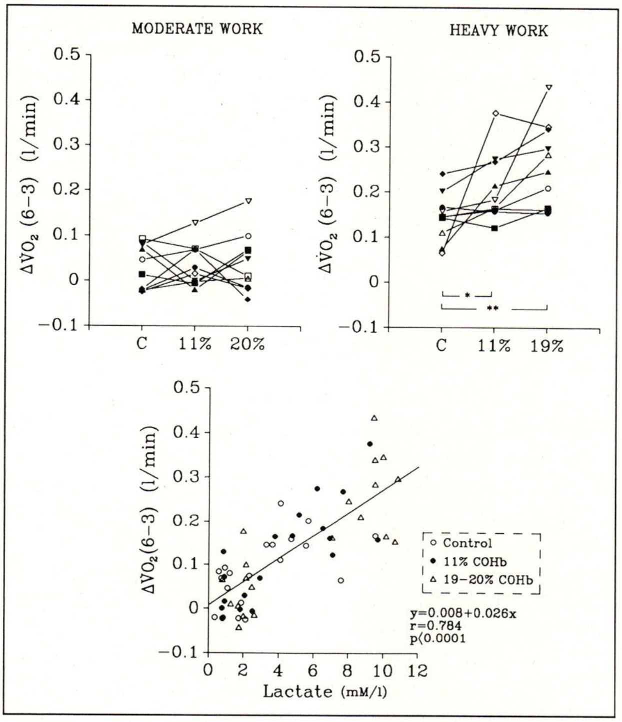

Fig. 12. Difference between $\dot{V}O_2$ at 6 min and 3 min of exercise ($\Delta\dot{V}O_2$6—3) in 10 normal subjects performing two constant work rates estimated to be of moderate and heavy intensity for three levels of carboxyhemoglobin (COHb) (upper panel). The $\Delta\dot{V}O_2$ 6—3 min values are plotted as a function of each subject's respective forearm vein lactate concentration at the end of 6 min of exercise at two work rates and for three levels of COHb. (From Koike et al [9], with permission)

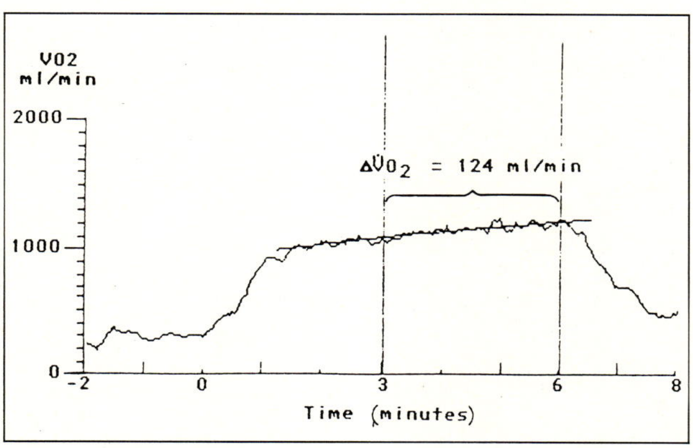

Fig. 13. Method illustrating the measurement of the difference in oxygen uptake ($\dot{V}O_2$ between 6 and 3 min of exercise ($\Delta\dot{V}O_2$ 6—3)) in a patient with cardiac disease (70 watts). The smooth line drawn on the plot between 3 and 6 min was determined by the best square fit for the breath-by-breath data. The difference in $\dot{V}O_2$ at the 6 min and 3 min points is calculated from the regression determined values.

min) indicates that the work is being performed above the subject's anaerobic threshold.

From the circulatory coupling of oxygen uptake at the lungs to oxygen consumption at the cells, it is clear that the oxygen uptake kinetics at the lungs is highly dependent on the functional capacity of the circulation. Therefore a very important determination in assessing cardiovascular function is the mean response time (or time constant) for $\dot{V}O_2$ in response to a work rate stimulus. Because patients with cardiovascular disease often exhibit cyclic fluctuations in breathing and may not tolerate multiple repetitions of exercise transitions, we have adopted the method of summing oxygen uptake during a 6 min exercise test and, from this, calculating the total oxygen consumed above the resting value. From the difference between this value and the calculated 6 min $\dot{V}O_2$, an oxygen deficit can be computed for the 6-min exercise period. Dividing the oxygen deficit by the $\dot{V}O_2$ above rest at 6 minutes, the time constant is obtained. Using this time constant, an exponential curve fit between 0 time and 6 min gives a good curve fit through the actual data as illustrated for the patient in Figure 14.

Control of Breathing During Exercise: The Training Factor

Many theories have been evolved with respect to ventilatory control in response to exercise, but none have specifically addressed the striking decrease in ventilation that occurs following exercise training. Figure 15, from Casaburi et al. [5], shows the change in the ventilatory response resulting from endurance training, for four different work rates in a single subject. The lowest work rate was below the subject's AT so there was no change in lactate consequent to exercise training, and there was no change in ventilation for that work rate. In contrast, ventilation was systematically reduced at the work rates above the lactic acidosis threshold, and the decrease in ventilation was well correlated with the decrease in lactate (Fig. 16). Each lmEq/L decrease in lactate was associated with approximately 7 liters per minute decrease in ventilation at the end of 15 min of work, after training. This translates into a sensitivity of ventilation change relative to hydrogen ion of approximately 3 liters

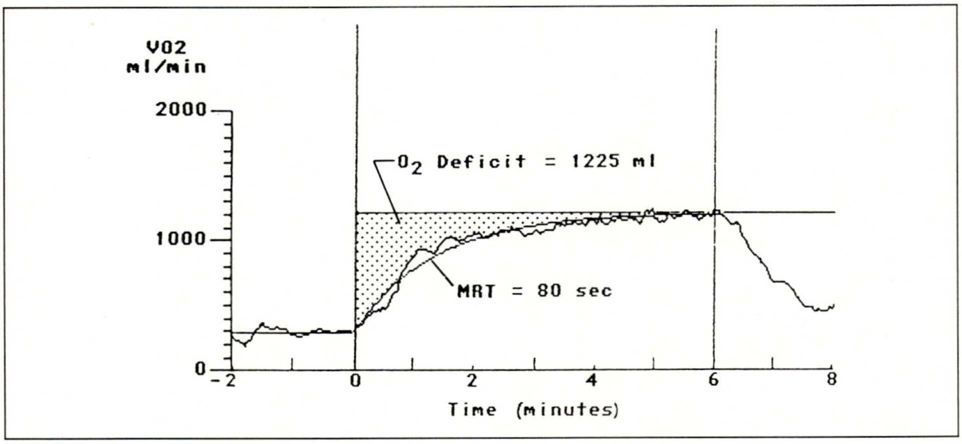

Fig. 14. Method for determining the mean response time or (time constant) of a patient with heart failure from breath-by-breath data. Exercise started at 0 time and was completed at 6 min. While the data for the subject (irregular curve) is an 8 breath moving average, the time constant was determined from the breath-by-breath measurements, as described in the text. The smooth curve was drawn by the computer through the data from rest to 6 min, from the calculated time constant, assuming a single exponential rise.

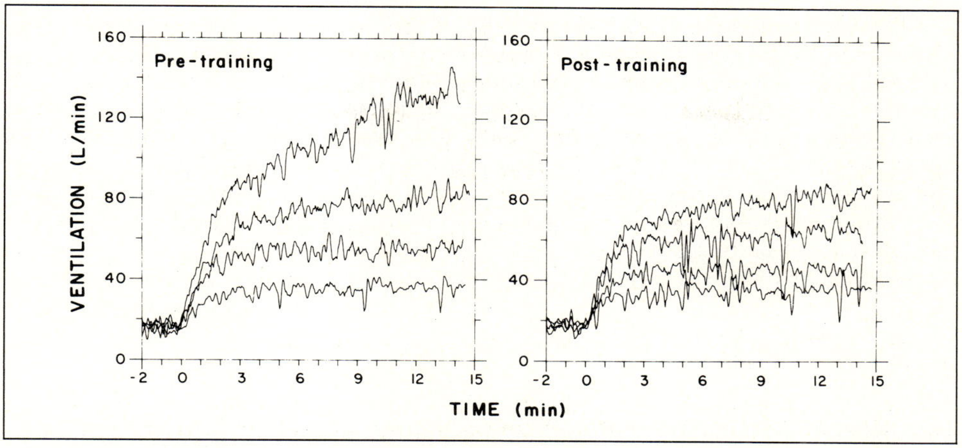

Fig. 15. Exercise ventilation in a normal male subject before and after intense endurance exercise training. Ventilation was significantly reduced only at those work rates for which there was an accompanying reduction in lactate. (From Casaburi et al. [5])

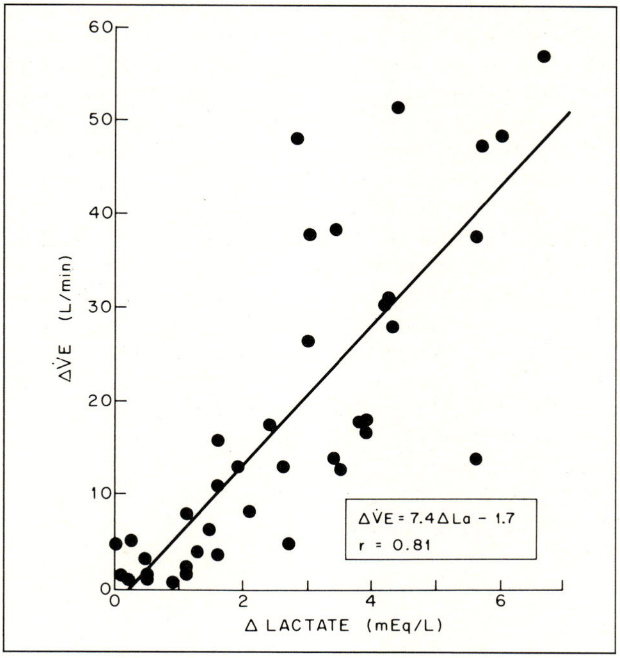

Fig. 16. Relationship between the decrease in lactate and ventilation in response to exercise training. Each of 10 subjects performed 4 work rates before and after training. Each point shows the decrease in end-exercise ventilation and the simultaneous decrease in end-exercise blood lactate following training. (From Casaburi et al. [5])

per minute per nanomole per liter decrease of H^+. Thus the striking change in ventilation consequent to training is compatible with the reduction of hydrogen ion production. This seems to be an excellent candid mechanism by which training alters the ventilatory response above the AT. There remains to be demonstrated another physiological stimulus which is modified by training, with as potent effect on ventilation as the homeostatic ventilatory mechanism regulating hydrogen ion.

In summary, a great deal of information about control mechanisms and cardiovascular function in response to exercise is learned from noninvasive measuring of gas exchange dynamics. While steady-state $\dot{V}O_2$ response to a given exercise work rate might be the same in patients with heart disease, normal sedentary subjects, and athletes, the dynamic changes in $\dot{V}O_2$ are very different. Adding an analysis of the simultaneous $\dot{V}CO_2$ kinetics, a great deal is also learned about the dynamics of the lactic acidosis of exercise. The exercise lactic acidosis, and the ability of the cardiovascular system to meet the O_2 requirement, appear to be functionally related.

Abstract

This paper addresses basic concepts concerning the interrelationship between oxygen consumption and work rate, the dependency of oxygen uptake kinetics on the work rate performed, and the implications of altered oxygen uptake and CO_2 output kinetics with respect to the exercise lactic acidosis. Apparent steady-states in $\dot{V}O_2$ are established at progressively longer times or not at all, the higher the work rate above the lactic acidosis threshold (LAT). Using low levels of carbon monoxide (CO) to increase the carboxyhemoglobin (CoHb) level to 10% and 20%, we demonstrated that $\dot{V}O_2$ is unaffected by the level of COHb for work rates below the LAT, but is reduced for work rates above the LAT during a progressively increasing work rate test. These studies support the hypothesis that the LAT is the anaerobic threshold (AT). $\dot{V}O_2$ kinetics, in response to a constant work rate stimulus, has been shown to be sensitively affected by alterations in cardiovascular function. Useful measurements reflecting altered $\dot{V}O_2$ kinetics include the time constant (T.C.) and the difference between $\dot{V}O_2$ at 6 minutes and 3 minutes of constant work rate exercise ($\Delta\dot{V}O_2$ 6—3). Both the T.C. and the $\Delta\dot{V}O_2$ 6—3 are well correlated with the magnitude of lactate increase at the end of 6 minutes of exercise. The influence of lactate increase on ventilatory control was studied analyzing the simultaneous changes in ventilation ($\dot{V}E$) and lactate in response to exercise training. The decrease in $\dot{V}E$ is correlated with the decrease in lactate consequent to training. Training does not significantly affect $\dot{V}E$ below the AT. The decrease in exercise $\dot{V}E$ resulting from training is closely correlated with the decrease in hydrogen ion with a sensitivity slope of approximately 3 L/min/nanomole of H^+. These studies demonstrate that the dynamic coupling of external to cellular respiration during exercise plays an important role in determining $\dot{V}O_2$ and $\dot{V}CO_2$ kinetics, the oxygen cost of work, the exercise lactic acidosis, and the ventilatory response to exercise.

Reference

1. Beaver WL, Wasserman K, Whipp BJ (1985) Improved detection of lactate threshold during exercise using a log-log transformation. J Appl Physiol 59: 1936—1940
2. Beaver WL, Wasserman K, Whipp BJ (1986) A new method for detecting anaerobic threshold by gas exchange. J Appl Physiol 60: 2020—2027
3. Beaver WL, Wasserman K, Whipp BJ (1986) Bicarbonate buffering of lactic generated during exercise. J Appl Physiol 60: 472—378

4. Brouha L, Radford EP, Jr. (1960) The cardiovascular system in muscular activity. In Science and Medicine of Exercise and Sports, edited by W.R. Johnson. New York Harper, 182—183
5. Casaburi R, Storer TW, Wasserman K (1987) Mediation of reduced ventilatory response to exercise after endurance training. J Appl Physiol 63: 1533—1538
6. Casaburi R, Spitzer, Haskell R, Wasserman K (1988) Effect of altering heart rate on gas exchange at exercise onset. Chest 95: 6-12
7. Casabure R, Barstow TJ, Robinson T, Wasserman K (1989) Influence of work rate on ventilatory and gas exchange kinetics. J Appl Physiol 67: 547—555
8. Hansen JE, Casaburi R, Cooper DM, Wasserman K (1988) Oxygen uptake as related to work rate increment during cycle ergometer exercise. Eur J Appl Physiol 57: 140—145
9. Koike A, Wasserman K, McKenzie DK, Zanconato S, Weiler-Ravell D. Evidence that diffusion limitation determines O_2 uptake kinetics during exercise in man. J Clin Invest (submitted for publication)
10. Koike A, Weiler-Ravell D, McKenzie DK, Zanconato S, Wasserman K (1990) Evidence that the metabolic acidosis theshold is the anaerobic threshold. J Appl Physiol
11. Krogh A, Lindhard J (1913) The regulation of respiration and circulation during the initial stages of muscular work. J Physiol (London) 47: 112—136
12. Linnarsson D (1974) Dynamics of pulmonary gas exchange and heart rate changes at start and end of exercise. Acta Physiol. Scand. Suppl. 415: 1—68
13. Moore-Ede, MC (1986) Physiology of the circadian timing system: predictive versus reactive homeotasis. Am J Phyiol 250 (Regulatory Integrative Comp. Physiol. 19): R 735—R752
14. Roston WL, Whipp BJ, Davis JA, Cunningham DA (1987) Effros RM, Wasserman K (1987) Oxygen uptake kinetics and lactate concentration during exercise in humans. Am Rev. Respir. Dis. 135: 1080—1084
15. Sietsema KE, Daly JA, Wasserman K (1989) Early dynamics of O_2 uptake and heart rate as affected by exercise work rate. J Appl Physiol 67: 2535—2541
16. Stringer W, McKenzie D, Casaburi R, Wasserman K (1990) Acid base regulation during exercise and recovery in man. Am Rev Respir Dis 141: A 119
17. Wasserman K, Van Kessel A, Burton GG (1967) Interactions of physiological mechanisms during exercise. J Appl Physiol 22: 71—85
18. Wasserman K, Whip BJ, Casaburi R (1986) Respiratory control during exercise. In: Handbook of Physiology, Section 3: The respiratory system, Volume 2: Control of Breathing, Part II. Eds.: A. P. Fishman, N. S. cherniack, J. G. Widdicombe and S. R. Geiger. Amer Physiol Soc., Bethesda, Maryland 595—619
19. Wasserman K, Beaver WL, Whipp BJ (1990) Gas exchange theory and the lactic acidosis anaerobic) threshold Circulation 81 (Suppl II): II-14-II-30,
20. Whipp BJ, Wasserman K (1972) Oxygen uptake kinetics for various intensities of constant load work. J Appl Physiol 33: 351—356

Author's address:

K. Wassermann, M.D., Ph. D.
Respiratory Medicine, A-15
Harbor-UCLA Med. Center
1000 W. Carson Street
Torrance, CA 90509, USA

Determination of $\dot{V}O_2$ Kinetics by Means of Spectral Analysis: A New Method for Evaluation of Endurance Capacity

J. Stegemann, U. Hoffmann, and D. Eßfeld

Physiologisches Institut der Deutschen Sporthochschule Köln, FRG

Tests for the assessment of aerobic capacity can be divided into three categories according to the exercise intensity required from the subjects:

1) Maximal tests, e.g.: determination of maximal oxygen consumption ($\dot{V}O_2$ max), maximal power or maximal exercise duration;

2) Tests requiring intermediate efforts, e.g.: determination of "thresholds" beyond which lactate accumulates in the blood, measurement of heart rate-$\dot{V}O_2$ relationship;

3) Low-intensity tests leading to decreased or unchanged blood-lactate conditions.

The first two groups comprise several standardized testing procedures widely used in sports medicine. Standardized methods are presently not available for low-intensity exercise tests. This means that subjects with low exercise tolerance or subjects in poor health condition are practically excluded from endurance performance tests. A major disadvantage resulting from this is that there is no systematic way of developing exercise-training regimens for these subjects. The lack of low-intensity tests is also unsatisfactory with healthy subjects. Maximal tests require a certain amount of motivation and cooperation from subjects. Moreover, maximal tests only indicate that one element of a variety of factors has reached its limits, they do not tell which one. Tests depending on increased concentrations of blood lactate require less, but still considerable effort. They will yield erroneous results when glycogen stores are depleted and, like maximal tests, they may induce endurance training effects, which is undesirable when exercise training prescriptions are to be studied. Tests operating within the range of "everyday" exercise intensities would therefore constitute a desirable expansion of the tests already existing. Methods of breath-by-breath $\dot{V}O_2$ determination may open this field for medical routine.

A starting-point for the development of such low-intensity tests is the observation that the rate of $\dot{V}O_2$ adjustment following changes in exercise intensity is faster in endurance-trained subjects [3, 6, 8, 9, 13, 14, 16, 17]. The method most frequently applied consists of step changes in exercise intensity such as changes from rest to low exercise intensities, or between two exercise levels within the aerobic range. Generally, the $\dot{V}O_2$ responses are fitted by explicit models, e.g. monoexponential functions. For that purpose, a linear relationship between workload (WL) and $\dot{V}O_2$ response dynamics is frequently implied, though this seems critical in the case of rest-exercise transitions because of particular changes in venous return and cardiac output. Moreover, several repetitions and an averaging process are necessary to obtain a characteristic $\dot{V}O_2$ response of a single subject. This is mainly due to two reasons:

– The resolution of $\dot{V}O_2$ responses is limited by breathing frequency. Fast $\dot{V}O_2$ step responses will provide only few $\dot{V}O_2$ values;

— Net oxygen uptake during single breathing cycles shows considerable fluctuations which are, among other factors, induced by intra-breath differences between inspired and exspired volumes.

$\dot{V}O_2$ kinetics can also be studied by means of sinusoidal changes in exercise intensity [2, 4]. This will generally lead to a sinuosidal $\dot{V}O_2$ responses of the same frequency. The relation between input (workload) and output ($\dot{V}O_2$) can then be described in terms of amplitude ratio and phase shift for each forcing frequency. Such analyses in the frequency domain require no explicit modeling; theoretically, they provide descriptions equivalent to step response analyses in the time domain. Other aspects of the selection of adequate approaches are practicability and feasibility. Testing single frequencies over a wide range is very time-consuming. On the other hand, these analyses will give insight into the range of higher frequencies that will not be reached when using monoexponential fittings of step responses.

If the assumption of dynamic linearity between workload and $\dot{V}O_2$ is justified, frequency analyses can be speeded up by simultaneous application of several testing frequencies. One type of multifrequent analysis uses randomized switching between two intensities (pseudo random binary sequence (PRBS)). This minimizes the test duration and it can be measured very easily with common ergometers. However, adequate application and interpretation of this approach need some theoretical background of frequency analysis.

The PRBS protocol

In our workload protocol (Fig. 1), intensities are randomly changed between two levels during a time interval of 450 s. The minimum duration of each level is 30 s. For cycle ergometry in young healthy subjects, we prefer steps between 20 W and 80 W at a pedalling frequency of 1 Hz. This PRBS signal is a multifrequent stimulus from which $\dot{V}O_2$ responses to the fundamental frequency of 450 s and to the higher harmonics can be computed by means of spectral analysis. In the standard experiment the basic 450 s-sequence is repeated twice. Before and after the PRBS interval constant levels of workload are added for the determination of steady-state responses at both exercise intensities. We confine the dynamic analysis to the first six harmonics (periods from 450 s down to 75 s). In this range cardiovascular effects have only a minor influence on the results [5]. A detailed description of the applied algorithms and the theoretical background is given by Eßfeld et al. [7].

Example

In Fig. 1 the $\dot{V}O_2$ kinetics of one highly endurance-trained subject and one untrained student are compared. The middle panel shows the $\dot{V}O_2$ responses to the PRBS protocol which are then transformed into the frequency domain for the first six harmonics.

The frequency responses are presented as Bode plots which consists of two parts. First, in a double logarithmic plot, are the quotients of $\dot{V}O_2$ and WL amplitudes vs. the frequencies tested. To compensate for differences in mechanical efficiency and respiratory quotients, each amplitude ratio (ml O2/(min · W)) is expressed as percentage of the static ratio obtained from the $\dot{V}O_2$ steady state values. Second, the

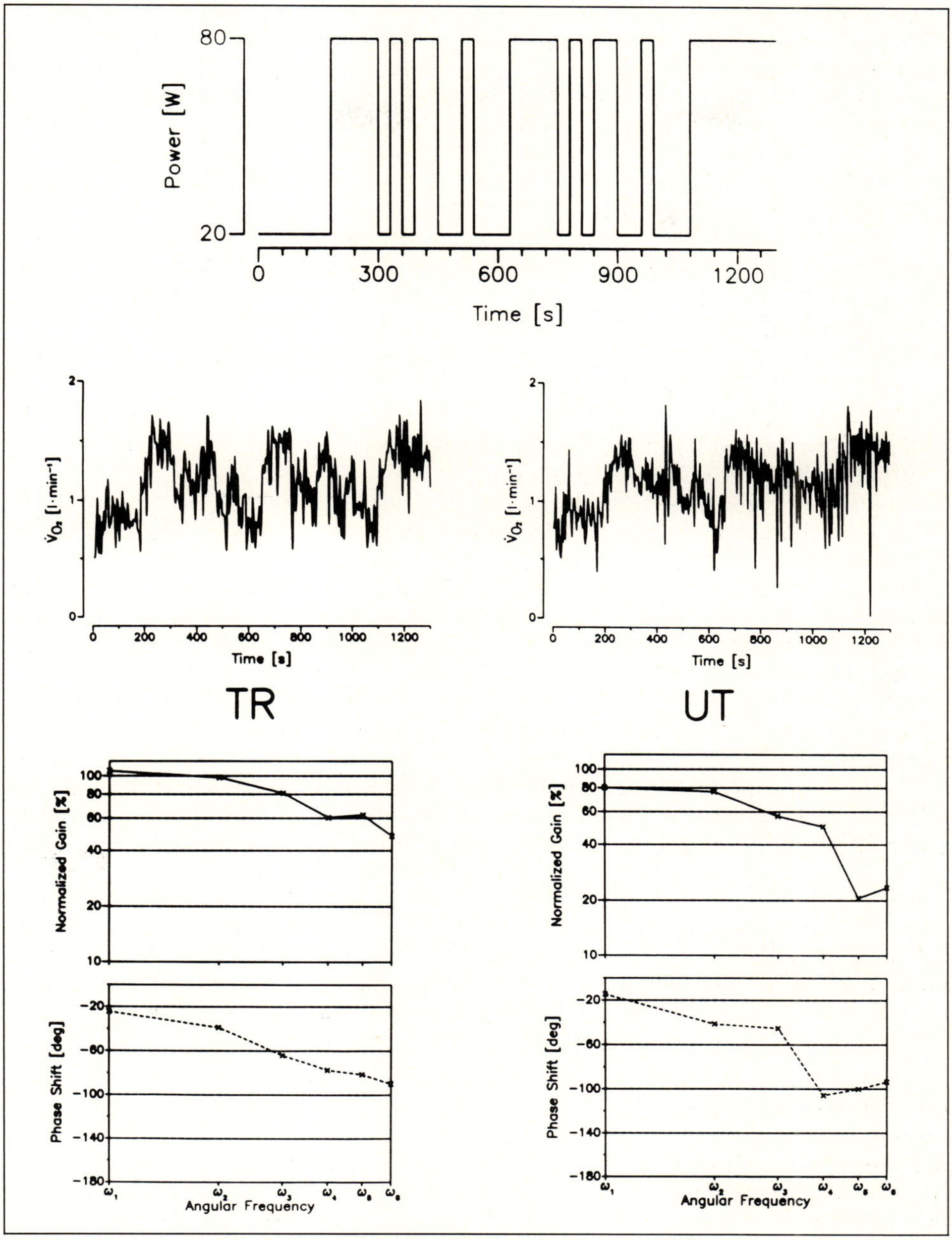

Fig. 1. Determination of $\dot{V}O_2$ kinetics in one endurance-trained (TR) and one untrained (UT) healthy subject. Top: PRBS protocol switching between 20 W and 80 W. The sequence from 180 s to 630 is repeated twice. Middle part: Time series of breath-by-breath $\dot{V}O_2$ responses. Bottom: Resulting frequency responses (Bode plots) for the first six harmonics (i = i × 14 mrad/s; periods: 450 s to 75 s). Dynamic gains are expressed as percentage of steady-state gains.

phase shifts between $\dot{V}O_2$ and WL signals vs. the logarithmic frequencies. The major difference between the two subjects of Fig. 1 is that the amplitude ratios of the trained subject assume higher values over a wider range of frequencies. This means that changes in exercise intensity lead to faster adjustment of $\dot{V}O_2$ in the trained subject.

Experience with the PRBS protocol

We have applied the PRBS protocol in various experimental contexts to study the effects of:
- 500 ml blood withdrawal [1];
- fluid losses induced by 6 h of head-out of water immersion [10];
- different levels of ventilation [7];
- a 7-day bedrest [15];
- supine vs. upright body position during exercise [12];
- different relative $\dot{V}O_2$ max values [6];
- day-by-day variations (reproducibility) in single subjects [11];
- isolated changes in venous blood volume and muscle perfusion kinetics (analysis by means of a computer model [5]).

The studies generally show that periods down to 75 s yield reproducible results which are mainly influenced by the endurance capacity of the working muscle group. For higher frequencies (periods less than 75 s) there is an increasing distortion through non-linear factors, in particular, cardiac output and muscle perfusion kinetics. In contrast to $\dot{V}O_2$ max measurements the PRBS data are not significantly affected by changes in blood volume. Further comparisons of endurance tests are summarized in Table 1.

The present experience with the PRBS approach suggests that this method qualifies as a test for the determination of local endurance capacity. The current technique allows for further reductions in exercise intensity or working muscle mass.

Table 1: Qualitative comparison of different endurance tests (+++: high, ++: intermediate, +: low, 0: absent effects or influences).

	$\dot{V}O_2$ max	Lactate-dependent tests	PRBS
Demands on instrumentation	++	+	+++
Required exercise intensity	+++	++	+
Short-term effects on other physiological parameters	+++	++	+
Training effects	+++	++	+
Influence of:			
— Motivation	+	0	0
— Blood volume	+++	++	+
— Muscle perfusion	+++	++	+
— Mass of working muscle	+++	+++	+

Therefore, this test in combination with optimal breath-by-breath techniques provides a means for assessing the aerobic capacity of patients, which could, as yet, not be subjected to exercise tests.

One problem that still has to be solved is to condense the complex information in such a way that users can interpret the data without previous familiarization with frequency-response techniques.

References

1. Baum K, Hoffmann U, Eßfeld D, Stegemann J (1990) Time courses of endurance performance parameters following 500 ml of blood withdrawal. Fourth European Symposium on Life Sciences Research in Space (ESA Sp-307): (in press)
2. Casaburi R, Whipp BJ, Wassermann K, Beaver WL, Koyal SN (1977) Ventilatory and gas exchange dynamics in response to sinusoidal work. J Appl Physiol: Respirat Environ Exercise Physiol 42: 300—311
3. Cerretelli P, Pendergast D, Paganelli WC, Rennie DW (1979) Effects of specific muscle training on $\dot{V}O2$ on-response and early blood lactate. J Appl Physiol: Respirat Environ Exercise Physiol 47: 761—769
4. Chang KS, Snellen JW (1982) The use of sinusoidally changing workloads as an aid to identify dynamic properties of physiological systems. Eur J Appl Physiol 49: 97—109
5. Eßfeld D, Hoffmann U, Stegemann J (1991) A model for studying the distortion of muscle oxygen uptake patterns by circulation parameters. Eur J Appl Physiol (in press)
6. Eßfeld D, Hoffmann U, Stegemann J (1987) $\dot{V}O2$ kinetics in subjects differing in aerobic capacity: Investigation by spectral analysis. Eur J Appl Physiol 56: 508—515
7. Eßfeld D, Hoffmann U, Stegemann J (1990) Ventilatory effects of hypercapnic end-tidal PCO2 clamps during aerobic exercise of varying intensity. Eur J Appl Physiol 60: 412—417
8. Hagberg JM, Hickson RC, Ehsani AA, Holloszy JO (1980) Faster adjustment to and recovery from submaximal exercise in the trained state. J Appl Physiol: Respirat Environ Exercise Physiol 48: 218—224
9. Hickson RC, Bomze HA, Holloszy JO (1978) Faster adjustment of O2 uptake to the energy requirements of exercise in the trained state. J Appl Physiol: Respirat Environ Exercise 44: 877—881
10. Hoffmann U, Baum K, Baer FM, Eßfeld D, Stegemann J (1987) Influence of a 6 h head-out water immersion on different tests of endurance performance capacity. Third European Symposium on Life Sciences Research in Space (ESA SP-271): 51—54
11. Hoffmann U, Baum K, Eßfeld D, Stegemann J (1990) Intraindividual variability of $\dot{V}O2$ frequency responses in physically active subjects. Fourth European Symposium of life sciences research in space (ESA SP-307) (in press)
12. Hoffmann U, Eßfeld D, Stegemann J, Schütze H (1990) Comparison of $\dot{V}O2$ kinetics in upright and supine position. Acta Astronautica (in press)
13. Powers SK, Dodd S, Beadle RE (1985) Oxygen uptake kinetics in trained athletes differing in $\dot{V}O2$ max. Eur J Appl Physiol 54: 306—308
14. Sietsema KE, Daly JA, Wassermann K (1989) Early dynamics of O2 uptake and heart rate as affected by exercise work rate. J Appl Physiol 67: 2535—2541
15. Stegemann J, Eßfeld D, Hoffmann U (1985) Effects of a 7-day head-down tilt (6 °) on the dynamics of oxygen uptake and heart rate adjustment in upright exercise. Aviat Space Environ Med 56: 410—414
16. Weltmann A, Katch V (1967) Min-by-min respiratory exchange and oxygen uptake kinetics during steady-state exercise in subjects of high and low max $\dot{V}O2$. Res Quart 47: 490—498
17. Whipp BJ, Wassermann K (1972) Oxygen uptake kinetics for various intensities of constant-load work. J Appl Physiol 33: 351—356

Author's address:

Prof. Dr. med. J. Stegemann,

Physiologisches Institut der Deutschen Sporthochschule Köln, Carl-Diem-Weg 6, 5000 Köln 41

The Importance of Lactate Measurement for the Determination of the Anaerobic Threshold

H. Heck

Institute for Cardiology and Sports Medicine, German University of Sports Sciences, Cologne, FRG (Director: Prof. Dr. R. Rost)

Introduction

In 1976, Mader et al. (14) introduced the terms "lactate threshold" and "aerobic-anaerobic threshold" as important parameters for the diagnosis of performance capacity. Since then, these terms have undergone several modifications [2, 11, 18, 20].

Threshold was defined by Mader et al. as: "The field of transition between the mere aerobic and the partially anaerobic muscular energy metabolism performance under production of lactate, is called "aerobic-anaerobic threshold". An increase of lactate up to 4 mmol/l in peripheral blood can be rated as a criterion for the assessment of the aerobic-anaerobic threshold, for example, by a gradual increase of work rates".

Frequently, the theoretical and experimental proof of the 4 mmol/l threshold was questioned by for example, Tesch et al. [21]: "The rationale for using a concentration of 4 mmol/l to define onset of lactate accumulation may be questioned."

In the following, findings are given which prove the 4 mmol/l threshold by experimental data; some of them have already been published [6—10]. (Concerning the theoretical proof of the threshold we refer the reader to [16]). In addition, it will be demonstrated that threshold determination at 4 mmol/l lactate is only valid when a defined test protocol is used. Any variations or differences will cause a change of the value of lactate threshold.

It can be derived from the threshold definition that, in a prolonged duration of work, threshold is identical with that load which causes "maximum lactate steady state". By the term "maximum lactate steady state" (maxLass), that load is defined when lactate production and lactate removal are just in balance. Any higher load intensity causes a continuous increase of blood lactate.

MaxLass covers energy metabolism at the borderline completely aerobically, since the anaerobically produced lactate is equally removed and the removal by aerobic means is mostly performed by the skeletal and heart musculature and the liver. Accordingly, total metabolism of energy supply is purely aerobic from the viewpoint of balance.

Therefore, maxLass is a suitable parameter for the validity of the different threshold concepts.

The following questions were examined by treadmill and bicycle ergometry:

1) At which lactate level does maxLass occur?
2) Which lactate level corresponds with the load of maxLass in graded tests?
3) What influence does load increase have, and what influence does test protocol have on threshold lactate?

Methods

Three different investigations are described. The first was performed with adults on a treadmill, the other two with adults and children by bicycle ergometry.

First investigation

Subjects: The subjects were 16 normal, healthy males with varying endurance capacities. Four subjects were long-distance runners (two of them among the nations top runners). All of the subjects were experienced treadmill runners and had frequently participated in treadmill tests. Anthropometric data: height: 179.3 cm (± 5.0), weight: 71.7 kg (± 8.0), age: 29.8 years (± 6.0).

Experimental procedure: Each subject participated in two graded tests and five constant work load tests on the treadmill. The first graded test was begun at a speed of 2.6, 3.0, or 3.4 m/s, depending on endurance capacity, and was increased by 0.4 m/s every 5 min to exhaustion. Following each loading level, the test was interrupted for 30 s to take blood samples for determination of lactate. The second test differed from the first only in that the loading duration was 3 min.

The prolonged exercise tests were composed of a 3-min warm-up (60 % of lactate threshold) and a 25-min exercise phase at a constant speed. The loading level of the first continuous exercise corresponded to the 4 mmol/l threshold in the graded test with loading duration of 5 min. Depending on the lactate values of the first or the previous tests, the continuous exercise test running speed was increased or decreased by 0.1 or 0.2 m/s. At least one, and preferably two experiments had to be conducted above the loading level to indicate a steady state of lactate. For the purpose of determining lactate, the exercise was interrupted at the end of the warm-up phase and after every 5-min interval.

Second investigation

Subjects: We examined 22 male subjects, two of them were practicing endurance sports athletes (triathlon, cycling). The others practiced leisuretime sports. Anthropometric data: height: 181.3 cm (± 4.4), weight: 74.5 kg (± 6.9), age: 25.9 years (± 4.8)

Experimental procedure: Each subject performed four graded tests and five constant work load tests on the cycle ergometer.

Graded tests:

Test	Input load (watts)	Step (watts)	Step duration (min)	Load increase (watts/min)
A	70 100 130	30	5	6.0
B	25	25	2	12.5
C	50	50	3	16.7
D	50	50	2	25.0

Test schemes C and D are procedures recommended in the FRG for testing of top athletes. Test scheme B is often used for persons with low performance capacity and children. Test scheme A corresponds approximately in its load increase to treadmill exercise with a 0.4 m/s grading and 5-min step duration related to equal oxygen uptake and a body weight of 70 kg.

Tests with constant load

After the graded tests the first examination was done with a load corresponding to 4 mmol/l lactate in test A. Depending on the registered lactate levels, in the next examination the load was increased by 10 W (sometimes by 5 W). There was a 3-min-warm-up at 60 % of threshold load in test A before the 30-min constant load test.

Third investigation

Subjects: We examined 18 children (8 girls, 10 boys) ranging in age from 8 to 15 years. Anthropometric data: height: 148.6 cm (± 9.9), weight: 39.4 kg (± 8.9), age: 11.3 years (± 1.6).

Experimental procedure: Each subject passed one graded test and five constant work load tests on a bicycle ergometer. The load scheme of graded test was 25 W/2 min with starting load of 25 W. The constant workloads were identical with those of adults (see above).

Lactate determination: Lactate determination was made by analysis of blood samples taken from earlobes (Finalgon salve hyperemic test) by calibrated capilette with a volume of 0.02 ml and emptied into an Eppendorf test tube filled with 0.2 ml of 0.6 N perchloric acid. Dietze et al. (4) stated that almost the same lactate values were gained from the earlobe and the finger pad, whereas the cubital venous values were significantly lower.

Measurement of lactate was made enzymatically using testing equipment from Boehringer Mannheim (FRG) according to the semimicro method described by Mader et al. [15]. When using a semi-automatic measurement, Mader et al. [15] found an analysis variation of 1.26 % at a low lactate level (3.4 mmol/l), and of 0.62 % at a high lactate level (18.7 mmol/l).

Testing equipment: The treadmill (Woodway Geres Co., Lörrach, FRG) has a running surface area of 230 cm × 70 cm. The speed is variable within the range of 0—7.4 m/s. The angle of incline can be adjusted from 0%—34%. We used an incline of 1%. The bicycle exercise was performed on an electrically braked ergometer (Elema-Schönander, Sweden).

Determination of load at 4 mmol/l lactate: In the graded test, the load at 4 mmol/l lactate was determined by linear interpolation. Kuipers [13] found an individual variation coefficient of 4—7% for the 4 mmol/l threshold when using bicycle ergometry. König et al. [12] indicate an average value of 4.1% at an individual variation of 2.8 to 5.4% (10 examinations/subject).

Determination of the maximum lactate steady state: To ascertain the maximal lactate steady state, only the values from the last 20 min were considered, since in some cases the lactate curve was still rising after 5 min. As a continuous increase

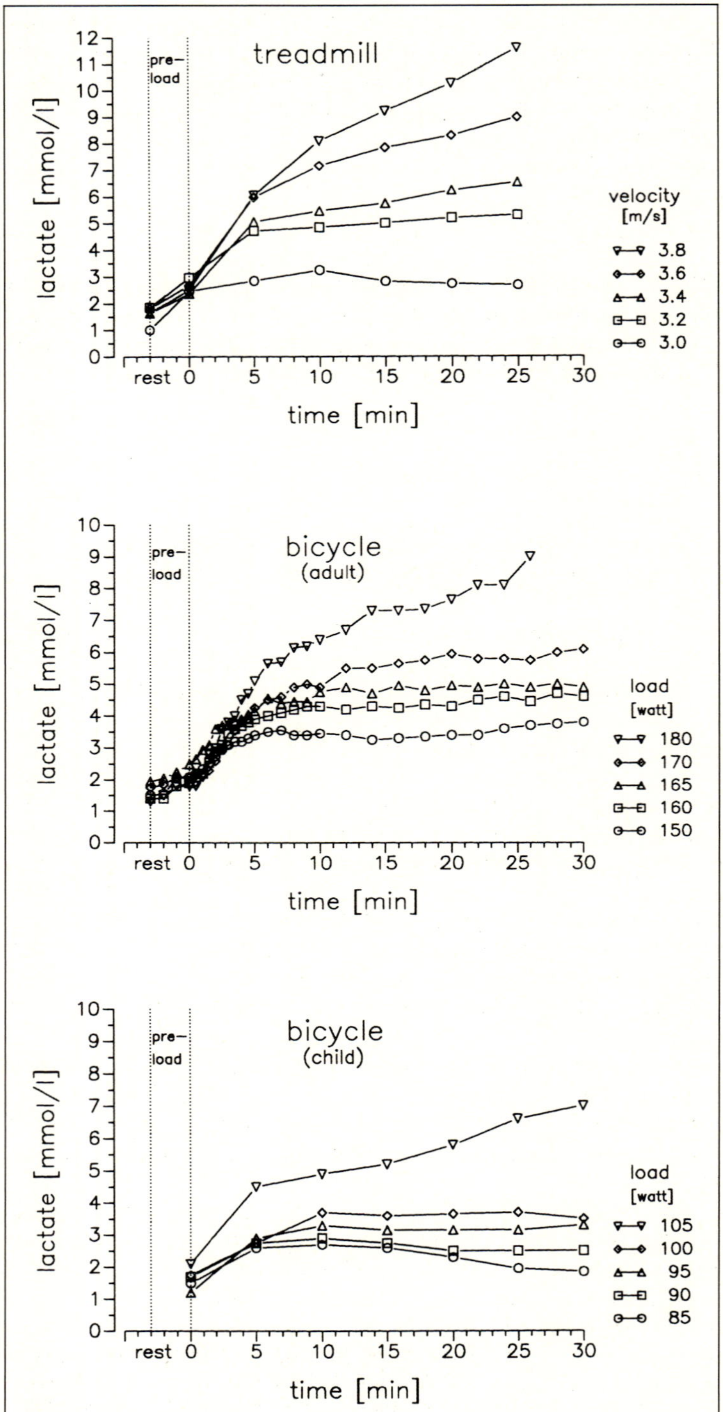

Fig. 1. Examples for lactate during continuous exercise tests at five different loads on the treadmill (upper) and bicycle (middle: adult, lower: child).

was observed in some subjects at low work loads and lactate concentrations, which did not increase more rapidly at higher workloads, we established the determination of maxLass as follows: The lactate value and the load are sought at which a maximal steady state of lactate is attained or when lactate level does not increase more than 1 mmol/l during the last 20 min of exercise. The mean value of the measurement of the last 20 min is considered to be the lactate value of maxLass and the corresponding load value as the load of maxLass.

Statistics: Standard statistical procedures were employed to calculate mean and standard deviation. The statistical significance of differences between paired samples was evaluated with the Wilcoxon test. A repeated analysis of variance (Anova) was made for comparison of mean values of the different test protocols. Relations of variables were examined by the linear one- or two-dimensional regression and correlation. In all statistical analyses the 0.05 level of significance was used.

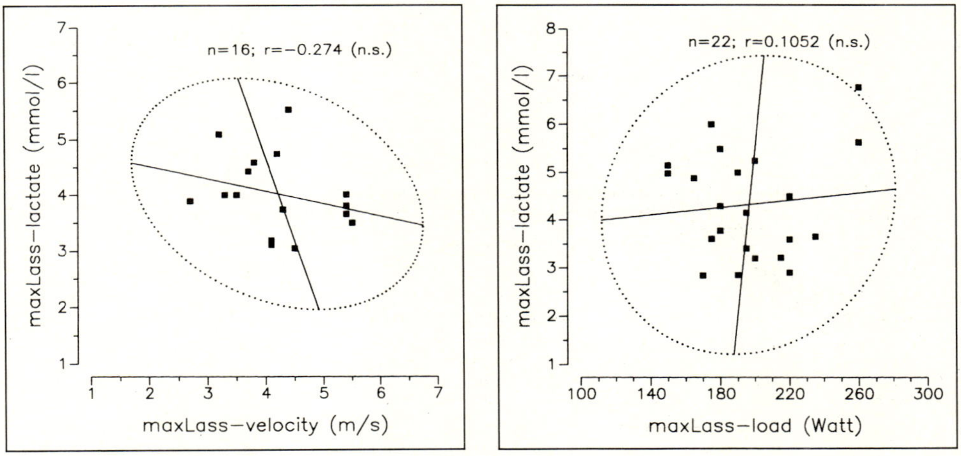

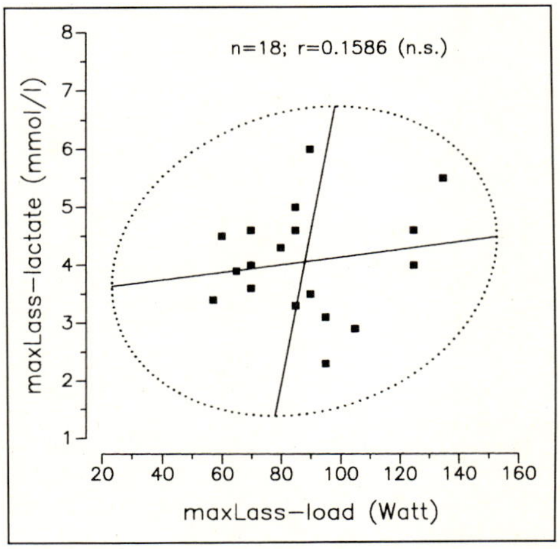

Fig. 2. Linear regression with 95%-confidence elipse and correlation between maxLass-lactate and maxLass-load (upper left: treadmill; upper right: bicycle-adults; lower: bicycle-children).

Results

Maximum lactate steady state

In all subjects maxLass could be determined. Figure 1 illustrates the lactate time curves for one subject in the three series.

On the average, maxLass-lactate was at 4.02 (± 0.70; min = 3.1; max = 5.5) for treadmill load, for bicycle ergometer at 4.32 (± 2.11; min = 2.9; max = 6.8) for adults, and at 4.06 mmol/l (± 0.83; min = 2.3; max = 6.0) for children. There was no dependence of maxLass-Lactate on maxLass-load and therefore not on endurance capacity (Fig. 2).

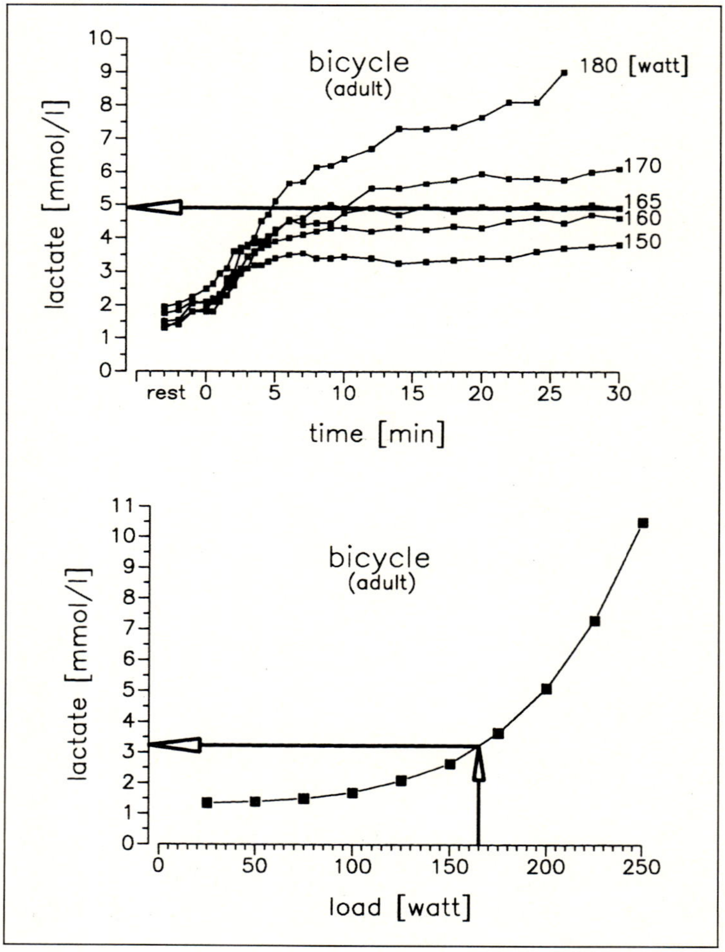

Fig. 3. Example for determination of lactate value of anaerobic threshold: upper: maxLass was found at 165 W and at a maxLass-lactate of 4.9 mmol/l; lower: in the graded test (25 W/2 min) a load of 165 W produced a lactate value of 3.25 mmol/l.

Anaerobic threshold

The lactate level of the anaerobic threshold was determined in the graded test by a load corresponding to that of maxLass by linear interpolation (see Fig. 3).

Mean, standard deviation, minimum, maximum, and statistical tests of threshold lactate for different test protocols are given in Table 1. In the treadmill test a re-

Table 1. Mean, standard deviation, minimum, maximum, and statistical tests of threshold lactate in graded tests with maxLass load for the different test protocols

Threshold lactate (mmol/l)							
Test	Load increase	n	$\bar{x}$	± s	Min	Max	Statistics
Treadmill	0.4 m/s/5 min	16	4.05	0.86	2.85	5.20	Wilcoxon
	0.4 m/s/3 min	16	3.50	0.60	2.50	4.35	$p < 0.01$
Bicycle: adults	30 watts/5 min	22	3.62	0.82	2.15	5.01	1-way Anova
	25 watts/2 min	22	3.11	0.66	1.94	4.28	$p < 0.01$
	50 watts/3 min	22	3.02	0.62	1.71	4.26	
	50 watts/2 min	22	2.79	0.67	1.31	3.78	
Bicycle: children	25 watts/2 min	18	3.03	0.56	2.00	4.10	

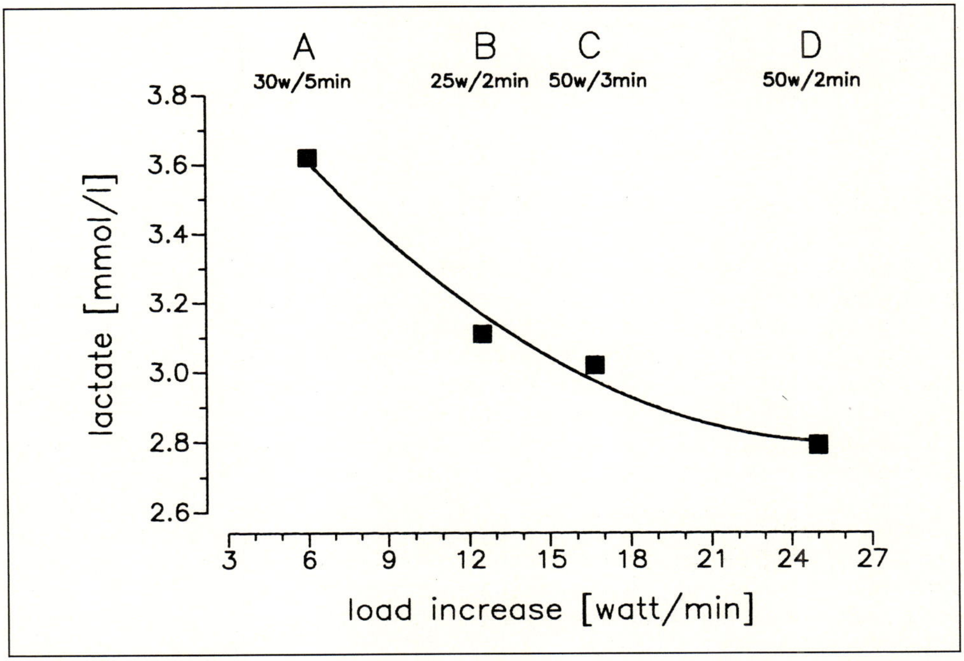

Fig. 4. Mean threshold lactate in relation to load increase in cycle ergometry. Quadratic regression: $Y = 4.17 - 0.106 \times X + 0.00205 \times X^2$.

duction of step duration from 5 to 3 min caused a reduction of threshold lactate from 4 to 3.5 mmol/l. In bicycle ergometry, an increasing workload causes a highly significant decrease of threshold lactate (Table 1, Fig. 4). For adults and children, threshold lactate (3.11 and 3.03 mol/l) is more or less equal when using the same test protocol.

A change of the test protocol causes highly significant effects on load levels at 4 mmol/l lactate (Table 2).

Table 2. Mean, standard deviation, minimum, maximum, and statistical tests of load at 4 mmol/l lactate for the different protocols

Load at 4 mmol/l lactate (m/s) or (watts)							
Test	Load increase	n	$\bar{x}$	± s	Min	Max	Statistics
Treadmill	0.4 m/s/5 min	16	4.20	0.88	2.35	5.46	wilcoxon
	0.4 m/s/3 min	16	4.34	0.85	2.63	5.58	$p < 0.001$
Bicycle:	30 watts/5 min	22	203.8	34.5	154.0	265.8	1-way anova
adults	25 watts/2 min	22	216.3	35.7	160.9	275.4	$p < 0.001$
	50 watts/3 min	22	218.7	36.5	157.6	287.4	
	50 watts/2 min	22	229.9	38.2	168.2	315.7	

No significant correlations between lactate at anaerobic threshold and maxLass-load were found (Figs. 5, 6 and 7).

Discussion

Lactate-steady-state

During constant work loads in submaximum intensity range, we found significant lactate increases in adults and children when using a treadmill or cycle ergometer.

In the past, this increase in lactate was attributed to the O_2-deficit resulting from the onset of work [5, 17]. Today, numerous publications illustrate that there is production of lactate at submaximum work. A review of literature can be found in [9].

Here, the level of lactate concentration is the result of lactate-production, -transport, -distribution, and -removal. The latter mostly takes place by lactate oxidation in resting and loaded musculature including heart muscle, and by gluconeogenesis in the liver [1]. On the assumption that the elimination depends on lactate concentration and load intensity, there is a lactate steady state as long as the rate of lactate production is higher than the maximum rate of removal [9, 16]. In bicycle or treadmill load, on the average, this maximum lactate steady state is about 4 mmol/l, independent of age and endurance capacity. When using cranking exercise the mean value was about 1 mmol/l higher (unpublished findings). Possibly, maxLass-lactate levels are higher when work has to be performed for more then 30 min. Partially, lactate curves show divergences above maxLass from linear increase.

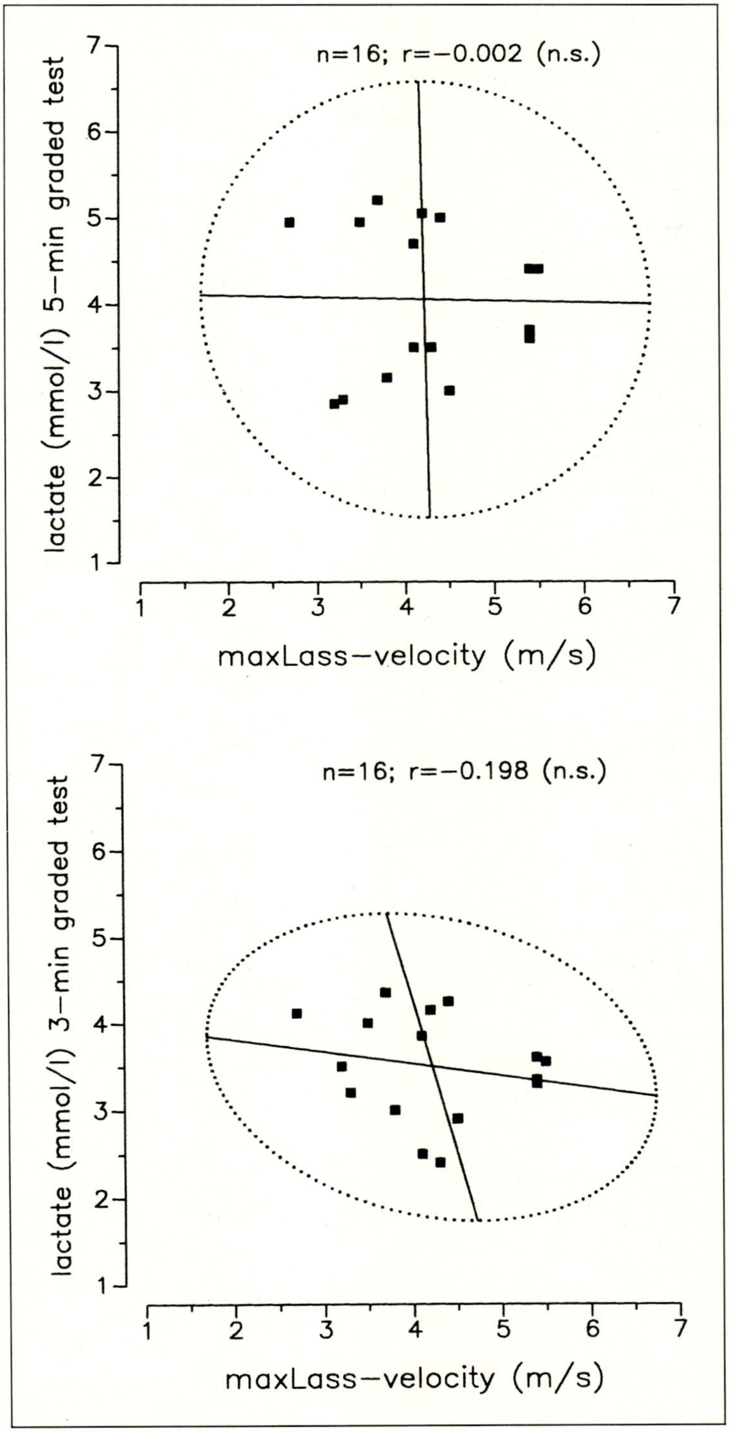

Fig. 5. Two-dimensional linear regression and correlation between anaerobic threshold lactate and maxLass-load on treadmill (upper: 5-min graded test; lower: 3-min graded test).

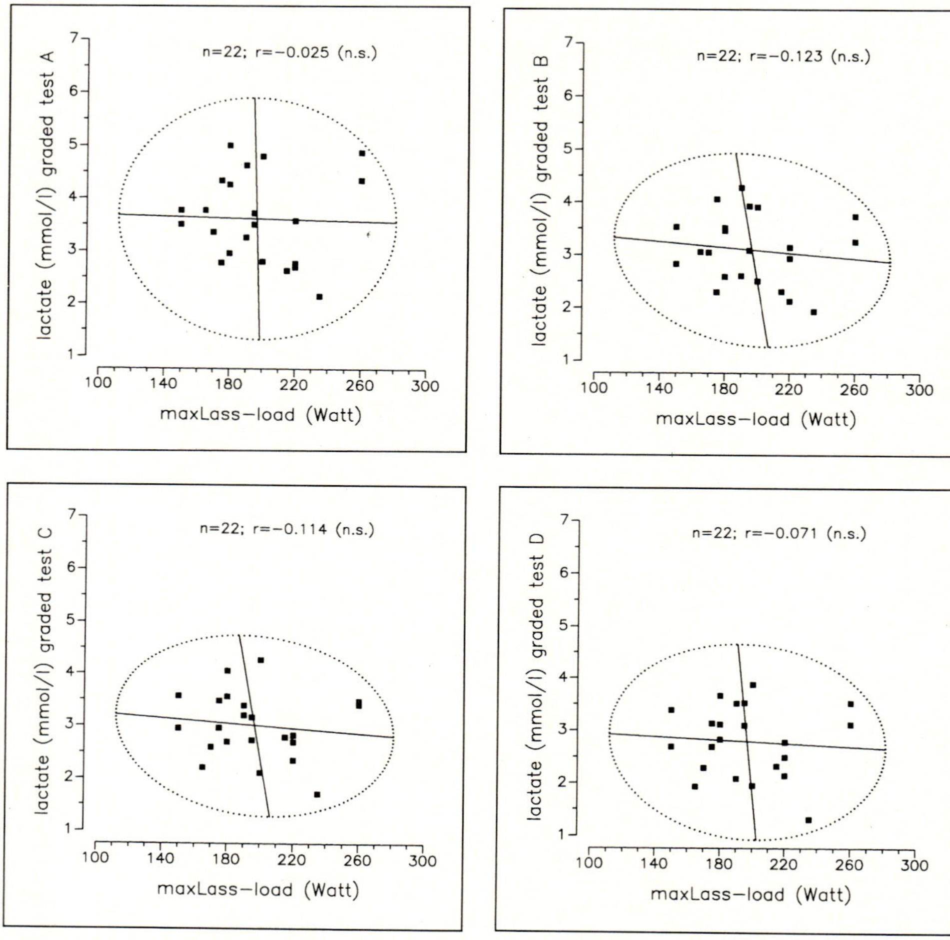

Fig. 6. Two-dimensional linear regression and correlation between anaerobic threshold lactate and maxLass-load in adults on bicycle ergometer (upper left: test A; upper right: test B; lower left: test C; lower right: test D).

Anaerobic threshold

On the average, load at a lactate level of 4 mmol/l in a graded treadmill test with a step duration of 5 min corresponds with lactate steady state. Therefore, the anaerobic threshold according to Mader et al. is a statistic value. In the individual test subject threshold will differ more or less from this value. The anaerobic threshold has nothing to do with a "breaking point" or a "turning point" of the lactate curve, as it is sometimes referred to in literature [3, 19]. It could be proved theoretically that such a breaking point does not exist [9, 16]. When breaking points in the lactate curve are observed, this is probably mostly due to faults in measuring.

A reduction of step duration from 5 to 3 min shifts the lactate curve to a higher velocity. Load at 4 mmol/l lactate increases on the average for about 0.14 m/s. Mean

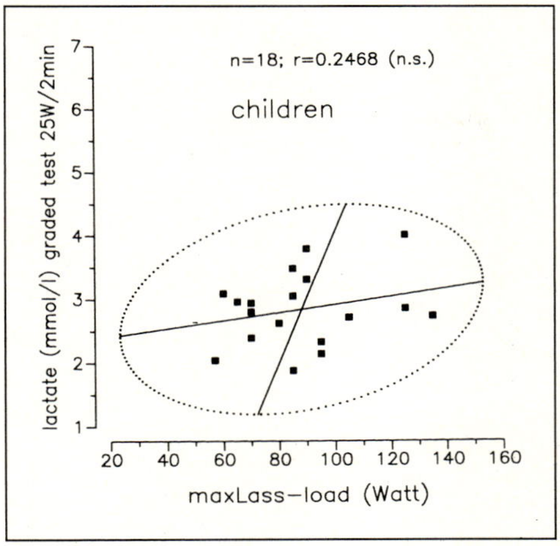

Fig. 7. Two-dimensional linear regression and correlation between anaerobic threshold lactate and maxLass-load in children on cycle ergometer (load increase 25 W/2 min).

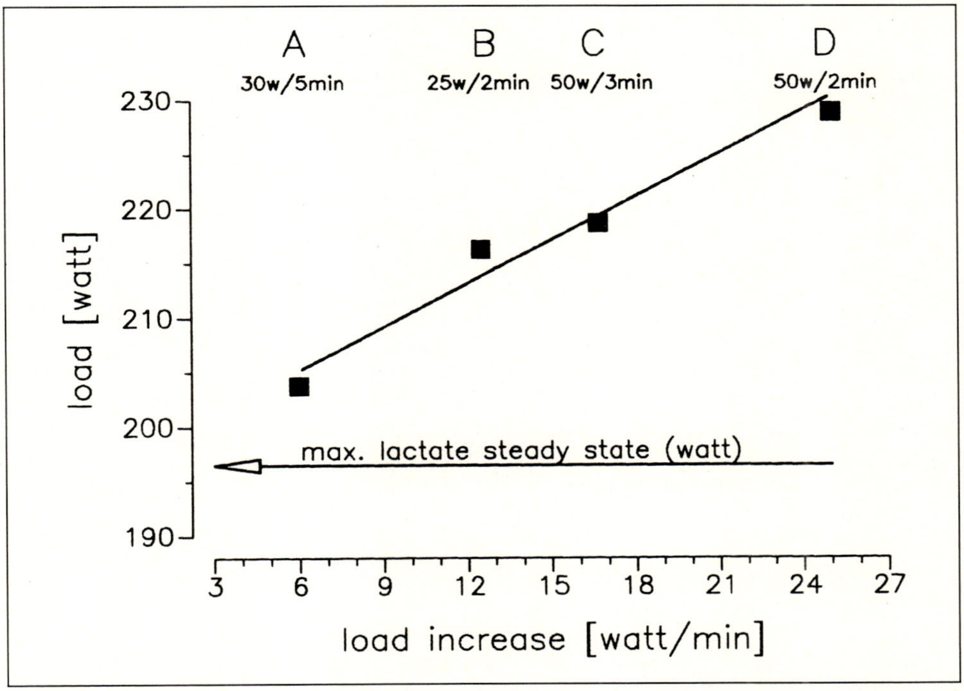

Fig. 8. Mean value of load at 4 mmol/l lactate for the four graded tests. The maxLass-load is at 196 W.

lactate level at corresponding maxLass velocity is 3.5 mmol/l in a 3-min graded test. This means that, on the average, load at 4 mmol/l lactate in a 3-min graded test is higher than maxLass load, and that anaerobic threshold is fixed at a too-high level.

In the usual bicycle ergometer test, divergences are even more distinct. At a load increase of 25 W/2 min and 50 W/3 min, load corresponds with maxLass (Fig. 4),

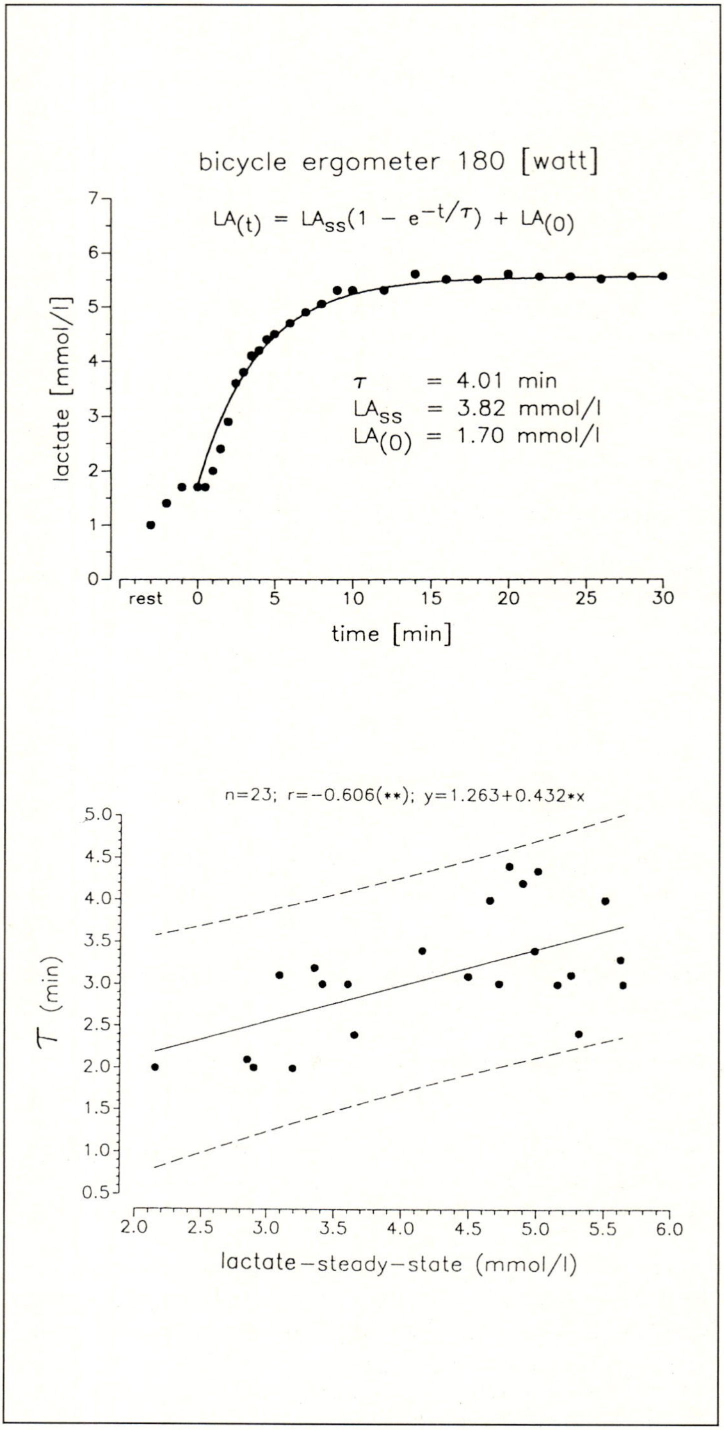

Fig. 9: Upper: example for the determination of velocity constant of lactate increase; lower: correlation and regression between velocity constant τ and steady state lactate.

which conforms to a lactate value of approx. 3 mmol/l. This signifies that threshold values normally stated at 4 mmol/l lactate are too high. With increasing load, at 4 mmol/l lactate differs increasingly from maxLass (Fig. 8). When increasing load by 1 W/min the 4 mmol/l threshold increases on the average by 1.3 W.

The reason for an increase of threshold values when increasing load is the kinetics of lactate. Heck et al. (9) investigated the time-course of steady-state lactate curves by exponential regression analysis. There is a significant correlation between steady-state lactate value and velocity constant of lactate increase (τ), so that τ per mmol/l maxLass increases of 0.43 min (Fig. 9). For a steady-state lactate of 2 resp. 4 mmol/l, a velocity constant of 2 resp. 3 min results. Consequently, only 63% resp. 78% of the final value are obtained by a step duration of 3 min. As a result, underestimation of steady-state lactate value is higher the shorter the step duration.

Conclusion

Mader et al. have defined anaerobic threshold at 4 mmol/l lactate by using treadmill ergometry and a defined load scheme. Changes of the test protocol or of the kind of load cause changes of threshold lactate value. In such cases, the term “anaerobic threshold” should be replaced by “4 mmol/l-load” by stating the test protocol. Only then can results of different investigators be correctly compared.

Summary: Mader et al. defined the aerobic-anaerobic threshold as field of transition between the mere aerobic and the partially anaerobic muscular energy metabolism performance.

Concerning continuous load the definition of the threshold is identical with the maximum lactate steady state (maxLass). It is the highest load under which a lactate steady state can still be stated; any higher load will cause a continuous increase of blood lactate.

We investigated at which lactate value maxLass occurs during bicycle ergometry or treadmill exercise. In addition, we examined lactate values at maxLass load in graded load tests with different rates of load increase.

The following important results were found:

1) On the average, lactate value of maxLass is at about 4 mmol/l for treadmill and cycle ergometer work.

2) In the treadmill test with a 0.4 m/s grading and a 5-min step duration, the load at a lactate value of 4 mmol/l corresponds on the average with maxLass. When reducing the step duration to 3 min, then the load at 3.5 mmol/l lactate corresponds with maxLass.

3) In graded tests on a bicycle ergometer there is a dependence between the increase of load and the lactate value corresponding with maxLass. An increasing load causes a decrease of threshold lactate values that correspond to the regression equation:

$Y = 4.17 - 0.106 \times X + 0.00205 \times X^2$

(Y = lactate (mmol/l), X = load increase (Watts/min))

The reason for the dependence of threshold lactate value on the rate of load increase is lactate kinetics. At a continuous load in the range of lactate steady state, the time constant τ is at 2—3 min.

Our findings show that the anaerobic threshold at 4 mmol/l lactate is only valid for a treadmill load with a load increase of 0.4 m/s/5 min. In common bicycle ergometer loads, such as 50 watts (W)/3 min and 25 W/2 min, the corresponding lactate value is at about 3 mmol/l.

References

1. Brooks GA (1985) Anaerobic threshold: review of the concept and directions for future research. Med Sci Sports Exerc 17 (1): 22—31
2. Bunc V, Heller J, Novak J, Leso J (1985) Determination of the individual anaerobic threshold. Acta Universitas Carolinae, Gymnica 21 (1): 73—81
3. Davis JA, Caiozzo VJ, Lamarra N, Ellis JF, Vandagriff R, Prietto CA, McMaster WC (1983) Does the gas exchange anaerobic threshold occur at a fixed blood lactate concentration of 2 or 3 mM Int J Sports Med 4 (2): 89—93
4. Dietze A, Donath R, Rockstroh K (1974) Vergleichende Untersuchungen der Laktatkonzentrationen in Blutproben aus verschiedenen Entnahmenstellen. Med u Sport 14 (12): 370—379
5. di Prampero PE (1973) Grundlagen der anaeroben Energiebereitstellung und der O_2-Schuld bei körperlichen Höchstbelastungen. Med u Sport 13 (1): 1—13
6. Heck H, Mader A, Hess G, Mücke S, Müller R, Hollmann W (1985) Justification of the 4-mmol/l lactate threshold. Int J Sports Med 6: 117—130
7. Heck H, Hess G, Mader A (1985) Vergleichende Untersuchung zu verschiedenen Laktat-Schwellenkonzepten. Dtsch Z Sportmed 36 (1): 19—25; (2): 40—52
8. Heck H, Reinhards G, Mader A, Hollmann W (1987) Maximales Laktat-steady-state und Laktatschwelle bei Kindern. In: Rieckert H (Hrsg): Sportmedizin-Kursbestimmung Springer, Berlin
9. Heck H (1987) Laktat in der Leistungsdiagnostik. Habilitationsschrift, Köln
10. Heck H, Börnert F, Müller T, Hollmann W (1989) Laktatkinetik bei konstanter und stufenförmig ansteigender Belastung auf dem Fahrradergometer. In: Böning D, Braumann KM, Busse MW, Maassen für die Gesundheit. Deutscher Ärzte-Verlag, Köln
11. Keul J, Simon G, Berg A, Dickhuth H.-H., Goerttler I, Kübel R (1979) Bestimmung der individuellen anaeroben Schwelle zur Leistungsbewertung und Trainingsgestaltung. Dtsch Z Sportmed 30 (7): 212—218
12. König U, Roßkopf P, Heck H (1991) Die Variabilität des Laktats bei ansteigender Fahrradergometerarbeit. 32. Deutscher Sportärztekongreß, 18.—21. 10. 1990 München (Kongreßband in Vorbereitung)
13. Kuipers H (1983) Variability of physiological responses to exercise. Vrieseborch, Haarlem
14. Mader A, Liesen H, Heck H, Philippi H, Rost R, Schürch P, Hollmann W (1976) Zur Beurteilung der sportartspezifischen Ausdauerleistungsfähigkeit im Labor. Sportarzt und Sportmedizin 27 (4): 80—88; (5): 109—112
15. Mader A, Heck H, Föhrenbach R, Hollmann W (1979) Das statische und dynamische Verhalten des Laktats und des Säure-Basen-Status im Bereich niedriger bis maximaler Azidosen bei 400- und 800-m-Läufern bei beiden Geschlechtern nach Belastungsabbruch. Dtsch Z Sportmed 30 (7): 203—211; (8): 249—261
16. Mader A, Heck H (1986) A theory of the metabolic origin of "Anaerobic Threshold". Int J Sports Med 7 (Suppl 1): 45—65
17. Margaria R, Edwards HT (1934) The removal of lactic acid from the body during recovery from muscular exercise. Amer J Physiol 107: 681—686
18. Pessenhofer H, Schwaberger G, Schmid P (1981) Zur Bestimmung des individuellen aerob-anaeroben Übergangs. Dtsch Z Sportmed 32 (1): 15—17
19. Skinner J, McLellan H (1981) The transition from aerobic to anaerobic metabolism. Res Q Exercise Sport 51: 234—248

20. Stegmann H, Kindermann W, Schnabel A (1981) Lactate kinetics and individual anaerobic threshold. Int J Sports Med 2 (3): 160—165
21. Tesch PA, Sharp DS, Daniels WL (1981) Influence of fiber type composition and capillary density on onset of blood lactate accumulation. Int J Sports Med 2 (4): 252—255

Author's address:

PD Dr. H. Heck,
Institut f. Kreislaufforschung und Sportmedizin,
Deutsche Sporthochschule Köln,
Carl-Diem-Weg 6,
5000 Köln 41

The Significance of Spirogergometry from the View-point of Sports Cardiology

R. Rost and H. Heck

Institut of Sports Medicine and Cardiology, German Sports University, Cologne, FRG

If a comment on the significance of spirogergometry (SEM) is made, it should be that sports cardiology considers SEM as its very own method. From the beginning of sports cardiology, the athlete's larger heart was of interest to physicians, who used to consider a large heart as indicative of disease. However, in contrast to the large diseased heart, the athlete's large heart demonstrates an enhanced, and not a decreased performance capacity. A crucial point in its assessment, therefore, is the comparison of the heart's size and power.

These facts were already well known to Henschen, who was the first to describe the athlete's heart near the end of the last century, when he made the statement that "the large heart will win the competition". He found that those athletes did win long distance skiing races in whom he found the largest heart size, identified only by percussion. Actually, the measurement of cardio-pulmonary capacity by success in athletic competition is only a rough one, since there are many other parameters which have to be taken into account, such as motivation, coordination, and peripheral metabolic factors. In search for more objective parameters in this comparison, the percutoric determination of cardiac size was replaced by radiological measurement of cardiac volume. The assessment of cardiac respiratory capacity occurred with measurement of maximal oxygen uptake ($\dot{V}O_2$ max). These results confirmed Henschens statement (Fig. 1). Therefore, the measurement of $\dot{V}O_2$ max (which,

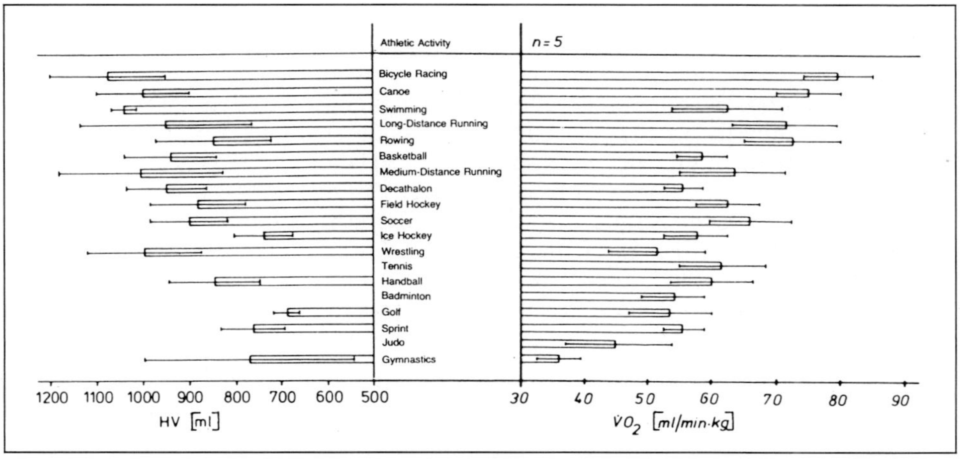

Fig. 1: Heart volume (HV) and $\dot{V}O_2$ performing different athletic activities.

Table 1. Publications in the German Journal of Sports Medicine (Deutsche Zeitschrift für Sportmedizin).

Period	$\dot{V}O_2$	Lactate
1959—1965	9	0
1966—1975	12	11
1976—1985	5	20
1986—1988	0	9

according to Hollmann, was a criterium of cardiorespiratory performance) became the "gold standard of sports medicine" in the 1960s and 1970s. Laboratories not equipped for this rather expensive technique were considered second class in the scientific opinion.

In sports medicine in the last decade SEM was, to a large extent, substituted by the measurement of metabolic parameters, particularly lactate levels. This is demonstrated by the number of publications on lactate release in athletes (Table 1). In the 1960s there were, in the German Journal of Sports Medicine, nearly exclusively papers on $\dot{V}O_2$, with no mention of lactate. In the last decade this has changed.

The reasons for this development arei:

1) Sportsmedical research and experience came to the conclusion that maximal performance depends only to a minor degree on maximal cardiac power. The cardiovascular system fairly rapidly reaches its maximum since the heart cannot increase unlimitedly. If the critical heart weight and thus the maximal cardiac output have been reached, further increase of performance can only be achieved by metabolic adaptation.
2) It could be shown that in the case of a known power-output a measurement of $\dot{V}O_2$ is not necessary, since the mechanical efficiency is constant under all conditions known up to now, even in diseased vs. healthy subjects, or trained vs. untrained subjects. This is particularly true in bicycle ergometry (Fig. 2). A large number of comparisons demonstrate that there is, on the average, an oxygen demand of 11.5 per kg $\times$ min $\times$ W. A load of 100 W, for example, demands an oxygen uptake of $100 \times 11.5 + 300$ ml for the basic metabolism = 1450 ml. Therefore, the measurement of this $\dot{V}O_2$ is not necessary.

On the contrary, the measurement of $\dot{V}O_2$ brings about disadvantages rather than benefits regarding the methodological errors. As an example, a comparison of the results from various highly qualified sports medical laboratories can be made. Figure 3 demonstrate considerable systematic deviations among these various laboratories [4]. Additionally, in the results of individual laboratories there are greatly varying standard deviations (Fig. 4). If there are already such large differences between highly specialized sports medical laboratories, it must be asked what significant errors can be expected in less experienced or exacting institutions. Therefore, it seems to be better to indicate the power in watts and to calculate $\dot{V}O_2$ from the power values.

Particularly in the United States, power is usually measured by $\dot{V}O_2$-values, using the treadmill test in contrast to Europe and its predominance of the bicycle test. In the treadmill test without a slope, a direct indication of power is not possible, therefore an indirect indication of energy consumption becomes necessary. This fact

Bicycle ergometer ($\dot{V}O_2$ in ml/min; Load (L) in watts)					
$\dot{V}O_2$ =	230	+	11.2 * L	Men	(Aigner)
$\dot{V}O_2$ =	-30	+	11.0 * L	Women	(Aigner)
$\dot{V}O_2$ =	320	+	11.3 * L		(Berg, Keul)
$\dot{V}O_2$ =	300	+	12.0 * L		(Rost)
$\dot{V}O_2$ =	435	+	10.8 * L		(Reiterer)
$\dot{V}O_2$ =	368	+	12.1 * L	Cyclists	(Schwaberger)
$\dot{V}O_2$ =	360	+	11.0 * L	Cyclists	(Bachl)

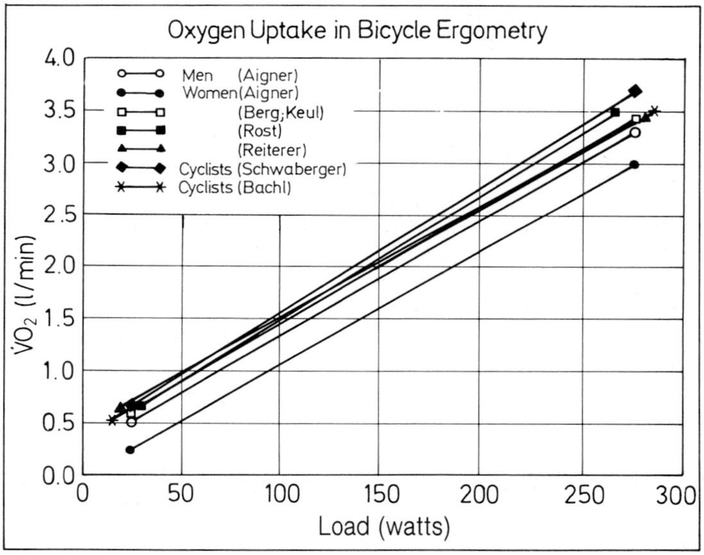

Fig. 2. Relation between oxygen uptake and work intensity in various working groups.

has also led to the american use of metabolic equivalents (MET's) to characterize intensity of load (equals to 3.5 ml $\dot{V}O_2$/kg/min), a parameter which in most cases cannot be measured directly, but has to be taken from tables or must be estimated according to e.g. the Astrand-Rhyming nomogram.

Actually, in SEM the measurement of $\dot{V}O_2$ is less important than its relation to other parameters such as ventilation or $\dot{V}CO_2$, as far as obtaining parameters of relative exhaustion and for assessing aerobic anaerobic threshold (AT) by respiratory quotient or respiratory equivalent. Meanwhile, it has been shown that the same result can be achieved more easily, comfortably, and ecommically by measuring lactate acid concentration. Up to now, it has not been shown that there is any systematic difference between the performance measurements and the lactate acid AT. The major importance of lactic acid AT is that it can be easily measured outside the laboratory, e.g. on the playing field. These considerations are also applicable to cardiac patients, allowing measurement out of hospitals under daily routine conditions.

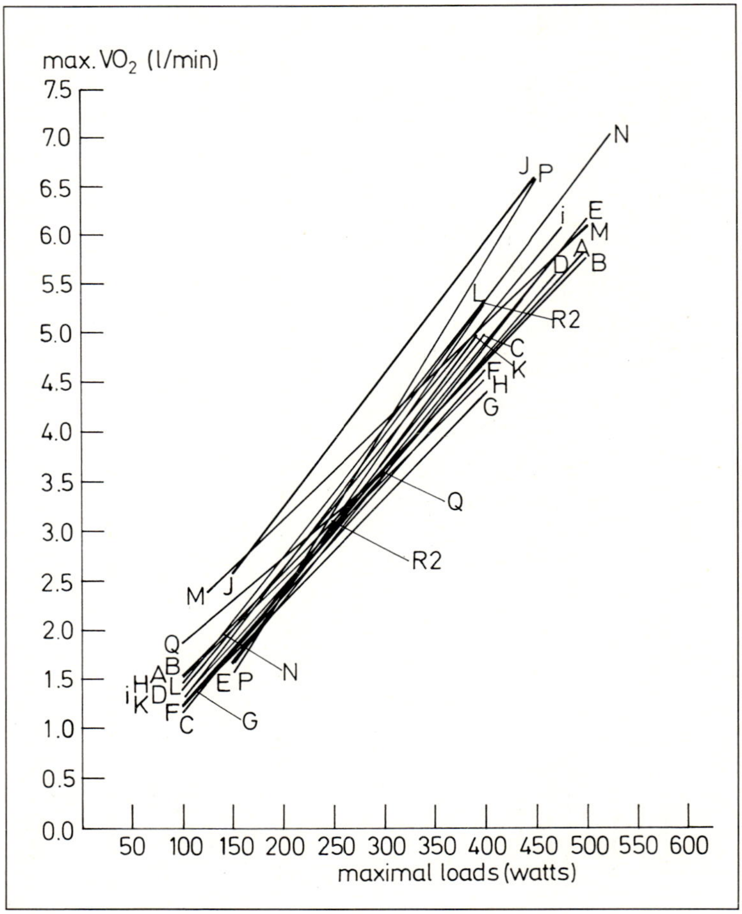

Fig. 3. Regression lines between oxygen uptake and work intensity in the results of sportsmedical investigation centers in the FRG. Each letter respectively each line represents one center.

On the other hand, the new computerized SEM-systems provide (in contrast to the older models) the possibility of easy measurement, not only of the absolute amount of $\dot{V}O_2$, but also of parameters regarding the dynamics of oxygen uptake. This needs to be further investigated as to its benefit in the evaluation of patients.

In summing up the advantages of computerized SEM in sports cardiology, we should stress that our present assessment is more hypothetical than factual. Further study is necessary, with the following considerations:

1) Is there really a maintenance of energy efficiency in cardiovascular patients?

2) Is there a systematic difference between metabolic and respiratory AT, and if so, what is its clinical relevance?

3) What is the clinical significance of oxygen uptake dynamics?

4) Will a combination of metabolic and respiratory factors allow a complete description of energy release (particularly important in forms of ergometry where there is no constant mechanical efficiency, e.g. in treadmill tests, rowing-ergometers, and others)?

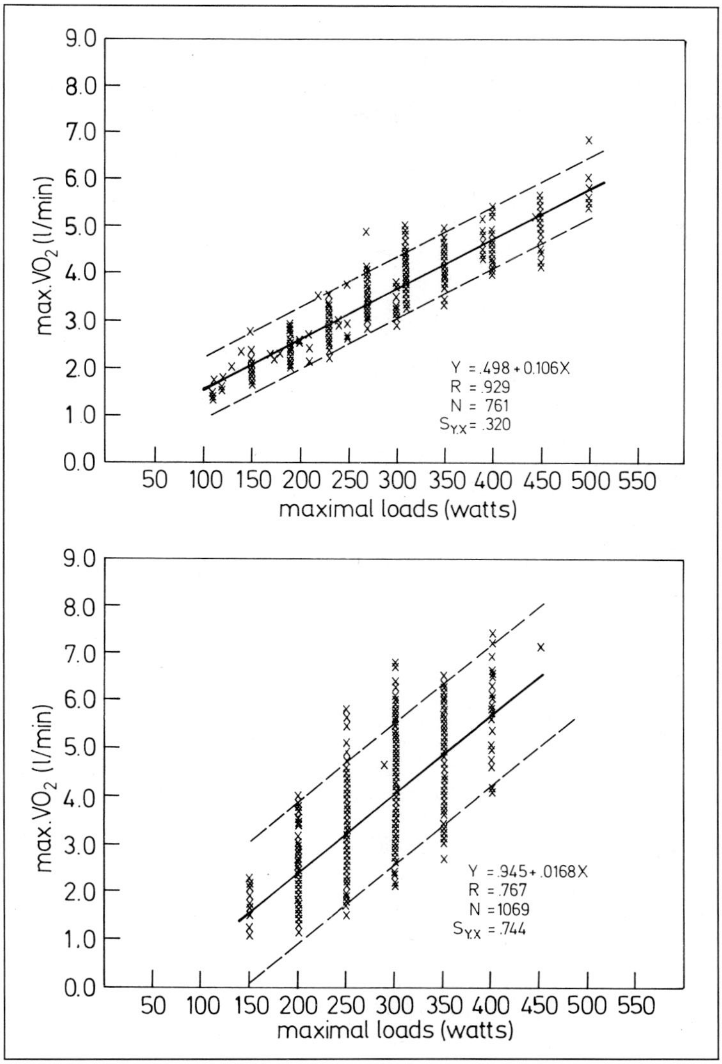

Fig. 4. Intralaboratorial standard deviations in the relation between oxygen uptake and work intensity. The upper figure represents our own laboratory (which was fairly good, not the best), the lower a large center with a rather high deviation.

5) To elucidate the expected significance of SEM in the evaluation of pulmonary disease.

6) SEM for indirect calorimetric assessment of energy release has been important when mechanical efficiency factors were not known. Measuring lactate acid levels is only in assessment of the patient's exhaustion, not of his objective performance. SEM has been primarily used for stress testing under laboratory conditions, but we expect portable, telemetric units to provide valuable in formation on patients during their daily routines.

Summary: Sports cardiology considers spiroergometry (SEM) as "its own method", since it was the gold standard in the evaluation of cardiovascular training effects from the 1950s to the 1970s. It has since been largely replaced by measurement of metabolic parameters, particularly that of lactic acid concentration (LA) because: oxygen uptake ($\dot{V}O_2$) is strongly correlated to work intensity, e.g. it can be calculated nomogrammatically if the load is known; measurement of $\dot{V}O_2$ in absolute terms was less important than its correlation to other parameters such as ventilation, $\dot{V}CO_2$, and respiratory equivalent (R) in order to get parameters of relative exhaustion. All these parameters are dependent on aerobic-anaerobic-threshold (AAS) which can be much more easily measured by LA. Up to now, no clinically significant difference has been shown between respiratory and metabolic thresholds. The new computerized SEM systems may challenge this conclusion, since the time-dependent analysis of oxygen uptake may elucidate new aspects and different results under physiologic and pathophysiologic conditions. This hypothesis remains to be investigated.

References

1. Aigner A, Muss N, Femminger H (1981) Berechnung der maximalen Sauerstoffaufnahme anhand von Regressionsgleichungen. Österreich J Sportsmed: 11, 3
2. Bachl N (1985) Normwertsystem zur Beurteilung der Leistungsfähigkeit in Freizeit-, Breiten- und Leistungssport — unveröffentl. Ergebnisse, In: Aigner A: Sportmedizin in der Praxis, Springer Berlin, Heidelberg, New York, Tokyo
3. Berg A, Keul J (1982) Physiology and metabolism responses of female athletes during laboratory and field exercise. Congress on Women and Sports, Karger Basel
4. Heck H, Emirkanian O (1979) Messung der maximalen Sauerstoffaufnahme bei ABC-Kaderuntersuchungen, Präzision und Richtigkeit der Sauerstoffaufnahmemessung in den einzelnen Untersuchungszentren. In: Fleischer H (Hrsg) Sportmedizinische Untersuchungen im Breitensport, 1974—1977
5. Henschen S (1989) Skilanglauf und Skiwettlauf — eine medizinische Studie Mitt med Klin Upsala, Jena
6. Reiterer W, Bachl N (1977) Kriterien der körperlichen Leistungsfähigkeit — limitierende Faktoren und diagnostische Kriterien des Ausdauerleistungsvermögens. Wien med Wschr Suppl: 42
7. Rost R, Hollmann W (1982) Belastungsuntersuchungen in der Praxis. Thieme, Stuttgart
8. Schwaberger G, Pessenhofer H, Schmid P, Wolf W, Sauseng N (1982) Grundlagen der aeroben Leistungsdiagnostik. Österreich J Sportmed: 12, 3

Author's address:

Prof. Dr. R. Rost
Direktor des Institutes für Kreislaufforschung und Sportmedizin
Lehrstuhl für Kardiologie u. Sportmedizin
Deutsche Sporthochschule Köln
Carl-Diem-Weg 6
5000 Köln 41

Thoracic Electrical Bioimpedance — Alternative or Complement in Cardio-pulmonary Exercise Testing?

R. K. Klocke, A. Kux, G. Mager, U. J. Winter, J. Klüppelberg, H. W. Höpp, and H. H. Hilger

Third Clinic of Internal Medicine University of Cologne, FRG

Introduction

The noninvasive determination of hemodynamic parameters at rest and during physical stress is increasingly gaining importance, since invasive measurements for the observation of large patient collectives, particularly follow-ups, are very expensive technically and furthermore not ethically justifiable. Various existing clinically utilized methods, such as e.g. echocardiography, have methodological limits. Thoracic beat-to-beat electrical impedance cardiography (IG) is an indirect, noninvasive method for the determination of stroke volume and cardiac output. The examination is quickly and easily performed, without danger to the patient, and is repeatable as often as desired; it requires only the passive participation of the patient. The ICG is based upon the measurement of thoracic electrical resistance change synchronous with the cardiac rhythm. Using the derived base impedance and the resistance changes resulting from intrathoracic volume shifts during systole and diastole, one can calculate the stroke volume of the left ventricle. The impedance fluctuations are derived simply by means of attached ECG electrodes (Ag/AgCl).

In this overview, we shall show the theory, its validity, possible clinical applications, and a comparison with simultaneously utilized computerized spiroergometry (CPX).

Theory of the bioimpedance method

The fundamentals of ICG were studied by Atzler and coworkers in 1932. Nyboer then took up the method in 1940 [4, 16] and developed a formula for calculation of the stroke volume:

$$SV = \frac{Q \cdot L^2 \cdot \Delta Z}{{Z^2}_o}$$

where
SV = stroke volume of left ventricle (ml);
Q = specific resistivity of blood (ohm-cm);
L = distance between two inner electrodes (cm);
Z_O = base impedance between both inner electrodes (ohm);
ΔZ = impedance change during systole (ohm).

The method was significantly improved by Kubicek and coworkers in the late 1960s as part of a NASA research project.

Kubicek introduced the ventricular ejection time T and the first derivative of the impedance change, dZ/dt into Nyboer's formula [16]:

$$SV = \frac{Q \cdot L^2 \cdot T \cdot dZ/dt}{Z^2_o}$$

where
SV = stroke volume of left ventricle;
Q = specific resistivity of blood (ohm-cm);
L = distance between both inner electrodes (ohm);
Z_o = thoracic base impedance between both inner electrodes (ohm);
T = ventricular ejection time (s);
dZ/dt = impedance change during ejection (ohm/s)

Kubicek carried out the first clinical studies with this method on healthy subjects and obtained good results [16]. Nonetheless, for routine clinical use the ICG fell back into oblivion.

In the early 1980s, Sramek [22] and coworkers improved the clinical applicability in that they introduced simple ECG electrodes (Ag/AgCl) instead of the previously common band electrodes. Furthermore, more individual patient data were incorporated into the formula propounded by Kubicek. The newly developed formula was entered into the software of the NCCOM3-R7 impedance computer (BoMed Medical Manufacturing, Irvine, Calif., USA). Operation of the NCCOM3-R7 is controlled by the QRS signal. For every heartbeat the following values are measured and recorded: heart rate (HR), thoracic fluid index (TFI), ventricular ejection time (VET), and ejection velocity index (EVI). The value of the volume of electrically participating thoracic tissue (VEPT) is assumed empirically. From the above parameters the stroke volume is calculated as follows:

$$SV = VEPT \times VET \times \frac{EVI}{TFI}$$

where
SV = stroke volume of left ventricle (ml);
VEPT = (thorax length L)^3/4.25 (cm^3);
VET = ventricular ejection time
EVI = ejection velocity index (ohm/s);
TFI = thoracic fluid index.

Finally, cardiac output (CO) is calculated from the formula CO = HR × SV and simultaneously recorded.

Numerous research groups have carried out comparative studies with invasive procedures and have found good correlations [2, 3, 6].

For clinical purposes, the determination of cardiac output is sufficiently accurate. Intraindividual variations are more reliably and accurately registered than interindividual variations. Above all, qualitative predictions are made possible by ICG.

Some accompanying illnesses make interpretation of the ICG measurement more difficult, e.g. pulmonary edema, heart valvular insufficiency, shunts, and gram-negative sepsis. This shows the importance of a thorough case history and clinical examination for the interpretation of the measured values obtained by ICG.

CDDP software for processing the bioimpedance signal

The bioimpedance data obtained with the NCCOM3-R7 cardiac output monitor can be printed out on line, beat-to-beat. However, there is also the possibility of digital data processing with a CDDP-2 system (Cardio Dynamic Data Processing System, BoMed). The program runs on DOS 3.2 using a conventional personal computer. After every 16 cardiac cycles the bioimpedance data are entered into the computer. The CCDP program evaluates the data and displays two different graphs on a monitor. The recording of the cardiac index (CI) and the stroke index (SI) make some other derived cardiovascular parameters available. These are mentioned here only for the sake of completeness. The peak flow index (PFI) is the maximal blood-flow velocity in the descending aorta during the expulsion period, and is considered to be a contractility parameter (ml/s/m^2). The ejection fraction (EF) can be calculated from the systolic time relationships (given as %). The enddiastolic index (EDI) arises from the relationship of the stroke volume and ejection fraction with respect to the body surface (given in ml/m^2). The thoracic fluid index (TFI) corresponds to the total base impedance of the thorax (ohms). The contractility index (CI) is the relationship of maximal impedance change to the base impedance (s^{-1}). The acceleration index (ACI) gives acceleration of blood flow during the first 20 ms after opening of the aortic valve (s^{-2}). Using the additional simultaneous determination of the median arterial blood pressure, which we obtain with the Dynamap oscillation blood-pressure measurement system (Critikon), the software calculates the systemic vascular resistance index (SVRI). However, for this purpose, the central venous pressure is assumed to be 3 mmHg, if not known to be otherwise (systemic vascular resistance index unit is ohm/m^2). Furthermore, the left-ventricular work index (LCWI) can be calculated, although one also assumes the PCW to be 6 mm Hg (kgm/m^2). The data can be visualized as a bar graph on a so-called diagnostic sheet (see Fig. 1). There is also the possibility of transferring to a so-called therapeutic diagram, from which one can read the actual condition of the patient with respect to a defined therapeutic goal. This is obtained from the values for the cardiac index, the median arterial blood pressure, SVRI, and LCWI, as shown in Fig. 2.

Investigation of the validity of bioimpedance

The improvement of the determination of stroke volume and cardiac index with thoracic bioimpedance according to the method of Sramek (22) offers the advantages of a continuous beat-to-beat recording of the measured values using a simple application of electrodes. In comparison with the method of Kubicek (16), however, it lacks the possibility of recording an analogous curve of the thoracic fluid index and the impedance change with time by simultaneous ECG recording. The computerized calculation of cardiac index from recorded digital values thus cannot be duplicated with certainty. A further possible disadvantage of the otherwise simple and rapidly performed examination may be the shape of the chosen electrodes. In

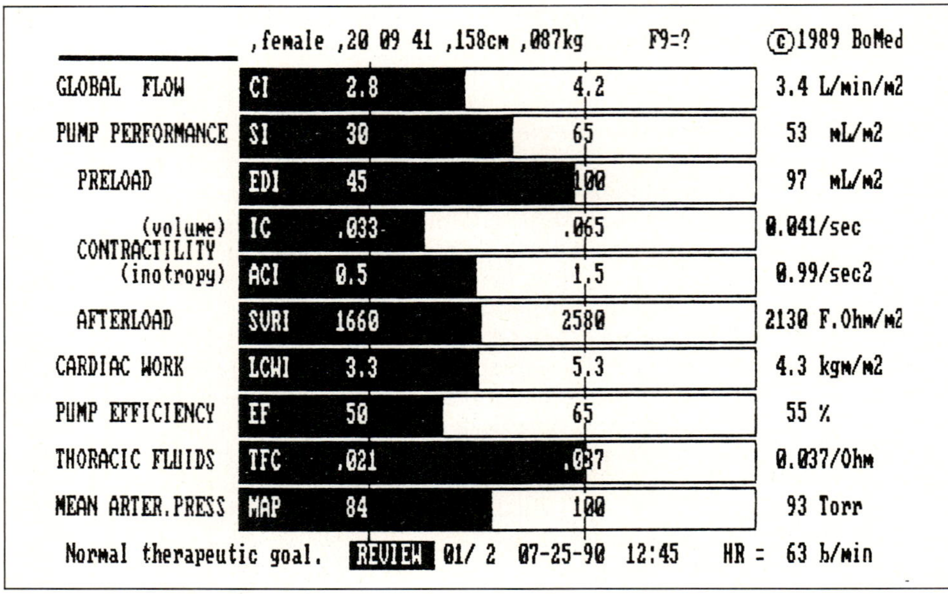

Fig. 1. CDDP software — diagnostic sheet

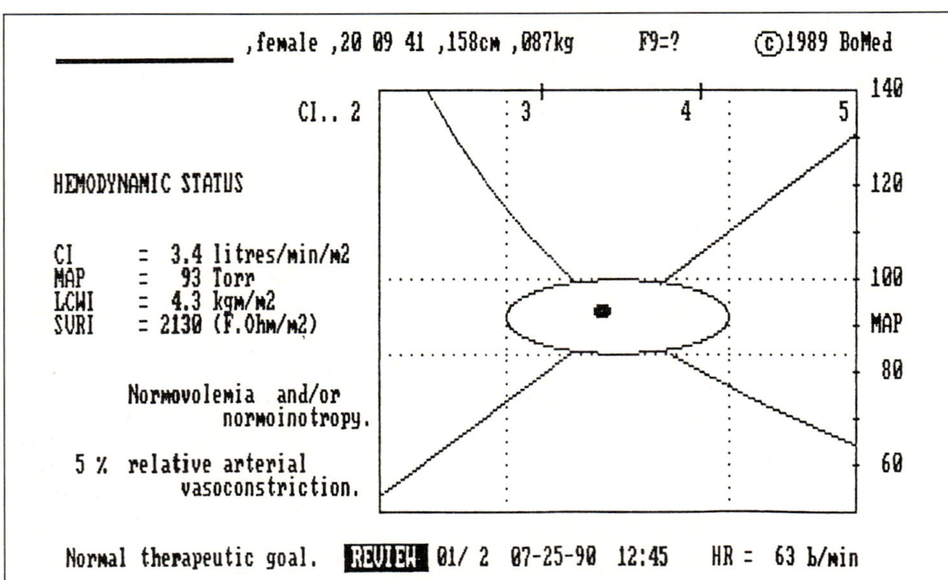

Fig. 2. CDDP software — therapeutic diagram

comparison to the awkward metal bands, there is difficulty of possible electric field effects which cannot be definitely distinguished.

Furthermore, there is no option of making hematocrit-related adjustments of the data, since Sramek assumes that the fluid index is unchanged for hematocrit values between 26% and 66% and he enters it into his formula as an invariable. In addition, the length of the thorax L is determined only on the basis of sex, height, and weight, yet the length of the thorax has an important influence on the calculation of the stroke volume.

In order to utilize a noninvasive measurement system for determination of cardiac index, one must be able to obtain comparative invasive measurement values. However, the fundamentally correct approach to validating the system is restricted by limitations of the method. The measured thoracic impedance variations with the inferred transported fluid volume do not correspond quantitatively to the invasively measured cardiac output obtained by the Fick method or the thermodilution technique. We have nevertheless undertaken a comparison with the invasive cardiovascular data in order to test the validity [15]. For the evaluation of our results, however, one must also note that we did the examination on patients with relatively stable cardiovascular conditions without notable valvular defects, in particular, no valvular insufficiencies, without shunts, and without clinically relevant thoracic fluid accumulation such as pulmonary edema. In the comparison of the measured cardiac index values with the Fick method there was a good correlation, given the expected fluctuations of biological measurement methods ($n = 109$, $r = 0.82$, ≤ 0.001), (details in [15]). Likewise, comparison of the impedance method with the determination of cardiac index by thermodilution in intensive care patients at rest with simultaneous measurement gave a clinically useful and reliable correlation, given the above-mentioned assumptions ($n = 28$, $r = 0.90$, $p \leq 0.001$). In the course of a dynamic examination, patients with coronary heart disease or cardiomyopathy were examined on a resting ergometer by simultaneous impedance cardiography and thermodilution technique. Here again there was a sufficiently exact correlation between the two techniques ($n = 108$, $r = 0.87$, $p \leq 0.001$). Furthermore, the intraindividual fluctuations achieved on the ergometer under stress were well documented ($r = 0.84$, $p \leq 0.001$). The particular changes of the cardiac index were thus shown to be measurable with considerable sensitivity. In reviewing all simultaneous absolute measurements of the cardiac index, one observes an adequate agreement between the invasive techniques and bioimpedance.

The other noninvasive hemodynamic data given in the CDDP software are invariably dependent upon the cardiac output determinations reported above. Detailed discussion of individual parameters cannot be presented here. However, one should note that the method used for calculating the peripheral resistance and the left-ventricular work index contains several possibilities for error which should be kept in mind when interpreting the results. The median pressure determined by the oscillating blood-pressure method must still be entered manually. Furthermore, standardized values are assumed for central venous pressure and the PCW. These can be altered, however, if the values are known. Despite the mentioned methodological deficiencies, the very simple and rapid operation of the NCCOM3-R7 beat-to-beat impedance systems is convincing. Continuous recording of the cardiac index gives a cardiac output determination sufficiently accurate for clinical purposes, while quickly and reliably recording individual variations. Altogether, the measurement method satisfies qualitative considerations rather than presenting an accurate quantification of cardiac output.

Simultaneous spiroergometry (CPX) and bioimpedance studies

At rest and during stress the oxygen uptake ($\dot{V}O_2$) as well as carbon dioxide output ($\dot{V}CO_2$) of the lungs are measurable parameters; from these, together with the tidal volume and mechanics of breathing, one can deduce the overall condition of the cardio-respiratory system. The exercise tolerance of the organism is limited by the cardiovascular system. Increasing physical stress requires an elevated cardiac index (CI), which can be greatly increased through the heart rate and stroke volume index in order to supply sufficient oxygen to peripheral tissues. But the peripheral oxygen utilization of working musculature can also be increased. It therefore seems tempting to acquire simultaneously obtained information about the particular cardiac index and cardiac output, as well as O_2-uptake and CO_2-output. For this purpose, we have applied cardio-pulmonary exercise testing (CPX) parallel to the bioimpedance technique at rest and during stress on the resting ergometer. In this way, one can noninvasively measure the basic hemodynamics, gas exchange, and peripheral oxygen utilization. The unique condition of the patient can thus be determined in relation to the above-mentioned values. Both methods complement each other with respect to their information about the patient's cardio-pulmonary capacity. Furthermore there is, naturally, a certain relationship between increased oxygen uptake and an increased cardiac index under stress. Invasive examinations by Weber had already shown a certain correspondence of the changes in cardiac index and oxygen

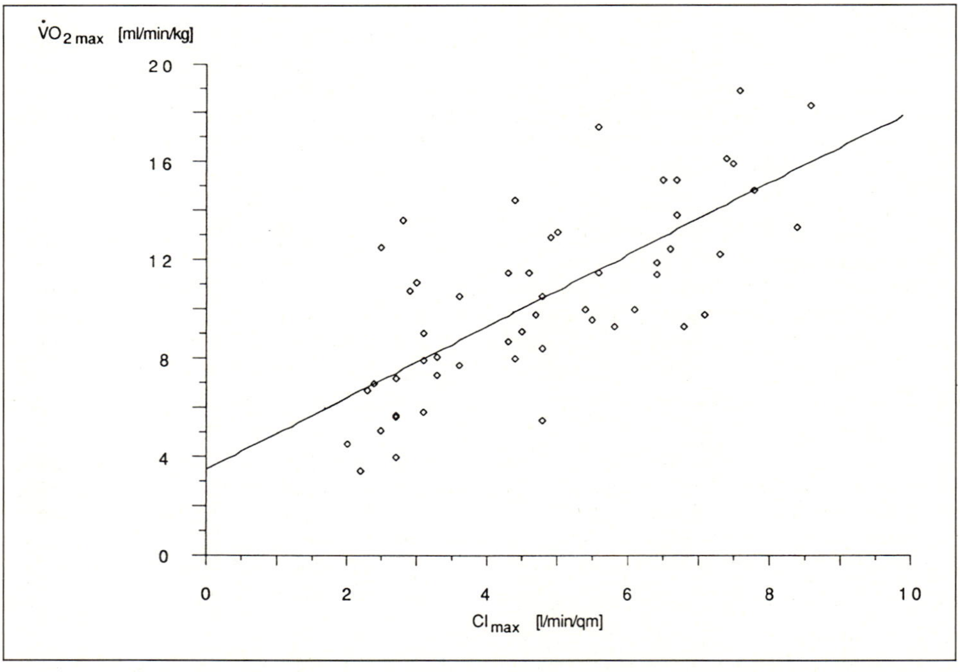

Fig. 3. Correlation between maximum oxygen uptake and maximum cardiac index in patients with heart failure NYHA II + III ($n = 57$; $r = 0.853$)

uptake. In a consecutive series of patients with left-ventricular failure, we found a correlation between maximum oxygen uptake and attained cardiac index; the correlation coefficient was r = 0.853. As one can see from Fig. 3, there are nonetheless large individual differences between increased cardiac index and increased oxygen uptake. However, this is precisely what makes the individual interpretation of the results possible. When our results are assigned to the individual classifications, our noninvasive data are also found to be similar to those of Weber.

Conclusion

In summary, we believe that for clinical purposes, measurement of cardiac index by the digital beat-to-beat thoracic impedance technique of Sramek (22) allows an adequate determination of this circulatory factor and qualitative aspects at rest and under stress. When applied simultaneously with spiroergometry (CPX), the bioimpedance technique offers a clear insight into the basic hemodynamic condition of the patient. Appropriate linear relationships between attained oxygen uptake and the determined cardiac index could be shown. Bioimpedance cardiography thus is a complementary technique to be useful during cardiopulmonary exercise testing.

References

1. Alt E, Wirtzfeld A, Klein G (1983) Hämodynamische Ergebnisse bei ventrikulärer und physiologischer Stimulation. Herz/Kreislauf 2: 31—36
2. Appel PI, Bernstein DP, Curtis DL, Shoemaker WC, Kram HB, Fleming AW (1987) Evaluation of a continuous, on-line real-time noninvasive cardiac cardiac output and ejection fraction measurements by electrically bioimpedance in critically ill patients. Crit Care Med 15: 364
3. Appel PI, Kram HB, Mackabee J, Fleming AW, Shoemaker WC (1986) Comparison of measurements of cardiac output by bioimpedance and thermodilution in severely ill surgical patients. Crit Care med 14: 933—935
4. Atzler E, Lehmann G (1932) Über ein neues Verfahren zur Darstellung der Herztätigkeit. Arbeitsphysiologie 5: 636—680
5. Bergbauer M, Sabin G (1983) Hämodynamische Langzeitresultate der bifokalen Schrittmacherstimulation. DMW 108: 545—549
6. Berntein DP (1986) Continuous noninvasive real-time monitoring of stroke volume and cardiac output by thoracic electrical bioimpedance. Crit Care Med 14: 898—901
7. Betz R, Batanier CK, Mocellin R (1977) Die Impedanzkardiographie als Methode zur quantitativen Bestimmung des Herzzeitvolumens? Vergleichende Messungen mit dem Fickschen Prinzip. Basic Res Cardiol 72: 46—56
8. Braunwald E (1964) Comments on the hemodynamic significance of atrial systole. Am J Med 37: 665—669
9. Fananapazir I, Bennett DH, Monks P (1983) Atrial synchronized ventricular pacing: Contribution of the chronotropic response to improved exercise performance. PACE 6: 601—608
10. Fülle P, Weinhold C, Wenke K, Bach P (1988) Vergleichende Studie mit fünf verschiedenen frequenzadaptiven Schrittmachersystemen. Z Kardiol 78 2: 218
11. Fujinami T, Nakano S, Nakayama K, Takada K (1979) Impedance cardiography for the assessment of cardiac function during exercise. Japan Circulation J 43: 215—223
12. Kappenberger L (1983) Hämodynamische Ergebnisse der Schrittmacherbehandlung mit unterschiedlichen vorhofbeteiligenden Systemen. Herzschrittmacher 3: 243—245
13. Knapp E (1976) Die Impedanzkardiographie. Wiener klin Wochenschr, Suppl 58: 1—15
14. Knapp K, Gmeiner R, Hammerle P, Raas E (1976) Der Einfluß der Vorhofkontraktion auf das Schlagvolumen bei Schrittmacherstimulation. Z Kardiol 65: 783—789

15. Klocke RK, Hein A, Mager G, Höpp HW, Hilger HH (1989) Kontinuierliches nichtinvasives real-time-monitoring des Herzzeitvolumens mittels der neuen beat-to-beat Bioimpedanztechnik (BoMed NCCOM 3). Theorie — Validität — klinische Anwendungsmöglichkeiten. Intensivmed 26: 161—167
16. Kubicek WG, Karnegis JN, Patterson RP, Witsoe DA, Mattson RH (1966) Development and evaluation of an impedance cardiac output system. Aerospace Med 37: 1208—1212
17. Lang E, Durst OE, Weikl A, Denkl P, Kessel R, Wieluch W, von Niedner K (1974) Die Impedanzkardiographie. Münch Med Wschr 39: 1661—1666
18. Lüderitz B (1986) Therapie und Diagnostik kardialer Rhythmusstörungen. 2. Auflage, Springer, Berlin, Heidelberg, New York
19. Miles DS, Sawka N, Wilde SW, Doerr BM, Frey MAB, Glaser RM (1981) Estimation of cardiac output by electrical impedance during arm exercise in women. J Appl Physiol 51: 1488—1492
20. Nechwatal W, Bier P, Eversmann A, König E (1976) Die unblutige Bestimmung des Herzzeitvolumens mit der Impedanzkardiographie. Vergleichende Untersuchungen mit der Thermodilutionsmethode. Basis Res Cardiol 71: 542—552
21. Schuster CJ, Schuster HP (1984) Application of impedance cardiography in critical care medicine. Resuscitation 11: 225—274
22. Sramek BB (1983) Electrical bioimpedance. Med Electron 14: 95—103
23. Wirtzfeld A (1981) Klinische Gesichtspunkte der Schrittmachertherapie bei bradykarden Rhythmusstörungen. Verh Dtsch Ges Kreisl Forsch 47: 98—110

Author's address:

Dr. med. R. K. Klocke
Klinik III für Innere Medizin
Universität zu Köln
Josefph-Stelzmann-Str. 9
5000 Köln 41 (Lindenthal), FRG

2. Clinical Value in Coronary Heart Disease and Myocardial Failure

Role of Spiroergometry in Clinical Exercise Testing

H. Löllgen, P. Dirschedl and U. Fahrenkrog

Med. Clinic, Dept. of Cardiology and Pneumology, Community Hospital, Remscheid, Ruhr-University, Bochum, FRG

Introduction

Exercise testing is widely used for examination of healthy and diseased subjects. Indications for exercise testing range from diagnosis of special diseases to evaluation of functional capacity in athletes, normals, and patients (Table 1). In addition, exercise testing is needed to get objective information on the patient's status. It is well-established that subjective symptoms and signs, including New York Heart Association (NYHA) classification do not necessarily correlate with parameters obtained during exercise testing. This holds true for patients with cardiomyopathy (Fig. 1) and valvular heart disease as well [15, 18, 25]. Further, hemodynamics at rest do not predict hemodynamic response during exercise. These latter findings are of utmost significance for those studies using interventional procedures such as pharmacotherapy or revascularization (Table 1).

Spiroergometry as a part of exercise testing has been used for some time [1, 2, 4, 6, 11, 23, 26, 30] and it is a well established method for studying cardiopulmonary function [6, 11, 12, 20, 24, 26—30]. The role of spiroergometry critically depends on indications and underlying problems evaluated by the exercise test. The increased interest in spiroergometry is mainly due to improved methodological approaches with computer-supported analysis.

This paper deals with four aspects:

— indications for exercise testing and spiroergometry;
— methodological problems with regard to spiroergometry and exercise testing;
— recommendations for exercise testing in cardiac and pulmonary diseases with special reference to concurrent methods;
— Critical assessment of the role of spiroergometry

Table 1. Indications for exercise testing.

Diagnostic Indications:
— evaluation of functional capacity;
— evaluation or provocation of symptoms and severity of a disease;
— Screening for suspected or latent diseases

Therapeutic Indications:
— control of therapy (drug, surgery, PTCA);
— rehabilitation or conditioning program

Prognostic Indications:
— prognosis of a disease (constancy or progression);
— risk stratification.

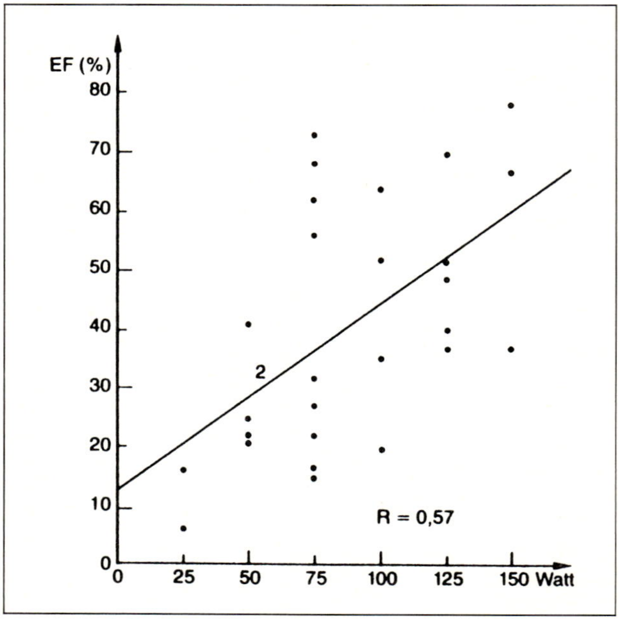

Fig. 1. Ejection fraction in relation to exercise capacity in 33 patients with dilated cardiomyopathy [18].

Indications for exercise testing

Ergometry is performed for diagnostic purposes to detect suspected or latent diseases that do not present symptoms or signs at rest [19].

Indications for diagnostic ergometry are:

- evaluation of functional capacity of healthy subjects, patients;
- evaluation of physical fitness for special tasks or special occupations;
- investigations on aspects of physical fitness (for research purposes);
- evaluation or provocation of symptoms to determine the severity of a disease;
- screening for suspected latent diseases such as coronary artery disease, hypertension, hyperkinetic circulation, exercise-induced asthma, disturbed respiratory gas exchange, and left-heart failure or latent pulmonary hypertension;
- exercise testing soon after myocardial infarction (risk stratification);
- screening for suspected diseases in apparently healthy subjects or in those with an increased number of risk factors or with high prevalence of a disease.

Therapeutic indications for ergometry as control of therapy are:

- control of drug therapy (coronary artery disease, heart failure etc.);
- control after revascularization by aorto-coronary bypass surgery or percutaneous transluminal coronary angioplasty (PTCA) or cardiac surgery other than bypass;
- control after pacemaker implantation, especially for rate-adaptive systems;
- control after heart transplantation;
- control of rehabilitation and conditioning programms.

Prognostic indications for ergometry are [19, 20]:

- prognosis of a disease according to the result of acute exercise testing, constancy or progression of the disease;

— risk stratification which leads to a diagnostic procedure.

Special parameters have to be used for diagnosis of coronary artery disease, hypertension, or disturbed respiratory gas exchange. Spiroergometry or gas exchange measurements provide information on aerobic capacity, functional impairment, and cardio-pulmonary reserve. Spiroergometry gives additional or differential diagnostic information with regard to special diseases.

Diagnosis of certain diseases by ergometry requires specific test approaches such as exercise ECG and thallium scintigraphy for detecting ischemic heart disease, right-heart catheterization for analysis of left-ventricular failure or pulmonary hypertension, blood-pressure measurements for hypertension, and blood and alveolar gas analysis for determination of impaired respiratory gas exchange due to obstructive lung disease of the disturbed diffusion capacity.

Methodological aspects

Ergometry and spiroergometry raise many methodological problems. Some aspects of quality control (Table 1) and standardization (Tables 2, 3) have been addressed

Table 2. Quality control in exercise testing.

Equipment and laboratory	
Ergometer	Type/producer; date of first calibration; data of latest calibration; mean deviation of power output
Blood pressure	Date of calibration
ECG recorder	Date of control check; zero drift; response time; chart speed; linearity
Electrodes	Date of control; impedance
Exercise (ECG)	Registration qualitiy
Air flow receptor	Range of linearity, stability of baseline and gain; response time
Oscilloscope	Data of control
Defibrillator	General check; date of latest instruction; date of training
Laboratory	Humidity/temperature (daily protocol)
Staff	
Examinations before testing; physical examination, history, resting ECG; current therapy, informed consent	
Continuing education and training of the laboratory staff	
Physician present during testing	
Repeated calibrations of ergometer every two years; ECG recorder, scope, education once a year; defibrillator, emergency procedure, respiratory gas receptor every three months	
Emergency	
Control of equipment, drugs, procedures (date)	
Date of latest training (including cardiopulmonary reanimation (CPR))	
Written protocol of emergency procedure	
Telephone number of 'EMT' of EM doctor, and of next hospital/next intensive care unit (ICU)	
Patients	
Exercise program: prescripted?; definition of start and endpoints of exercise testing; guidelines for stopping the test?; documentation of signs and symptoms of exercise testing	

Table 3. Recommendations for an exercise testing program (bicycle).

Field of application	Initial workload (W)	Increment
GP office, clinic; 'routine ergometry'	50	
Occupational medicine	75—100 (good fitness!)	10 or 20 W min^{-1} or
Nuclear coardiology	50	25 W per 2 min
Reduced fitness	25	
Pneumology	(25) 50	
(in case of right heart catheterization and blood analysis)		
Paediatric stress testing	1 W kg^{-1} bodyweight	0—5 W kg^{-1} (3 min)
Sports medicine	50 (♀)	50 W per 2 or 3 min
	100 (♂) of 150	25 W in the range of exhaustion

Table 4. Recommendations for an exercise testing program (treadmill).

Field of application	Initial workload	Increment
Clinic, offic	4 km h^{-1} (2.5%) of 4—6 km h^{-1} (0%) walking; from 7 km h^{-1} (0%) running	2.5% per 3 min 1 km h^{-1} per 3 min
Sports medicine	8—12 km h^{-1} (2—2.5 m s^{-1} (1—1.5% or 5% resp.), or 8 km h^{-1} (2.5%)	2 km h^{-1} per 3 min (0.5 m s^{-1}) 2.5% per 2 min*
Angiology	3.6 km h^{-1} (12·5%) of 4.0 km h^{-1} (10.0%)	until pain
Pneumonology	4—6 km h^{-1} (5%) or 8—10 km h^{-1} (0%)	until dyspnea

Table 5. Criteria of exhaustion.

Work load	< 90% of predicted
Heart rate:	220 — age
Base excess:	< 9 mmol/l
Lactate:	> 9 mmol/l
pH:	< 7.25
RPE:	> 16
RQ:	> 1.0
REq:	< 35

in previous meetings [16, 17, 19], and only in a few publications [7—9, 11, 13, 21, 22, 24, 26—28]. However, accuracy of recorder and analyzers have to be checked regularly. Not only is it necessary to know the time constant of the O_2 and CO_2 analyzers, but also that of the whole system, from mouthpiece to analyzers (Table 5). Some recommendations on precision and accuracy are given in Table 2.

Factors affecting oxygen uptake and $\dot{V}O_{2max}$ are (according to the literature): age, body mass, height, sex, method of measurement, body position, exercise program, state of training, smoking habits, pregnancy, and altitude [20]. Physiological factors well-known to influence $\dot{V}O_{2max}$ are given in Fig. 2.

Spiroergometry is closely related to maximum and submaximum performance of ergometry. However, even in this context, recommendations and procedures differ

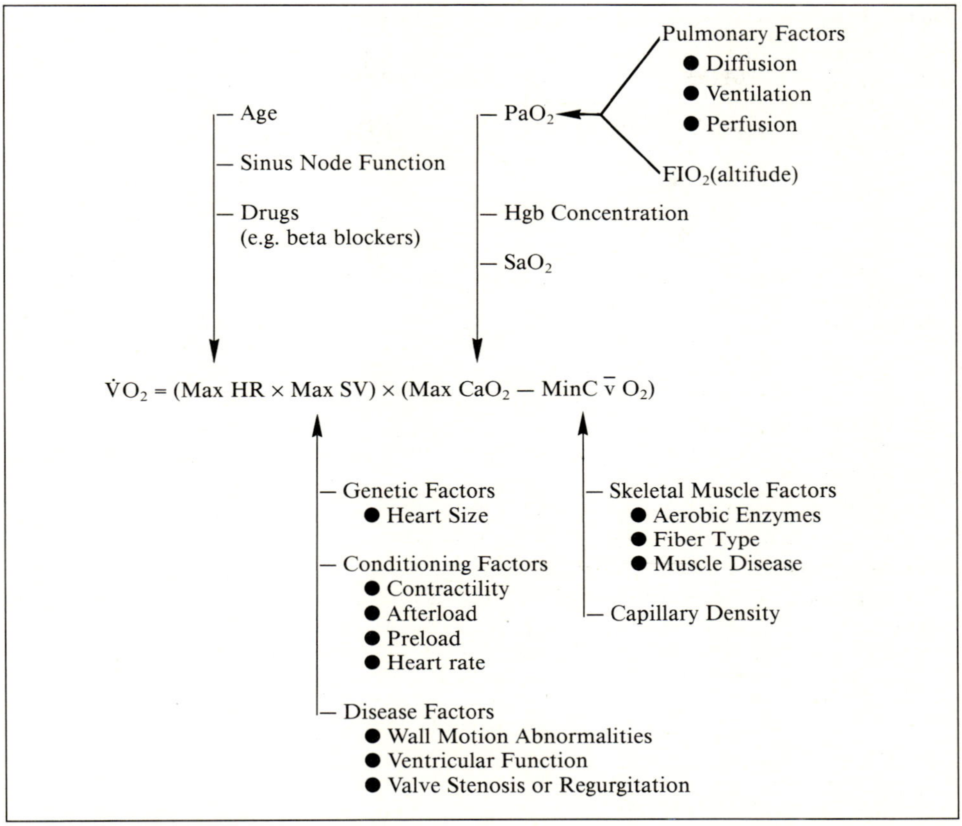

Fig. 2. Contributing and modifying factors of $\dot{V}O_{2max}$ and anaerobic threshold (modified from [8]).

widely in recent reports. Maximal exercise testing is mostly related to $\dot{V}O_{2max}$. $\dot{V}O_{2max}$ is defined by the classic description of Astrand with a leveling off, i.e. a constant $\dot{V}O_2$ despite further increments of work load. Some more objective criteria of exhaustion or $\dot{V}O_{2max}$ are given in Table 6 [20]. All exercise tests not fulfilling these criteria may be called peak exercise tests. Symptom-limited exercise tests are maximal exercise tests with a stop due to ischemia, arrhythmia, dyspnea, or fatigue. Investigators rarely report true $\dot{V}O_{2max}$, in the severely ill patient [27], because it is unlikely that patients with severe and symptomatic diseases can reach a plateau for $\dot{V}O_2$ [13, 14, 17, 24].

Even defining $\dot{V}O_{2max}$ as a failure of oxygen intake to increase by more than 1 ml/kg/min with increasing workload, such a $\dot{V}O_{2max}$ is often difficult to obtain. Further, definition of peak $\dot{V}O_2$ is vague. Reproducibility and objective characterization has low reliability. Some authors claim that changes of up to 25% have to be reported to get significant changes [3, 16, 20, 25]. Furthermore, information on maximum exercise capacity is not applicable to patients daily routine activities.

Studies often use maximal workload or maximal working time (e.g. treadmill time); these parameters are very weak, unreliable, and prone to subjective influences either by the patients and/or by the investigators. Reproducibility is poor [15, 16].

To summarize, measurement of $\dot{V}O_{2max}$ in patients is possible, but difficult to obtain if cardiopulmonary function is severely compromised. Submaximal testing may be an alternative approach.

Submaximal testing has gained much interest due to measurement of aerobic-anaerobic threshold. Again, there are many problems with this parameter. Lactate and ventilatory threshold may be different. Determination of ventilatory threshold is critically dependent on the manner of evaluation (V-slope), and the ventilatory equivalent for oxygen or carbon dioxide. Some authors raised objections on the reliability of detecting the threshold [3, 4, 14, 15, 20, 25, 28]. Lactate threshold may be difficult to read if the working capacity in patients is very low as in severe ischemic heart disease or cardiac failure [14, 15, 18].

However, from a practical point of view, the ventilatory threshold seems to be more appropriate to use for analysis of functional capacity in patients than is $\dot{V}O_{2max}$.

These criticisms are further supported by the problems inherent in reference values. As mentioned above, reference values for $\dot{V}O_{2max}$ or anaerobic threshold vary widely due to numerous factors.

Heck et al. compared reference values from different laboratories in the FRG [10]. They found a large variability of $\dot{V}O_{2max}$ among exercise testing laboratories. With regard to the discrepancies of reference values, comparability of data is limited. A

Table 6. Variability of parameters of exercise testing.

$\dot{V}_E$ (l/min)	Variability of			
	global reference values (whole collective)		individual reference values (11 probands)	
Rest:	$\overline{X}$: 8 l/m SD: 1.9 V%: 24.6		$\overline{V\%_p}$: 20.6 ± 3.1	
150 W:	$\overline{X}$: 69 l/min SD: 15.1 V%: 21.9		$\overline{V\%_p}$: 9.8 ± 3.2	
	Aerobic threshold (2 mmol/l)	Anaerobic threshold (4 mmol/l)	Individual anaerobic threshold	Individual compensation threshold
$\overline{x}$ $WATT_1$	151.8	219.0	144.3	227.0
s	29.0	26.8	21.8	20.2
V %	19.1	12.2	15.2	8.9
$\overline{x}$ V $\%_2$	15.6	7.7	12.7	5.3
s	7.8	3.8	7.1	3.4
Range V $\%_2$	6.0—34.1	3.1—18.4	3.6—25.3	2.2—14.1

Abbreviations: $\overline{x}$ = mean; SD = Standard deviation; V % = coefficient of variation in percent; W = Work load in watts; Index: 1 = Group mean values, Index: 2 = Intra individual values

Table 7. Value of spiroergometry in clinical exercise testing.

Coronary artery disease		+
Valvular heart disease		++
Hypertensive heart disease		(+)
Dilated cardiomyopathy		++
Left-heart failure		++
Chronic obstructive lung disease		++
Pulmonary hypertension		(+)
Lung diseases		+
Pacemaker therapy		++
Diagnosis:	(+)	
Function:	++	
Therapy:	+++	
Prognosis:	+	
Abbreviations:	(+) + important ++ very important +++ extremely important	

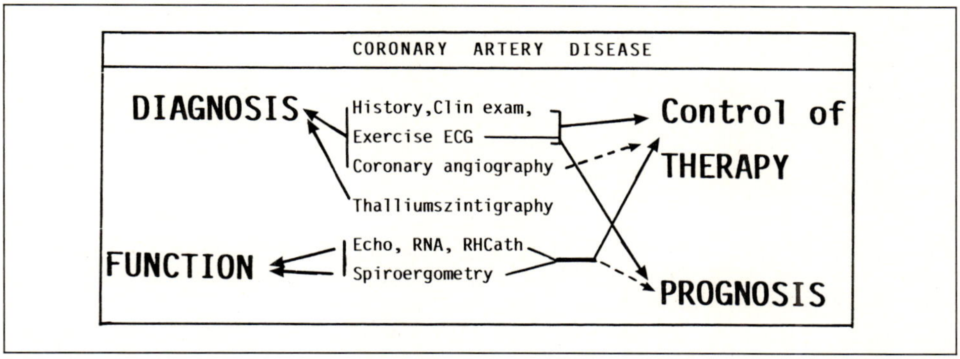

Fig. 3. Scheme of the role of diagnostic procedures in coronary artery disease. Broken arrows indicate a weak or missing significance only.

more useful approach may be a meta-analysis with pooling of data, though this is only partly reliable from a statistical view. Detailed information on the methodological approach is even necessary in order to make data from different investigators comparable. Perhaps, comparing data within a study, and before and after intervention, constitutes the only valid way to analyze results. However, as methodology and software for spiroergometry both have improved within the last years, results from different laboratories and different locations should agree and be identical. Nonetheless, quality control of ergometry is a permanent requirement in the exercise testing laboratory.

Furthermore, no general agreement exists on recommendations for reference values for $\dot{V}O_{2max}$, although much data have been published [6, 12, 16—20]. Some recommendations on aerobic-anaerobic threshold were recently published [19, 20].

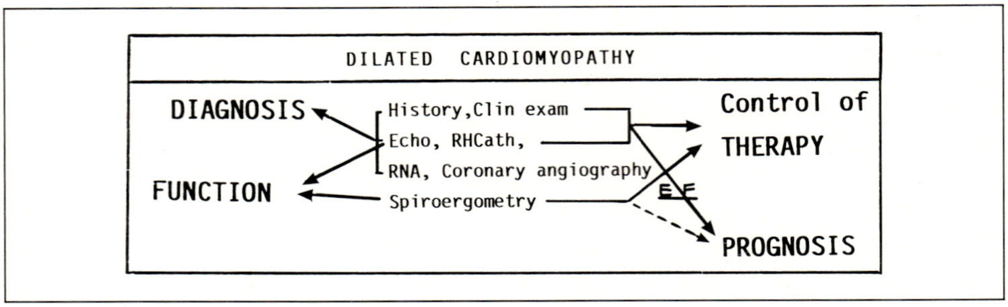

Fig. 4. Diagnostic procedures in dilated cardiomyopathy

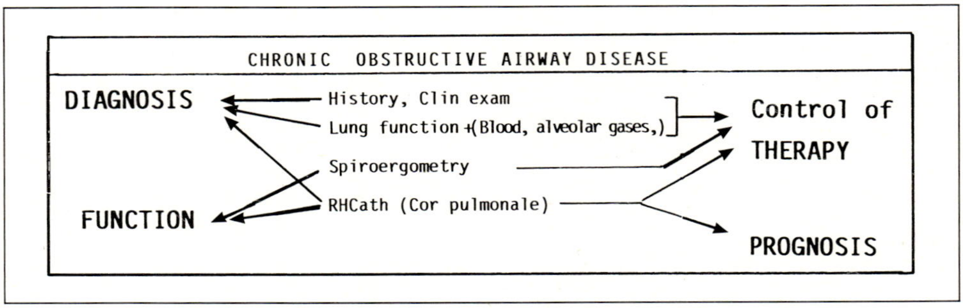

Fig. 5. Diagnostic procedures in chronic obstructive lung disease

Invasive Studies

Invasive hemodynamic measurement may overcome the problems with spiroergometry. However, right-heart catheterization cannot be performed in most cases. Short-term reproducibility is of limited reliability [23, 25]. The invasive character of this procedure may influence parameters, such as total peripheral resistance. Repeated measurements may be biased by spontaneous fluctuations due to training or drug effects. Initial drug response may not correspond to long-term drug effects [20, 25].

Hemodynamic reactions at rest in acute testing do not necessarily indicate and predict results during exercise testing. Increase of cardiac output after drug administration does not correlate to clinical status and vice versa. Decrease of capillary wedge pressure has to surmount certain values (e.g. up to $\pm$ 5 mmHg) to indicate significant changes. These are some of the objections to right heart catheterization during exercise testing for measurement of interventional effects.

Nonetheless, central hemodynamics as assessed by catheter are the standard for basic evaluation of drugs or comparable interventions in heart disease with respect to the critical remarks given above. This procedure is a basic approach in heart failure for establishing diagnosis and for measuring the effects of therapy in acute or chronic treatment. Right-heart catheterization is also the definitive method for demonstrating pulmonary hypertension secondary to lung disease. Doppler echocardiography may be a future approach to evaluate pulmonary hypertension.

Criticism may also be applied to determination of ejection fraction (EF) at rest and during exercise. Changes of EF depend on pre- and afterload; they are not clearly indicative in mitral or aortic regurgitation and do not necessarily reflect diastolic properties of the left ventricle. The EF is accepted as a marker of impaired left-ventricular function and of cardiac prognosis.

Besides, nuclide angiography cannot be repeated very often due to radiation exposure.

However, changes or constancy of EF do not closely correlate to clinical status, functional capacity, or central hemodynamics. There are reports on deterioration of clinical state despite increase of EF [14, 15, 18, 25]. In summary, EF as a noninvasive parameter gives one aspect of left-ventricular function, but it is not a first-choice parameter.

Of the parameters characterizing functional capacity and heart function, none of these measurements alone give sufficient valid information. Each approach offers only certain aspects of heart function and clinical symptoms. Taken together, all parameters may provide a clearer insight into the mechanism of heart disease and the effects of drugs and interventions.

Ergometry and spiroergometry to evaluate cardiac and pulmonary diseases

The following gives some diagnostic procedure guidelines on several diseases:

The basic methods used in this context are:

- exercise ECG;
- echocardiography at rest and at exercise (including Doppler technique);
- right-heart catheterization;
- thallium scintigraphy, radionuclide angiography (RNA);
- blood and alveolar gases, diffusion capacity;
- spiroergometry, lactate analysis.

Coronary artery disease:

Diagnosis: history, exercise ECG, coronary angiography;
Left-ventricular function: RNA, echocardiography, angiography;
Arrhythmia: ECG, Holter monitoring, late potentials, electrophysiological testing (EPS);
Functional capacity: spiroergometry (less significant, but useful for long-term observation);

Arterial Hypertension:

Diagnosis: blood pressure at rest and during exercise. Echocardiography;
Functional capacity: Spiroergometry of limited value, additional information possible.

Dilated Cardiomyopathy:

Diagnosis: History, clinical findings. Echocardiography, right-heart catheterization, coronary angiography;

Left-ventricular function:

Functional capacity: Important role of spiroergometry (therapy, prognosis).

Congenital and acquired valvular heart disease:

Diagnosis: Clinical findings, echocardiography. Right and left heart catheterization;
Functional capacity: critical and important role of spiroergometry.

Chronic obstructive lung disease:

Diagnosis: Clinical findings, history, pulmonary function including blood and alveolar gases (rest, exercise), diffusing capacity;
Functional capacity: Spiroergometry of significant supplemental value;
If cor pulmonale is suspected: Right-heart catheterization.

Heart failure of different etiology:

Diagnosis: History, clinical findings, x-ray echocardiography. Right-heart catheterization, possibly, coronary angiography. Radionuclide angiography.
Functional capacity: high significance of spiroergometry.

Value of Spiroergometry in clinical exercise testing

Diagnosis in cardiac and pulmonary diseases is mostly based on history and clinical findings. Echocardiography is a basic approach for further diagnosis, as are some other procedures such as radionuclideangiography, catheterization, and threshold measurements or $\dot{V}O_{2max}$ are other supplemental indicators toward the entire, unique picture. Spiroergometry is very sensitive to $AVDO_2$ and cardiac output; thus, this method is a very reliable and informative procedure for evaluating functional capacity, but it is of less significance for disease-related diagnosis.

Spiroergometry is useful for control and observation of effects of intervention such as drug therapy, training, or revascularization, pacemaker therapy, or cardiac transplantation. Other uses for spiroergometry are in occupational and sports medicine as this approach is highly objective. Spiroergometry is an old but reliable method and relatively inexpensive, although experienced physicians are required to interpret the results. A critical interpretation with respect to quality control is strongly recommended.

Finally, clinical state and quality of life, defined by the patient's ability to remain functionally active, are additional aspects to be considered in addition to laboratory data obtained by exercise testing and ECG measurements.

References

1. American College of Sports Medicine: Guidelines for exercise testing and prescription. Lea & Febiger, Philadelphia, 1986
2. Astrand, PO, Rodahl K (1974) Textbook of work physiology. McGraw Hill, New York, 1977
3. Bachl N (1984) Specificity and test precision of the anaerobic threshold. In: Löllgen H, Mellerowicz H (eds) (1984): Progress in Ergometry. Quality control and test criteria. Springer, Heidelberg, p 92—105
4. Bachl N, Graham T, Löllgen H (eds) (1991) Advances in Ergometry. Springer, Heidelberg New York
5. Cohn JN (ed) (1987) Quantitative exercise testing for the cardiac patient: The value of monitoring gas exchange. Circulation II, Suppl VI: 76
6. Ellestad MH (1986) Stress testing. 3. Aufl. Davis Comp, Philadelphia
7. Fardy PS, Yanowitz FG, Wilson PK (1988) Cardiac Rehabilitation, Adult Fitness, and Exercise Testing. Lea & Febiger, Philadelphia
8. Franklin BA, Gordon S, Timmis GC (1989) Exercise in modern medicine. Williams and Wilkins, Baltimore
9. Froehlicher VF (1987) Exercise and the heart. 2. Aufl. Year Book, Chicago
10. Heck H, Liesen H, Otto M, Hollmann W (1983) Das Verhalten spiroergometrischer Meßgrößen im Ausbelastungsbereich bei ABC-Kader-Untersuchungen. In: Mellerowicz, M, Franz, IW: Standardisierung, Kalibrierung und Methodik in der Ergometrie. Perimed. Erlangen, p 154—162
11. Hollmann W, Hettinger T (1990) Sportmedizin — Arbeits- und Trainingsgrundlagen. Schattauer, Stuttgart III. Aufl
12. Jones NL (1988) Clinical exercise testing, 3. Aufl. Saunders, Philadelphia
13. Karpman VL (1987) Cardiovascular System and Physical Exercise CRC Press, Boca Rayton, Florida
14. LeJemtel TH, Mancini D, Gumbardo D, Chadwick B (1985) Pitfalls and limitations of maximal oxygen uptake as an index of cardiovascular functional capacity in patients with chronic heart failure. Heart Failure 1: 112—124
15. Likoff MJ, Hare T, Gumbardo D, Chadwick B (1986) An assessment of the response in oxygen uptake and exercise duration in patients with chronic cardiac failure. Heart Failure 2: 164—175
16. Löllgen H, Mellerowicz H (1984) Progress in Ergometry, Quality control and test criteria. Springer, Heidelberg
17. Löllgen H, Ulmer HV (1985) Ergometrie-Empfehlungen zur Durchführung und Bewertung ergometrischer Untersuchungen. Klin Wschr 63: 651—677
18. Löllgen H, Wollschläger H, Samstag Y, Just H (1987) Belastungsdyspnoe bei Herz-Kreislauferkrankungen — Übersicht und Probleme. In: Wylicil P (Hrsg) Belastungsdyspnoe bei Herz-Kreislauf-Erkrankungen. München, Gedon und Reuss, p 51—74
19. Löllgen H, Ulmer HV, Crean P (Hrsg) (1988) Recommendations and standard guidelines for ergometry. Europ Heart J, Suppl K 9: 1—37
20. Löllgen H (1990) Kardiopulmonale Funktionsdiagnostik, 2 Aufl Doc Geigy/Editio Ciba Wehr
21. McArdle WD, Katch FI, Katch VL (1985) Exercise Physiology 2nd Ed Lea & Febiger, Philadelphia
22. MacDougall JD, Wenger HA, Green HJ (1982) Physiological Testing of the Elite Athlete. Mouvement Publicationsithaca, NY
23. Mellerowicz H, Franz IW (1983) Standardisierung, Kalibrierung und Methodik in der Ergometrie. Perimed, Erlangen
24. Naughton J (1988) Exercise testing: Physiological, Biochemical and Clinical principles. Futura Publishing Comp, New York

25. Packer M (1987) How should we judge the efficacy of drug therapy in patients with chronic congestive heart failure? The insights of six blind men. J Am Coll Cardiol 9: 433—438
26. Reindell H u Mitarb (1988) Funktionsdiagnostik des gesunden und kranken Herzens. Thieme, Stuttgart
27. Skinner JS (1987) Exercise testing and exercise prescription for special cases. Lea & Febiger, Philadelphia
28. Weber KT, Janicki JS (1986) Cardiopulmonary exercise testing. Saunders, Philadelphia
29. Willens HJ, Bievins RD, Wrisley D, Antonishen D, Reinstein D, Rubenfire M (1987) The prognostic value of functional capacity in patients with mild to moderate heat failure. Am Heart J 114, 1377—382
30. Wasserman K, Hansen JE, Sue DY, Wipp BJ (1987) Principles of exercise testing and interpretation. Lea & Febiger, Philadelphia
31. Wasserman K (1988) New concepts in assessing cardiovascular function. Circulation 78: 1060—1071
32. Wasserman K (ed) (1990) measures of functional capacity in patients with heart failure. Circulation 81, 1990, Suppl 11
33. Zelis R, Sinoway LI, Musch TI (1988) Why do patients with congestive heart failure stop exercise? J Am Coll Cardiol 12: 359—361

Author's address:

H. Löllgen, MD,
Med. Klinik, Dept. Cardiology,
Burgerstr. 211,
D-5630 Remscheid

Evaluation of the Cardiopulmonary Exercise Tolerance in Patients with Coronary Artery Disease (CAD) and Chronic Heart Failure (CHF)

U. J. Winter, A. K. Gitt, G. Mager, R. Klocke, G. Pothoff, M. Sedlak, H. W. Höpp, H. H. Hilger

Clinic III of Internal Medicine, Cardiology (Director: Prof. Dr. H. H. Hilger)
University of Cologne, FRG

Summary

The O_2-uptake at the anaerobic threshold ($\dot{V}O_2$ AT), as detected by gas exchange measurements during an incremental exercise test on a semi-supine bicycle, is an objective parameter for the estimation of cardiopulmonary exercise capacity. It was used to assess the severity of cardiopulmonary and cardiovasculary diseases in patients with coronary heart disease (CAD, N = 22, mean age 54.05 ± 7.88 years) and chronic heart failure (CHF, n = 15, mean age 57.73 ± 12.61 years). According to $\dot{V}O_2$ AT, we found a high distinction between the subjective and the objective evaluation of exercise capacity, using the Weber- and the NYHA-classes. The NYHA-classes provide insufficient criteria for exercise capacity (i.e. 14 CAD-patients NYHA II were individually assigned to very different Weber-classes: 2/14 Weber A, 2/14 Weber B, 4/14 Weber C, 5/14 Weber D, 1/14 Weber E). Our investigations showed that the O_2-uptake of every pedaled watt ($\Delta \dot{V}O_2/\Delta WR$) should be a parameter to estimate the exercise capacity, but seems to be very insufficient in patients with severe heart failure and low values of maximum work rate (WR). Oscillations of the respiratory variables during rest, exercise, and recovery were reported in 4/22 CAD-patients (18.2%) and in 9/15 CHF-patients (60%). A constant value for O_2-pulse, the O_2-uptake of every heart beat ($\dot{V}O_2/HR$), was reached in 10/22 CAD-patients (45.5%) and in 8/15 CHF-patients (53.3%). The computerized ergospirometry is a feasible, secure, accurate, and well-tolerated method to objectively evaluate the functional disability of patients with CAD of CHF. The present study offers new insights in the evaluation of critically ill patients using non-invasive procedures.

1. Introduction

Incremental ergospirometric exercise testing is a non-invasive procedure and allows the evaluation of cardiopulmonary and cardiovascular exercise capacity in patients during both peak and submaximal exercise performance. In contrast to the peak exercise level, the submaximal exercise performance and also the non-invasive respiratory determined anaerobic threshold (AT) cannot be influenced by the patient's motivation and, therefore, are more suitable parameters for the objective evaluation of the severity of cardiopulmonary and cardiovascular diseases. Consequently, incremental cardiopulmonary exercise testing can be a valuable tool in the clinical assessment of functional capacity, especially in patients with CAD and CHF.

2. Objective

The purpose of this study was to evaluate cardiopulmonary exercise testing in the assessment and classification of the severity of cardiopulmonary and cardiovascular diseases in patients with coronary heart disease and chronic heart failure. The responses to the stress tests were also used to evaluate the practicability and safety of cardiopulmonary exercise testing in comparison with the conventional stress test in which only the electrocardiogram is evaluated.

3. Results

3.1. Methodical aspects

Exercise testing equipment

We used a computerized cardiopulmonary exercise test (Table 1) for the examination of our patients (Table 2). Heart rate (HR), cuff blood pressure, and the electrocardiogram were monitored. Exercise and gas-exchange data were collected continuously by using a computerized breath-by-breath gas-exchange analyser utilizing a rapidly responding O_2- and CO_2- analyzer-system and pneumotachometer (Medical Graphics Corp., St. Paul, Min., USA). The O_2-uptake ($\dot{V}O_2$,) the CO_2-output ($\dot{V}CO_2$), and the respiratory exchange ratio (RER = $\dot{V}CO_2/\dot{V}O_2$), minute-ventilation ($\dot{V}_E$), and the respiratory rate (RR) were measured breath-by-breath. A tight-fitting face-mask with a dead space of 145 ml (Rudolph mask) was used to collect expired gas. A wave-like behavior of the breath-by-breath measured gas-exchange parameters $\dot{V}O_2$, $\dot{V}CO_2$, and $\dot{V}_E$ with $\pm \Delta\dot{V}O_2$ and $\pm \Delta \dot{V}CO_2$ of at least 200 ml/min, $\pm \Delta\dot{V}_E$ of at least 5 l/min, and a duration of 30 to 60 s during rest, exercise, or recovery is defined as oscillation (Wasserman [23]). The gas-analyzers and the pneumotachograph were calibrated before every test using a 3-1 syringe and reference gas including 12.00% O_2, 5.50% CO_2. The measurements were also corrected for barometric pressure, room temperature, and humidity before every procedure. The respiratory instruments and the computerized, electronically braked bicycle (Ergoline 900, Bitz, FRG) were interfaced to a personal computer (Mitsubishi MP-2300).

Table 1. Methodology

Methods:
- Incremental exercise test (15 W/25 W ramp)
- Measurement of:
  - Respiratory parameter
  - ECG
  - Blood pressure
  - Work rate
- Slope analysis
- Predetermining end points

Table 2. Patient population; (VD = vessel disease; PTCA = percutaneous transluminal coronary angioplasty)

	CAD-patients	CHF-patients
Number	22	15
Age (years)	54±8 (39—75)	58±13 (23—77)
Post posterior infarction	10	
Post anterior infarction	8	—
Post posterior and anterior infarction	2	—
Post PTCA	6	—
1-VD	10	—
2-VD	7	—
3-VD	5	—
NYHA I—II	3	—
NYHA II	14	4
NYHA II—III	3	—
NYHA III	2	11

From the collected data, we determined the O_2-uptake at the anaerobic threshold ($\dot{V}O_2$ AT in ml/min/kg), the maximal O_2-uptake (max. $\dot{V}O_2$ in ml/min/kg) [21, 22, 23, 25], the O_2-uptake of every pedaled watt ($\Delta\dot{V}O_2/\Delta WR$ in ml/min/watt) [10, 11], the O_2-Pulse, and the O_2-uptake of every heartbeat ($\dot{V}O_2$/HF in ml/min/b) [21, 22, 23, 25]. A special program (Medical Graphics Corporation) allowed for additional computations and graphic presentation of $\dot{V}CO_2$ vs. $\dot{V}O_2$-V-slope-analysis of the $\dot{V}O_2$ AT according to Beaver [21], HR vs. $\dot{V}O_2$, $\dot{V}_E$ vs. $\dot{V}O_2$, $\dot{V}_E$ vs. $\dot{V}CO_2$, $\dot{V}O_2$ vs. work rate (WR), $\dot{V}_E$ vs. time, RR vs. time, etc. During exercise, the ECG and the HR were continuously monitored, whereas the cuff BP was automatically measured every 1 min. The patients were told to perform to their maximum stress.

In order to determine the anaerobic threshold by gas analysis, we used four criteria: the V-Slope-Method according to Beaver [21] as stage-I-criteria according to Wasserman et al. [22] (behavior of $\dot{V}CO_2$ as a function of $\dot{V}O_2$ during cardiopulmonary exercise testing using a ramp protocol), the two-stage-II-criteria according to Wasserman et al. [22]: the increase of the respiratory equivalent for $\dot{V}O_2$ ($\dot{V}_E/\dot{V}O_2$) and the increase in end-tidal PO_2 ($PETO_2$) and RER-values > 0.97. Using the $\dot{V}O_2$-values at the anaerobic threshold, we assigned the patients to the Weber-classes A-E [25] (Table 3)

Table 3. Functional classification according to Weber et al. (25) and Wasserman (23)*

	$\dot{V}O_2$ max.		$\dot{V}O_2$ AT*	
	[mlO_2/kg/min]	[MET]	[mlO_2/kg/min]	[MET]
Class A;	> 20	> 5.7	> 14	> 4
Class B:	16—20	4.6—5.7	11—14	6—8
Class C:	10—16	2.9—4.5	8—11	2.3—2.9
Class D:	6—10	< 2.9	4—8	< 2.3
Class E:	< 6	< 1.7	< 4	< 1.1

MET : Metabolic equivalent

In patients who did not reach the AT, we chose the peak $\dot{V}O_2$-values for this purpose.

Practicability

Computerized ergospirometry proved to be highly practical and safe in our routine clinical evaluation. This experience confirms previous results of Tristani et al [20], who tested 607 patients in the Veterans Administration Cooperative Study. In only 10/37 of our patients the exercise test had to be stopped because of arrhythmia, and in one patient because of hypotension. Sullivan et al. [16] characterized ergospirometry as a safe method of examination in CAD-patients.

3.2. Reproducibility

In a group of normal and trained persons, we could observe a high reproducibility of the respiratory determination of the AT (unpublished data: n = 20, r = 0.89). Weber et al. [24, 25] tested patients with chronic heart failure on the treadmill and ascertained a high reproducibility of the respiratory determined anaerobic threshold (test-retest-correlation: r = 0.87). A high day-to-day-reproducibility of the values of the respiratory determined anaerobic threshold and the peak $\dot{V}O_2$ could also be found by Simonton et al. [15] in normals and in patients with chronic heart failure. A test-retest-correlation with r = 0.72 for the respiratory determined anaerobic threshold was indicated by Davis et al. [4] in healthy individuals when tested on the treadmill.

3.3. O_2-uptake at the anaerobic threshold ($\dot{V}O_2$ AT)

Determination

Investigations of Metra et al. [14], Matsumara et al. [13], Lipkin et al. [12], Weber et al. [26], Simonton et al. [15], and Sullivan et al. [18] pointed out the high percentage of respiratory determinability of the anaerobic threshold in patients with chronic heart failure. Weber et al. [24] and Matsumara et al. [13] confirmed that with increasing severity of heart failure the values of $\dot{V}O_2$ AT progressively decreased (inverse relation). Itoh et al. [11] also described the dependence of $\dot{V}O_2$ AT on patient's age and sex. With increasing age the O_2-uptake physiologically decreases. Weber et al. [26] indicated that $> 90\%$ of the tested patients with chronic heart failure and peak $\dot{V}O_2 < 25$ ml/min/kg reached their AT. Itoh et al. [11] determined the AT by gas exchange measurements in 95 of 99 normals. In our study the anaerobic threshold could be determined in 20/22 CAD-patients (91%) and 13/15 CHF-patients (87%) using the gas exchange parameters as described above; 2/22 CAD-patients (9%) and 2/15 CHF-patients (13%) did not reach the AT. The attainment of the anaerobic threshold cannot be influenced by the will of the patients. Therefore, it is an objective parameter for the estimation of the cardiopulmonary exercise capacity of patients suffering from CHF or CAD.

$\dot{V}O_2AT$ according to the NYHA-classes

Investigations of Weber et al. [24] and Matsumara et al. [13] showed the relationship of decreasing $\dot{V}O_2$ AT and increasing severity of heart disease. The differences in $\dot{V}O_2$ AT among patients in each functional class should not be overestimated because the ages of the patients in the more severe classes were higher than the ages of those in normal and milder classes. Itoh et al. [11] pointed out the dependence of $\dot{V}O_2$ AT on age and sex of the patients. The $\dot{V}O_2$ AT values in the different NYHA-classes demonstrated a considerable variation, especially in CAD-patients NYHA II. The values ranged between 4.0 and 17.3 ml/min/kg. This suggests that the NYHA functional classification inadequately describes the real cardiopulmonary exercise capacity of the patients. Also, the comparison of the findings in the coronary angiogram with the values of $\dot{V}O_2$ AT indicated that the group of CAD-patients with defined two-vessel disease (VD) only reached low levels of AT. A concomitant chronic heart failure could be excluded by other investigations. The $\dot{V}O_2$ AT-values of the 15 CHF-patients decreased with progressively declining NYHA functional classes, but were highly variable within every class.

3.4. Maximum O_2-uptake (peak $\dot{V}O_2$)

Peak $\dot{V}O_2$ and $\dot{V}O_2$ AT were used to assign patients with different grades of restriction in functional cardiopulmonary capacity, according to the Weber-classification. The values of peak $\dot{V}O_2$ are dependent on the severity of the heart failure, but are also influenced by the patient's motivation. Therefore, we used the $\dot{V}O_2$ AT according to Wasserman et al. [22] to define the individual Weber-class. Taylor et al. [19] used peak $\dot{V}O_2$ for the description of cardiopulmonary capacity in patients. Davis et al. [4] indicated a high correlation between $\dot{V}O_2$ AT and peak $\dot{V}O_2$.

Itoh et al. [11], however demonstrated in patients with chronic heart failure that peak $\dot{V}O_2$-value could hardly be estimated by the value of $\dot{V}O_2$ AT. They also showed the greater dependence of the age of the patients on peak $\dot{V}O_2$ than $\dot{V}O_2$ AT. Buchanan et al. [2] recognized the dependence of $\dot{V}O_2$ on the exercise-protocol, on the kind of exercise (i.e. treadmill or bicycle), and on the severity of heart failure. The behavior of the $\dot{V}O_2$-values of the tested CAD- and CHF-patients according to the NYHA functional classes is the same at peak exercise as at anaerobic threshold. The individual patients of each NYHA-class (i.e. CAD-patients NYHA II) obtained very different values of peak $\dot{V}O_2$. This fact again demonstrates that the NYHA functional classification is insufficient in describing real cardiopulmonary exercise capacity in patients with heart diseases.

Weber et al. [26] showed that no extrapolation of the data of maximum HR or maximum work rate to values of peak $\dot{V}O_2$-value was possible.

3.5. Comparison of the Weber- and NYHA-classes

The main advantage of the Weber-classification is based on the high objectivity of the parameter, which is responsible for the assignment to the different classes. The 14 CAD-patients NYHA II, who were allocated to all Weber-classes A-E, and the nine CHF-patients NYHA III were examples for the insufficiency of NYHA-classification (Table 4A, 4B). Van den Broek et al. [1] observed a large overlap of peak

Table 4A. Comparison of Weber- and NYHA-classifications in patients with coronary artery disease (n = 22). Patients of NYHA II could be found in every Weber-class.

	n = 2	n = 4	n = 7	n = 8	n = 1	
NYHA I–II		●●	●			n =3
NYHA II	●●	●●	●●●●	●	●●●●●	n = 14
NYHA II–III			●	●●		n = 3
NYHA III			●	●		n = 2
	Weber A	Weber B	Weber C	Weber D	Weber E	

Table 4B. Comparison of Weber- and NYHA-classifications in patients with coronary artery disease (n = 22). Patients of NYHA III had very different functional capacities and therefore could be found in Weber-classes C, D and E.

	n = 0	n = 1	n = 3	n = 6	n = 5	
NYHA II		●	●	●●		n = 4
NYHA III			●●	●●●●	●●●●●	n = 11
	Weber A	Weber B	Weber C	Weber D	Weber E	

$\dot{V}O_2$-values in classes NYHA II and III and described a high distinction between the subjective and the objective evaluation of exercise capacity in 42/82 patients (51%) with heart failure. Itoh et al. [11] and Franciosa et al. [7] proved that the NYHA-classification does not represent an objective parameter for the evaluation of the severity of heart failure. Investigations of Dunselman et al. [5] showed in 32% of NYHA II-patients nearly normal peak $\dot{V}O_2$-values, whereas 29% of NYHA III-patients only reached very low peak $\dot{V}O_2$-values. As a consequence, they should be assigned to class NYHA IV. Thus, the NYHA-classes are an insufficiant evaluation of the exercise capacity in CAD- and CHF-patients.

With the help of the Weber-classes ideal patients for clinical studies (CAD, CHF) can be better identified in the future.

3.6. Comparison of Weber-classes and maximum work rate

The maximum work rate cirteria is not sufficiently accurate to describe the real exercise capacity of an individual. Like peak $\dot{V}O_2$, the maximum work rate is also influenced by the patient's motivation and, therefore, it is not an objective parameter of cardiopulmonary exercise capacity. Not only the CAD, but also the CHF patients reached variable maximum work rate values within the different Weber-classes. We observed that one CAD patient of Weber E class attained a maximum work rate of 100 watts, which was higher than the mean of all Weber D patients. Francis et al. [8, 9] already discussed the different neurohumoral and hemodynamic responses to exercise in patients with heart disease, compared to those in normal subjects with resulting decrease of O_2-uptake and maximum work rate in patients with increasing severity of heart failure.

3.7. $\Delta\dot{V}O_2/\Delta WR$

The Weber-classification does not consider either age or sex of the patients, but the O_2-uptake at the anaerobic threshold and at peak exercise decreases with age and is physiologically lower in women than in men [11]. Hansen et al. [10] and Itoh et al. [11] chose the ratio $\Delta\dot{V}O_2/\Delta WR$ [ml/min/watt] as a reference-parameter for the evaluation of the functional capacity in patients. The normal values of the several investigators are very different. Wasserman et al. [10] described normal values of about 10.3 ml/min/watt, Itoh et al. [11] found 12.3 ± 1.6 ml/min/watt, and Coutinho et al. [3] determined 11.1 ± 2 ml/min/watt. Itoh et al. [11] observed 11.3 ± 1.6 ml/min/watt in patients NYHA I, 10.8 ± 1.7 ml/min/watt in patients NYHA II, and 8.8 ± 1.8 ml/min/watt in patients NYHA III. Coutinho et al. [3] described patients of Weber A with 9.7 ± 1 ml/min/watt, Weber B with 9.5 ± 2 ml/min/watt, and Weber C with 7.5 ± 2 ml/min/watt. Our investigations of CAD-patients showed 9.65 ± 2.95 ml/min/watt for Weber A, 9.19 ± 1.48 ml/min/watt for Weber B, 8.71 ± 1.5 ml/min/watt for Weber C, 5.46 ± 1.1 ml/min/watt for Weber D, and 4.21 ml/min/watt for Weber E. The CHF-patients of our study reached the following values: Weber B 8.63 ml/min/watt, Weber C 7.45 ± 0.92 ml/min/watt, Weber D 11.27 ± 3.86 ml/min/watt and Weber E 8.6 ± 2.79 ml/min/watt. Hansen et al. [10] described the following cardiovascular diseases: 10.16 ± 0.85 ml/min/watt in patients with arterial hypertension (n = 10), 8.29 ± 1.17 ml/min/watt in patients with heart failure (n = 51), 8.26 ± 1.20 ml/min/watt in patients with CAD and changes in ST segment (n = 20), 8.39 ± 0.77 ml/min/watt in patients with arrhythmia (n = 11), 8.63 ± 1.25 ml/min/watt in patients with arrhythmia and changes in ST segment (n = 8), 7.53 ± 1.55 ml/min/watt in patients with obstructive vascular disease (n = 7), and 8.70 ± 0.88 ml/min/watt in patients with chronic obstructive pulmonary diseases (n = 5).

For the evaluation of functional capacity in patients with severe heart failure and low values of maximum work rate this parameter seems inadequate, especially because of the different dynamics of $\dot{V}O_2$ at the beginning of and at peak exercise. One CHF-patient, for example, reached only 15 watts and increased his $\dot{V}O_2$ from 207 to 481 ml/min and, therefore, obtained an unlikely value of 18.27 ml/min/watt.

3.8. Chronotropic incompetence

A chronotropic incompetence could be observed in both patient-groups, especially in patients of Weber D and E. This phenomenon has already been described by Francis et al. [8, 9].

3.9. Oscillations

Oscillations of the gas-exchange parameters have already been reported by Wasserman et al. [23] in some CHF-patients as a kind of periodical Cheyne-Stokes-respiration. The reasons for these oscillations are unknown. The oscillations remained in our patients who were given high doses of ACE-inhibitors (Mager et al. this volume).

3.10. O_2-pulse-plateau

The low constant values of the O_2-pulse in patients with heart failure have already been described by Wasserman et al. [22]. We observed low plateau values in O_2-pulse in 45.5% of the CAD- and in 53.3% of the CHF-patients.

4. Conclusion

Computerized ergospirometry is a practicable, secure, accurate, and well-tolerated method with only non-significant sacrifice of time as compared with conventional exercise-ECGs. It provides much more information about the cardiopulmonary capacity of patients than does the ECG alone. With it, the role of vascular and pulmonary limitations during exercise can be determined. The $\Delta\dot{V}O_2/\Delta WR$-values and the Weber-classification allow a better evaluation of the functional cardiopulmonary capacity than do the NYHA functional classification, the maximum work rate in watts, or the maximum heart rate in bpm. The present investigations showed that patients with chronic heart failure were predominantly assigned to classes Weber D and E.

References

1. Van den Broek SAJ, Landsman MLJ, Portegies MCM, Lie KI (1990) Relation between aerobic capacity and NYHA classification in the assessment of functional state in heart failure. Symposium on exercise testing in congestive heart failure, Brussels
2. Buchanan N, Myers J, Walch D, McAnley P, Kraemer M, Hamilton-Wesler M, Froelicher V (1990) Effect of protocol and disease status on the hemodynamic and gas exchange response to exercise. Symposium on exercise testing in congestive heart failure, Brussels
3. Coutinho M, Treese N, Erbel R, Meyer J (1990) Anaerobic threshold detection in congestive heart failure. Symposium on exercise testing in congestive heart failure, Brussels
4. Davis JA, Vodak P, Wiulmore JH, Vodak J, Kurtz P (1976) Anaerobic threshold and maximal aerobic power for three models of exercise. J. Appl. Physiol. 41: 544—550
5. Dunselman PHJM, van der Mark ThW, Lie KI (1990) Value of cardio-pulmonary exercise tests in the selection procedure of patients for heart failure studies. Symposium on exercise testing in congestive heart failure, Brussels
6. Eldridge JE, Ramsey-Green CL, Hossack KF (1986) Effects of the limiting symptom on the achievement of maximal oxygen consumption in patients with coronary artery disease. Am J Cardiol 57: 513—517
7. Franciosa F (1986) Epidemiologic patterns, clinical evaluation and long-term prognosis in chronic congestive heart failure. Am J Med 80 (Suppl 2B): 14—20
8. Francis GS, Goldsmith SR, Ziesche S, Nakajima H, Cohn JN (1985) Relative attenuation of sympathetic drive during exercise in patients with congestive heart failure. J Am Coll Cardiol 5: 832
9. Francis GS (1987) Hemodynamic and neurohumoral responses to dynamic exercise: normal subjects versus patients with heart disease. Circulation 76 (Suppl VI): VI—11
10. Hansen JE, Sue DY, Oren A, Wasserman K (1987) Relation of oxygen uptake to work rate in normal men and men with circulatory disorder. Am J Cardiol 59: 669—674
11. Itoh H, Taniguchi K, Koike A, Doi M (1990) Evaluation of severity of heart failure using ventilatory gas analysis. Circulation 81 (Suppl II): II-31—II-37
12. Lipkin DP, Perrins J, Poole-Wilson PA (1985) Respiratory gas exchange in the assessment of patients with impaired ventricular function. Br Heart J 54: 321

13. Matsumara N, Nishijima H, Kojimas S, Hashimoto F, Minami M, Yasuda H (1983) Determination of anaerobic threshold for assessment of functional state in patients with chronic heart failure. Circulation 68: 360
14. Metra M, Raddino R, Cas LD, Visioli O (1990) Assessment of peak oxygen consumption, lactate and ventilatory thresholds and correlation with resting and exercise hemodynamic data in chronic congestive heart failure. Am J Cardiol 65: 1127—1133
15. Simonton CA, Higginbotham MB, Cobb FR (1988) The ventilatory threshold; Quantitative analysis of reproducibility and relation to arterial lactate concentration in normal subjects and in patients with chronic heart failure. Am J Cardiol 62: 100—107
16. Sullivan M, Froelicher V (1983) Maximal oxygen uptake and gas exchange in coronary heart disease. J Cardiac Rehabil 3: 539—560
17. Sullivan M, Higginbotham MB, Cobb FR (1988) Increases exercise ventilation in patients with chronic heart failure: Intact ventilatory control despite hemodynamic and pulmonary abnormalities. Circulation 77: 552—559
18. Sullivan M, Cobb FR (1990) The anaerobic threshold in chronic heart failure: relation to blood lactate, ventilatory basis, reproducibility and response to exercise training. Circulation 81 (Suppl II): II-47-II-58
19. Taylor HL, Buskirk E, Henschel A (1955) Maximal oxygen intake as an objective measure of cardio-respiratory performance. J Appl Physiol 8: 73
20. Tristani FE, Hughes CV, Archibald DG, Sheldahl LM, Cohn JN, Fletcher R for the VA Cooperative Study (1987) Safety of graded symptom-limited exercise testing in patients with congestive heart failure. Circulation 76 (Suppl VI): VI-54
21. Wasserman K, Whipp BJ, Kogal SN, Beaver WL (1973) Anaerobic threshold and respiratory gas exchange during exercise. J appl Physiol 35: 236—243
22. Wasserman K, Hansen JE, Sue DY, Whipp BJ (1986) Principles of exercise testing and interpretation. Lea & Febiger, Philadelphia
23. Wasserman K, Beaver WL, Whipp BJ (1990) Gas exchange theory and the lactic acidosis (anaerobic) Threshold. Circulation 81 (Suppl II): II-14.-II-30
24. Weber KT, Kinasewitz GT, Janicki JS, Fishman AP (1982) Oxygen utilization and ventilation during exercise patients with chronic cardiac failure. Circulation 65: 1213
25. Weber KT, Janicki JS (1986) Cardiopulmonary exercise testing; Physiologic Principles and clinical Applications. WB Saunders Company, Philadelphia
26. Weber KT, Janicki JS, McElroy PA (1987) Determination of aerobic capacity and the severity of chronic cardiac and circulatory failure. Circulation 76 (Suppl VI): VI-40

Authors' address:
PD Dr. U.J. Winter
Klinik III für Innere Medizin
Kardiologie
Universität zu Köln
Joseph-Stelzmann-Str. 9
5000 Köln 41, FRG

Respiratory Gas Analysis in Patients with Chronic Heart Failure

H. Drexler

Medizinische Klinik III, University of Freiburg, Freiburg i. Br., FRG

Introduction

Traditionally, the clinical severity of chronic heart failure has been assessed by clinical symptoms and was graded according to the criteria of the New York Heart Association (NYHA). These criteria are by their nature subjective with a low reproducibility [16]. In order to detect any change in the functional state of patients with heart failure, e.g. improvement over time with specific treatment, it appears crucial to apply an objective, reproducible, and sensitive method. Except for advanced, severe chronic heart failure, symptoms occur with physical activity only. Therefore, exercise testing with determination of variables unaffected by patient motivation and the supervising physician, should be useful in the assessment of functional capacity of patients with chronic heart failure (Table 1). It is important to recognize that the determination of LV-function, although of major prognostic value, correlates poorly with functional classes [2, 12, 14, 18, 34]. Thus, among patients with similar degrees of LV-dysfunction, clinical symptoms may vary considerably and normal exercise capacity may be almost preserved despite substantial LV-dysfunction. Two patients with identical cardiac lesions will have different symptoms during exercise if the peripheral circulation of one adapts to the exercise better than that of the other. Heart failure during exercise occurs when the peripheral circulation does not adequately adjust to an inadequate cardiac output to keep pace with the metabolic requirements of the exercising muscle. Thus, although the primary defect is due to myocardial failure, the symptoms are not solely dependent on the behavior of the heart. Similarly, exercise hemodynamics do not relate closely to exercise capacity in patients with chronic heart failure; in addition, it remains an invasive procedure which cannot be repeated unlimitedly.

Respiratory gas analysis as objective assessment of exercise capacity

Measuring the systemic oxygen consumption during exercise, the O_2 utilized by the exercising muscle can be assessed non-invasively. Maximal oxygen consumption represents the physiologic limit of aerobic capacity of the body and thus is an objective assessment of exercise capacity. Unfortunately, maximal oxygen consumption defined by a plateau of O_2 consumption despite an increase in exercise load, cannot be obtained in many patients with chronic heart failure [21]. Therefore, several authors have referred to peak $\dot{V}O_2$ (max. $\dot{V}O_2$ or symptom-limited $\dot{V}O_2$) rather than true $\dot{V}O_2$ max. However, peak-$\dot{V}O_2$ is somewhat dependent on patient motivation and guidance of the supervising physician. Whereas the peak-$\dot{V}O_2$ is of limited value in an individual patient, it is useful in double-blind randomized trials. In the latter instance, motivation of patient and physician is equally distributed for patients receiving placebo or verum treatment (Table 2).

In an attempt to achieve an objective assessment without forcing the patient with severe heart failure to his maximal performance (which may pose more distress and even hazard to the patients), the concept of anaerobic threshold has received more attention in recent years.

The level of oxyen consumption ($\dot{V}O_2$) during exercise, above which aerobic energy production is accompanied by an aerobic mechanism that causes an increase in lactate and metabolic acidosis, is termed the anaerobic threshold. The $\dot{V}O_2$ at which the anaerobic threshold occurs is influenced by the factors that affect oxygen delivery to the tissues; it is increased when oxygen flow is enhanced and decreased when oxygen flow is diminished. Above the anaerobic threshold, in addition to the development of metabolic acidosis, exercise endurance is reduced, $\dot{V}O_2$ kinetics are slowed so that a steady-state is delayed, and minute ventilation increases disproportionately to the metabolic requirement and a progressive tachypnea develops. The anaerobic threshold can be measured directly from serial measurements of lactate concentration. As bicarbonate changes reciprocally with lactate, its measurement can also be used to estimate the lactate threshold. Alternatively, changes in gas exchange caused by the physical-chemical event of buffering of lactic acid by bicarbonate can be used to detect the anaerobic threshold during exercise [36].

Application and pitfalls of respiratory gas analysis in heart failure

Patients with severe heart failure develop a metabolic acidosis more quickly than normal individuals, that is an increased rate of muscle lactate production and a reduced rate of muscle oxygen utilization occurs [29, 46]. Recent data indicate that in heart failure, the major increase in lactate during exercise is due to increased production rather than to decreased removal, and that production is more pronounced when muscle O_2 supply is compromised [30, 31].

Recent advances in on-line computer-assessed analysis of breath-by-breath technique of respiratory variables have eased the determination of anaerobic threshold by respiratory gas analysis (for review see [39]).

Yet, it appears that the numerous criteria for the anaerobic threshold are in accordance with the clinical experience, and that it may be difficult at times to detect the anaerobic threshold in patients with chronic heart failure. Moreover, the theoretical concept has been challenged [43]. It has been shown that lactate production occurs in fully oxygenated conditions, and a rise in plasma lactate may not be linked to ventilatory anaerobic threshold. For example, in patients with McArdle syndrome a ventilatory anaerobic threshold has been observed despite the inability of lactate production in this disorder [17]. Recent data invited speculations that acid pH changes in the working muscle could stimulate ventilation during exercise independently of lactate acidemia [33].

Nevertheless, the gas exchange anaerobic threshold can be used as an important and highly reproducable point of submaximal exercise [28, 39]. Recently, Janicki et al. have demonstrated a good long-term reproducibility of respiratory gas-exchange measurements in patients with stable cardiac failure [19]. This is important when this approach is utilized to assess the long-term effect of newer pharmacologic therapy. The so-called V-slope method as delineated by Beaver et al. [1], and co-plotting of ventilation equivalents [28] of O_2 and CO_2 during exercise (for review see [7]) appear to be the most useful methods for determination in patients with chronic heart failure [28] (see Table 4).

Figure 1 illustrates the determination of anaerobic threshold by respiratory gas analysis using co-plotting of the ventilation equivalent for CO_2 and O_2 in a patient with chronic heart failure (peak $\dot{V}O_2$ 15.8 ml/min/kg).

Despite the wide-spread use of respiratory gas analysis in the United States, the exercise protocols, the methods of determining anaerobic threshold, and indexes for assessment of functional capacity differ in major centers of exercise testing in heart failure [3—5, 32, 37]. For example, the sampling interval can have a major impact on gas exchange data during exercise. Differences of as much as 20% in $\dot{V}O_2$ may occur because of the method of sampling gas exchange data (e.g. comparison of breath-by-breath values vs. 60-s sampling) [25, 27]. Therefore, it is important to specify the sample size used when reporting gas-exchange data.

Undoubtedly, the respiratory gas analysis in patients with chronic heart failure needs more standardization, and notably, sophisticated and expensive equipment is mandatory.

Arterial lactate for determination of anaerobic threshold

Given the controversy in the theoretical concept and lack of consensus in methodological aspects, some investigators have compared this approach with more simple techniques to determine anaerobic threshold [7, 38]. Based on excellent, long-standing experience in athletes, we used serial lactate measurements as a simple means to assess aerobic capacity in heart failure [26]. The anaerobic threshold determined by arterial lactate estimation correlated closely with the one assessed by respiratory gas analysis performed simultaneously. Moreover, our initial experience indicates that changes in anaerobic threshold (by lactate) occurring with long-term therapy are correlated with the changes in anaerobic threshold as determined by respiratory gas analysis. Given the high precision of arterial lactate measurements (± 3%), this approach may represent a practical method and avoid expensive and sophisticated equipment.

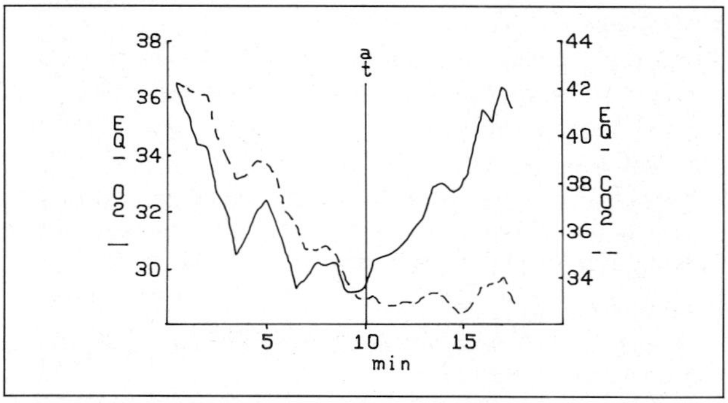

Abb. 1. Ventilation equivalents of O_2 and CO_2 during exercise (at = anaerobic threshold).

Clinical relevance

As stated above, respiratory gas analysis data have a good reproducibility in patients with chronic heart failure [19, 28, 39]. It appears that peak $\dot{V}O_2$ and $\dot{V}O_2$ at anaerobic threshold represent a useful method to assess the impact of therapy on the functional capacity of patients with heart failure. Indeed, the determination of peak $\dot{V}O_2$ has been frequently and successfully used to assess the effect of new therapeutic agents. Moreover, preliminary data suggest that a significant increase in peak $\dot{V}O_2$ (> 2 ml/min/kg) is accompanied by an improvement in quality of life [35].

Based on the data of the V-Heft study, Cohn et al. [6] have suggested that peak $\dot{V}O_2$ is an important measure of prognosis, e.g. if one uses a value of $\dot{V}O_{2max}$ of 10 ml/min/kg as a cut-off point, there is a poorer prognosis for patients with < 10 ml/min/kg. However, there is no continuous relationship when plotted against probability of survival. That is if the level of $\dot{V}O_{2max}$ is shifted to 13—14 ml/min/kg, the mortality of these groups (> 13 ml/min/kg vs < 13 ml/min/kg) is not significantly different [15].

Interestingly, the anaerobic threshold may be somehow coupled to the course of LV-ejection fraction during exercise. Koike et al. demonstrated that the anaerobic threshold occurs at a point when ejection fraction during exercise decreases [20]. Thus, respiratory gas analysis can detect the onset of LV-dysfunction during exercise. Clinically, respiratory gas analysis is most helpful for the differentiation of dyspnea due to pulmonary or cardiac disorders (see Table 3). It is important to emphasize that changes in central hemodynamics (e.g. secondary to effective therapy) are usually not immediately accompanied by appropriate improvement in peak $\dot{V}O_2$ or anaerobic threshold.

The muscle fatigue noted in exercising patients with congestive heart failure is probably related to increased muscular anaerobic activity and acidosis. It has been suggested that muscle acidosis and fatigue in patients with heart failure are related to reduction in nutritive flow to exercise muscle as a result of either impaired vasodilator capacity in the peripheral vasculature of such patients [44—47] or unfavorable distribution of increased available cardiac output [8, 30]. However, Wilson et al. [41] showed that increases in total limb blood flow induced by intravenous hydralazine failed to reduce femoral vein lactate concentration in patients with heart

Table 1. Respiratory gas analysis in chronic heart failure.

Methodological aspects

Bicycle ergometry (or treadmill) 15—25 watts per stage, 1—2 min per stage, determination of peak $\dot{V}O_2$, $\dot{V}O_2$ at anaerobic threshold, arterial lactate levels (e.g. by co-plotting $\dot{V}E/\dot{V}O_2$ vs. $\dot{V}E/\dot{V}CO_2$).

Clinical relevance

Objective measuring of functional capacity; Sufficient reproducibility in most patients; Indicator for quality of life (e.g. increase in $\dot{V}O_2$ of > 2 ml/min/kg); Relationship to LV-ejection fraction during exercise and to prognosis.

Value for follow-up

Assessment of long-term response and efficacy of medical therapy; Additional information on arterial lactate levels (?).

Table 2. Rationale for using anaerobic threshold.

1) No maximal stress test necessary in patients with chronic heart failure;
2) No influence by the patient motivation;
3) True $\dot{V}O_2max$ difficult to achieve in patients with chronic heart failure;
4) Correlation to endurance activity in athletes; daily activation in anaerobic range possibly a higher threshold for higher submaximal exercise (?).

Table 3. Pulmonary vs. cardiac dyspnea.

1) Decrease in arterial pO_2 during exercise if of pulmonary cause;
2) Anaerobic threshold difficult to achieve in pulmonary disease;
3) $\dot{V}E$ inappropriate in relationship to potential underlying disorders (e.g. respiratory muscle disease, thoracic surgery).

Table 4. Determination of anaerobic threshold in chronic heart failure.

1) Increase in $\dot{V}CO_2$ in relation to $\dot{V}O_2$, e.g. co-plotting or (better) V-slope-method (Beaver et al.);
2) Increase in $\dot{V}E$ and respiratory exchange ratio in relationship to $\dot{V}O_2$ or time;
3) $\dot{V}E/\dot{V}CO_2$ co-plotting to $\dot{V}E/\dot{V}CO_2$;
4) Serial arterial lactate determinations.

failure. Moreover, neither skeletal muscle oxygen delivery nor exercise capacity is improved in heart failure patients who are treated with hydralazine [40], isosorbide dinitrate [13], or the positive inotropic agents dobutamine [42] or milrinone [8]. Because an increase in blood flow to exercising skeletal muscle in patients with heart failure does not appear to be synonymous with a reduction in muscular acidosis and fatigue, it has been proposed that an intrinsic abnormality of skeletal muscle may account for impaired oxygen delivery and utilization and the resulting metabolic and clinical abnormalities observed in patients with heart failure [9, 22—42].

Importantly, ACE-inhibition does not alter exercise hemodynamics and peak $\dot{V}O_2$ acutely, but improves both central and peripheral hemodynamics, and peak $\dot{V}O_2$ after *long-term therapy* by increasing performance and oxygen extraction of skeletal muscle [10]. The latter is accompanied by a reversal of intrinsic alteration of skeletal muscle [11].

Summary: For the evaluation of the functional state of patients with heart failure, e.g. improvement over time with specific treatment, it appears crucial to apply an objective, reproducible, and sensitive method. Exercise testing with determination of variables unaffected by patient motivation and the supervising physician should be useful in the assessment of functional capacity of patients with chronic heart failure. Among patients with similar degrees of left-ventricular (LV)-dysfunction, clinical symptoms may vary considerably and normal exercise capacity may be almost preserved despite substantial LV-dysfunction. Maximal oxygen consumption represents the physiologic limit of aerobic capacity of the body and thus is an objective asessment of exercise capacity. Since the criteria for true maximal oxygen consumption are not obtained in the majority of patients with chronic heart failure, the determination of the anaerobic threshold has been applied, which provides an objective assessment of functional capacity without forcing the patient with heart failure to his maximal physical performance. The anaerobic threshold can be determined by respiratory gas analysis using the v-slope method and/or co-plotting of ventilation equivalents of O_2 and CO_2. Alternatively, serial lactate measurements may represent a useful and more inexpensive means for the determination of anaerobic threshold.

Since the reproducibility of respiratory gas analysis and arterial lactate measurements is excellent, these measurements can be used to assess the functional capacity of patients with chronic heart failure; in particular the effect of therapeutic interventions can be assessed. Moreover, the data obtained appear to provide prognostic information.

References

1. Beaver WL, Wasserman K, Whipp BJ (1986) A new method for detecting anaerobic threshold by gas exchange. J Appl Physiol 60: 2020—2027
2. Benge W, Litchfield RL, Marcus ML (1980) Exercise capacity in patients with severe left ventricular dysfunction. Circulation 61: 955—959
3. Buchfuhrer MJ, Hansen JE, Robinson TE, Sue DY, Wasserman K, Whipp BJ (1983) Optimizing the exercise protocol for cardiopulmonary assessment. J Appl Physiol 55: 1558—1564
4. Buller NP, Poole-Wilson PA (1988) Extrapolated maximal oxygen consumption: a new method for the objective analysis of respiratory gas exchange during exercise. Br Heart J 59: 212—217
5. Buller NP, Poole-Wilson PA (1990) Mechanism of the increased ventilatory response to exercise in patients with chronic heart failure. Br Heart J 63: 281—283
6. Cohn JN et al. (1987) Veterans administration cooperative study on vasodilator therapy of heart failure: influence of prerandomization variables on the reduction of mortality by treatment with hydralazine and isosorbide dinitrate. Circulation 75: IV-49
7. Dickstein K, Barvik S, Aarsland T, Snapinn S, Karlsson J (1990) A comparison of methodologies in detection of the anaerobic threshold. Circulation 81: II-38-II-46
8. Drexler H, Faude F, Hönig S, Jut H (1987) Blood flow distribution within skeletal muscle during exercise in the presence of chronic heart failure: effect of milrinone. Circulation 76: 1344—1352
9. Drexler H, Riede U, Schäfer H (1987) Reduced oxidative capacity of skeletal muscle in patients with severe heart failure. Circulation 76: IV-178
10. Drexler H, Banhardt U, Meinertz T, Wollschläger H, Lehmann M, Just H (1989) Contrasting peripheral short-term and long-term effects of converting enzyme inhibition in patients with congestive heart failure. A double-blind, placebo-controlled trial. Circulation 79: 491—502
11. Drexler H, Münzel T, Riede U, König H, Just H (1990) Effect of chronic heart failure on skeletal muscle: ultrastructural analysis of 55 cases. Europ Heart J (in press)
12. Franciosa JA, Ziesche S, Wilen M (1979) Functional capacity in patients with chronic left ventricular failure. Relationship of bicycle exercise performance to clinical and hemodynamic characterization. Am J Med 67: 460—466
13. Franciosa JA, Cohn JN (1979) Effect of isosorbide dinitrate on response to submaximal and maximal exercise in patients with congestive heart failure. Am J Cardiol 43: 1009—1014
14. Franciosa JA, Park M, Levine TB (1981) Lack of correlation between exercise capacity and indexes of resting left ventricular performance in heart failure. Am J Cardiol 47: 33—39
15. Franciosa JA (1987) Why patients with heart failure die: hemodynamic and functional determinants of survival. Circulation 75: IV-20-IV-27
16. Goldman L, Hasmoto B, Cook F, Lascalzo A (1981) Comparative reproducibility and validity of systems for assessing cardiovascular functional class. Circulation 64: 1227—1234

17. Hagberg JM, Coyle EF, Carroll JE, Miller JM, Martin WH, Brooke MH (1982) Exercise hyperventilation in patients with McArdle disease. J Appl Physiol 52: 991—994
18. Higginbotham MB, Morris KG, Conn EH, Coleman RE, Cobb FR (1983) Determinants of variable exercise performance among patients with severe left ventricular dysfunction. Am J Cardiol 51: 52—60
19. Janicki JS, Gupta S, Ferris ST, McElroy PA (1990) Long-term reproducibility of respiratory gas exchange measurements during exercise in patients with stable cardiac failure. Chest 97: 12—17
20. Koike A, Itoh H, Taniguchi K, Hiroe M (1989) Detecting abnormalities in left-ventricular function during exercise by respiratory measurement. Circulation 80: 1737—1746
21. Lipkin DP (1987) The role of exercise testing in chronic heart failure. Br Heart J 58: 559—566
22. Mancini DM, Ferraro N, Tuchler M, Chance B, Wilson JR (1988) Detection of abnormal calf muscle metabolism in patients with heart failure using phosphorus-31 nuclear magnetic resonance. Am J Cardiol 62: 1234—1240
23. Massie BM, Conway M, Yonge R et al. (1987) 31P nuclear magnetic resonance evidence of abnormal skeletal muscle metabolism in patients with congestive heart failure. Am J Cardiol 60: 309—315
24. Massie BM, Conway M, Yonge R et al. (1987) Skeletal muscle metabolism in patients with congestive heart failure: relation to clinical severity and blood flow. Circulation 76: 1009—1019
25. Matthews JI, Bush BA, Morales FM (1987) Microprocessor exercise physiology systems vs a nonautomated system. A comparison of data output. Chest 92: 696—703
26. Münzel T, Drexel H, Kurz S, Dickhut H (1989) Anaerobic threshold determination by serial lactate measurements: a simple means to assess aerobic capacity in heart failure. Circulation 80: II-56
27. Myers J, Walsh D, Sullivan M, Froelicher V (1990) Effect of sampling on variability and plateau in oxygen uptake. J Appl Physiol 68: 404—410
28. Simonton CA, Higginbotham MB, Cobb FR (1988) The ventilatory threshold: quantitative analysis of reproducibility and relation to arterial lactate concentration in normal subjects and in patients with chronic congestive heart failure. Am J Cardiol 62: 100—107
29. Solal AC, Chabernaud JM, Gourgon R (1990) Comparison of oxygen uptake during bicycle exercise in patients with chronic heart failure and in normal subjects. J Am Coll Cardiol 16: 80—85
30. Sullivan MJ, Higginbotham MB, Cobb FR (1989) Exercise training in patients with chronic heart failure delays ventilatory anderobie treshould and imperoves submaximal exercise performance. Circulation 79: 324—329
31. Sullivan MJ, Knight JD, Higginbotham MB, Cobb FR (1989) Relation between central and peripheral hemodynamics during exercise in patients with chronic heart failure. Muscle blood flow is reduced with maintenance of arterial perfusion pressure. Circulation 80: 769—781
32. Sullivan MJ, Cobb FR (1990) The anaerobic threshold in chronic heart failure. Relation to blood lactate, ventilatory basis, reproducibility, and response to exercise training. Circulation 81: II-47—II-58
33. Systrom DM, Kanarek DJ, Kohler SJ, Kazemi H (1990) 31P nuclear magnetic resonance spectroscopy study of the anerobic threshold in humans. J Appl Physiol 68: 2060—2066
34. Szlachcic J, Massie BM, Kramer BL, Topic N, Tabau J (1985) Correlates and prognostic implication of exercise capacity in chronic congestive heart failure. Am J Cardiol 55: 1037—1042
35. Tandon PK, Stander H, Dyke SH, Massey TJ, DiBianco R, Schwarz RP (1988) Assessment of the quality of life of patients with heart failure: a randomized, controlled drug trial. Heart failure 4: 3)—54
36. Wasserman K (1987) Determinants and detection of anaerobic threshold and consequences of exercise above it. Circulation 76: IV-29
37. Weber KT, Kinasewitz LGT, Janicki JS, Fishman AP (1982) Oxygen utilization and ventilation during exercise in patients with chronic cardiac failure. Circulation 65: 1213—1223
38. Weber KT, Janicki JS (1985) Lactate production during maximal and submaximal exercise in patients with chronic heart failure. J Am Coll Cardiol 6: 717—724
39. Weber KT, Janicki JS (1986) Cardiopulmonary exercise testing. WB Saunders Company, Philadelphia

40. Wilson JR, Untereker W, Hirshfeld J, Ferraro N (1981) Effects of isosorbide dinitrate and hydralazine on regional metabolic responses to arm exercise in patients with heart failure. Am J Cardiol 48: 934—938
41. Wilson JR, Martin JL, Ferraro N; Weber KT (1983) Effect of hydralazine on perfusion and metabolism in the leg during upright bicycle exercise in patients with heart failure. Circulation 68: 425—432
42. Wilson JR, Martin JL, Ferraro N (1984) Impaired skeletal muscle nutritive flow during exercise in patients with congestive heart failure: role of cardiac pump dysfunction as determined by the effect of dobutamine. Am J Cardiol 53: 1308—1315
43. Yeh MP, Gardner RM, Adams TD, Yanowitz FG, Crapo RO (1983) "Anaerobic threshold": problems of determination and validation. J Appl Physiol 55: 1178—1186
44. Zelis R, Mason DT, Braunwald E, Winterhalter M, King C (1968) A comparison of the effects of vasodilator stimuli on peripheral resistance vessels in normal subjects and in patients with congestive heart failure. J Clin Invest 47: 960—970
45. Zelis R, Mason DT, Braunwald E (1969) Partition of blood flow to the cutaneous and muscular beds of the forearm at rest and during leg exercise in normal subjects and in patients with heart failure. Circ Res 24: 799—806
46. Zelis R, Longhurst J, Capone RJ, Mason DT (1974) A comparison of regional blood flow and oxygen utilization during dynamic forearm exercise in normal subjects and patients with congestive heart failure. Circulation 50: 137—143
47. Zelis R, Nellis SH, Longhurst J, Lee G, Mason DT (1975) Abnormalities in the regional circulations accompanying congestive heart failure. Prog Cardiovasc Dis 18: 181—199

Author's address:

Dr. med. H. Drexler,
Medizinische Klinik III,
University of Freiburg,
Hugstetterstr. 55,
7800 Freiburg i. Br., FRG

Influence of Phosphodiesterase Inhibitors on Aerobic Capacity in Chronic Heart Failure

N. Treese, M. Coutinho, A. Werneyer, S. Rhein, R. Erbel, and J. Meyer

II. Medizinische Klinik Joh.-Gutenberg-Universität Mainz, FRG

Introduction

The diagnostic potential of exercise testing has been considerably enhanced by the concurrent measurement of respiratory gas exchange. The availability of rapidly responding gas analyzers together with linear air flow transducers have greatly facilitated the on-line monitoring of oxygen uptake ($\dot{V}O_2$), carbon dioxide production ($\dot{V}CO_2$), and minute ventilation ($\dot{V}E$) in the clinical exercise laboratory.

The objective of cardiopulmonary exercise testing in patients with chronic heart failure is to confirm the severity of symptoms, to classify the degree of heart failure, to predict prognosis, and to assess drug efficacy.

Maximal oxygen uptake ($\dot{V}O_2$ max) is generally considered to be the best available index for exercise capacity and can be used for precise and objective determination of cardiopulmonary fitness or disability [12, 29, 34].

Exercise capacity and peripheral circulation in CHF

Limitation of exercise tolerance is a major manifestation of chronic heart failure which carries independent prognostic significance [17, 25]. The reduced exercise capacity is not a simple consequence of depressed systolic left ventricular function, but reflects the complex compensatory peripheral response to the change of central hemodynamics. In normal subjects, maximal oxygen uptake is directly proportional to cardiac output. In chronic heart failure, however, exercise-induced dyspnea and fatigue are probably symptoms of the limited circulatory capacity to supply oxygen to the working muscle. Three general explanations are possible: 1) [12] lack of responsiveness of the failing heart to adrenergic or sympathetic stimulation; 2) [34] impaired ability of the peripheral circulation to increase blood flow in the working muscle; and 3) [29] intrinsic abnormalities of the muscle function and metabolism. Therefore, it is not surprising that in patients with more severe myocardial dysfunction the correlation between ejection fraction or other hemodynamic indices at rest and exercise capacity is poor [2, 11, 12, 13]. We compared peak oxygen uptake during exercise with left ventricular fractional shortening determined by 2D-echocardiography at rest. No correlation was found between the degree of left ventricular systolic impairment and the aerobic capacity (Fig. 1).

Other indices of exercise tolerance have a number of limitations. Symptom classification such as the New York Heart Association Functional Classes are subjective and inprecise, although attempts for a greater standardization have been made. Peak oxygen consumption has been correlated with symptom classification, however, a

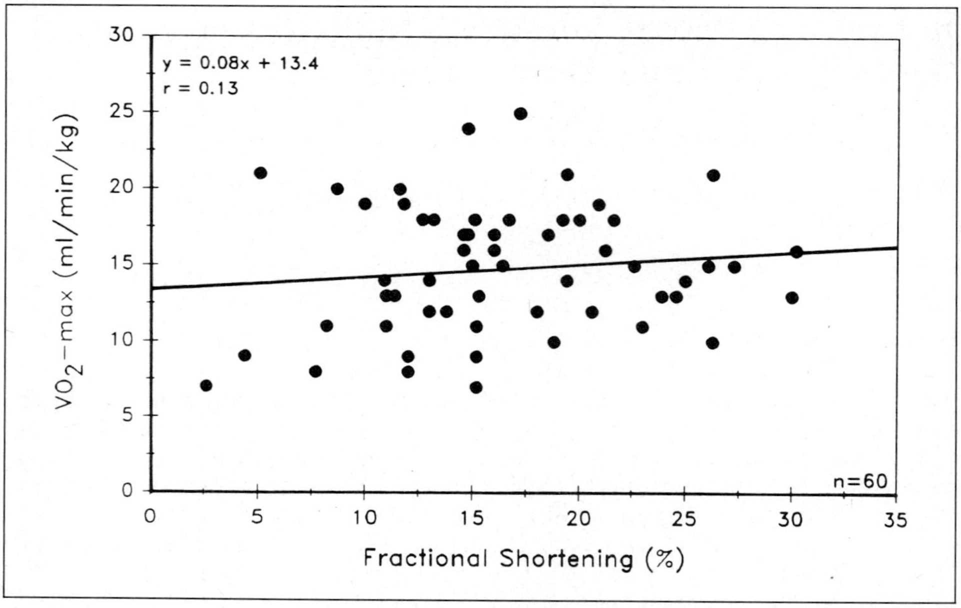

Fig. 1. Relation between fractional shortening determined by echocardiography and peak oxygen uptake ($\dot{V}O_2$ max) in patients with chronic heart failure treated with enoximone or captopril.

considerable overlap of $\dot{V}O_2$ max values in the different NYHA classes was obtained [6, 10]. Our findings similarly demonstrate that oxygen uptake at anaerobic threshold ($\dot{V}O_2$-AT) does not predict the NYHA functional class in chronic heart failure (Fig. 2). In contrast there was a very close correlation between peak oxygen uptake and maximal workload, independent of the degree of left ventricular function (Fig. 3).

Weber and Janicki [11] have shown that treadmill $\dot{V}O_2$ max correlated well with cardiac reserve as determined by simultaneous right heart catheterization. They described functional cardiac impairment as none or mild (Class A) in patients with a $\dot{V}O_2$ max above 20 ml/kg/min and as more severe (Class B to D) in patients with lower values. This classification appears particularly useful for risk stratification and evaluation of drug therapy.

The poor relationship between most indices of cardiac function at rest and exercise capacity underscores the importance of peripheral mechanisms in determining exercise tolerance. Zelis and coworkers have demonstrated a decreased forearm blood flow in patients with chronic heart failure following isometric and isotonic exercise [38]. These findings have been confirmed by other investigators, suggesting that exercise capacity is limited by the blood flow to the working muscle [24, 37].

Interestingly, it has been observed that therapy with inotropic or vasodilatory drugs that results in immediate improvement of central hemodynamics does not produce immediate changes of exercise capacity [15, 16]. Typically, it has been shown that captopril enhances exercise capacity after longterm treatment, however, without immediate effect on exercise performance, despite acute improvement of left ventricular function [17, 21]. Some drugs do not increase muscle blood flow. Redistribution of cardiac output towards non-muscular regions is proposed to explain these findings [18]. Furthermore, it has been observed that some drugs in-

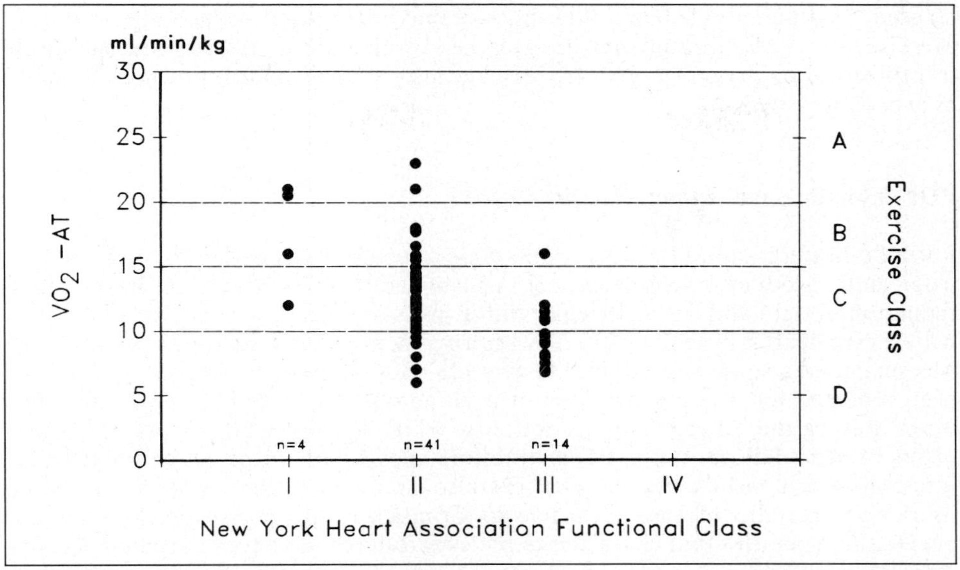

Fig. 2. Relation between NYHA functional class and oxygen uptake at anaerobic threshold ($\dot{V}O_2$-AT) and exercise classes: Weber classification [11] in patients with chronic heart failure treated with enoximone or captopril. Advanced NYHA functional class was associated with lower oxygen consumption; however, a wide range of anaerobic threshold values was observed in the different classes.

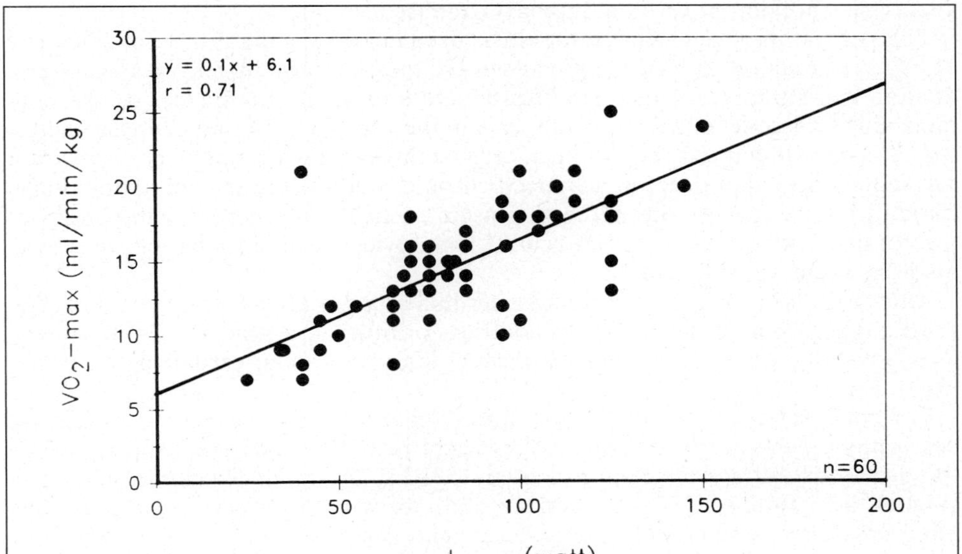

Fig. 3. Relation between maximal work load (ramp protocol with 10-watt increments of workload) and peak oxygen uptake ($\dot{V}O_2$ max) in patients with chronic heart failure treated with enoximone or captopril.

creased maximal muscle blood flow, but not maximal muscle oxygen uptake during exercise [19]. These finding may be explained by an inability of the working muscle to utilize the increased oxygen delivery because of abnormalities of muscle metabolism [20].

PDE inhibitors and aerobic capacity in CHF

Phosphodiesterase inhibitors are a new class of compounds with both positive inotropic and vasodilator properties [22]. A sustained increase of cardiac output and a reduction in right and left ventricular filling pressures has been observed in patients with severe heart failure [23—27]. The improvement of left ventricular performance was sustained also during exercise testing [28—30]. However, variable results have been reported for the improvement of peak aerobic capacity [31—36]. These findings may be due to the complex action of PDE inhibitors on peripheral mechanisms of heart failure. While PDE inhibitors consistently improve left ventricular function at rest and during maximal exercise, aerobic capacity appears only to be improved when the increase in cardiac performance results in a reversal of the peripheral abnormalities that characterize the syndrome of advanced chronic heart failure.

In our laboratory cardiopulmonary exercise testing is performed on a bicycle in semisupine position using a ramp protocol with increasing workload of 10 to 20 watts increment per minute. In contrast to treadmill exercise, true maximal oxygen uptake ($\dot{V}O_2$ max plateau) is rarely achieved on the bicycle (Fig. 3). Therefore, we use the ventilatory anaerobic threshold as submaximal level of total work capacity and as the endpoint of cardiopulmonary exercise testing.

The ventilatory anaerobic threshold has been defined as the disproportional rise of $\dot{V}CO_2$ in relation to $\dot{V}O_2$. At the anaerobic threshold the increasing lactate production will stimulate immediate bicarbonate buffering, thus increasing the non-metabolic CO_2 concentration that appears in the expired air. From exercise physiology it is known that only below the anaerobic threshold work can be performed for a sustained period of time. In advanced chronic heart failure the ventilatory anaerobic threshold can be considered as a useful, reliable, and reproducible index of the complex interaction between central hemodynamic alterations and its consequences in the working muscle.

Amrinone has been found to enhance aerobic capacity after 4 weeks, but not after acute drug administration [30]. In contrast, pirbuterol, a nonselective β-agonist, does not influence exercise capacity, despite improvement of cardiac performance [31].

In a small series of open-labeled studies, Weber and collegues have reported for both enoximone and piroximone a significant increase of aerobic capacity which was sustained during long-term treatment [33, 35]. Other investigatores have questioned these findings [15, 20]. Scriven and coworkers [23] performed a double-blind crossover comparison of enoximone and captopril over 4 weeks. Maximal oxygen uptake and cardiac output during exercise were determined in this study. Haemodynamic indices and maximal oxygen uptake improved to the same extent after both drugs.

Similarly, we performed a randomized study to assess the long-term efficacy of captopril and enoximone in chronic heart failure patients, using cardiopulmonary exercise testing and 2D-echocardiography. In some patients treated with enoximone anaerobic threshold and working capacity improved after 4 weeks but declined after a 6-months control period (Fig. 4). When compared to captopril, enoximone showed significant positive inotropic effects, as demonstrated by a typical change of the systolic time intervals. However, despite enhanced cardiac performance, aerobic capacity significantly decreased after 6 months in patients treated with enoximone compared to the captopril group. The study is limited by its design and its small size, but it appears that enoximone, in contrast to captopril, could not prevent the deterioration of heart failure in this study population [27].

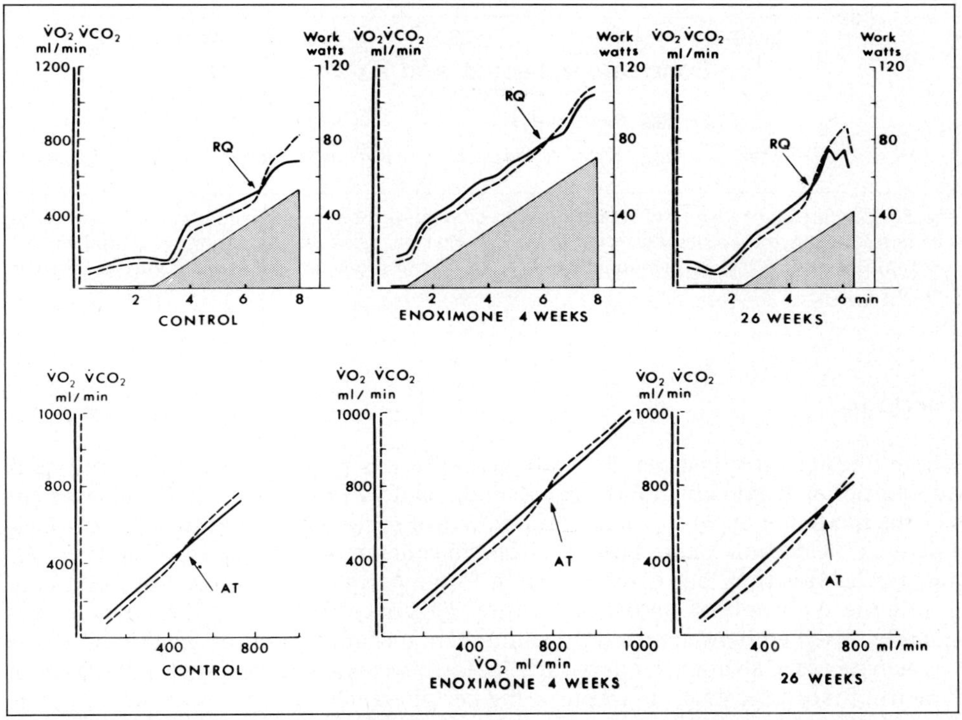

Fig. 4. Cardiopulmonary exercise testing in a patient with chronic heart failure NYHA Class III under long-term enoximone therapy. After 4 weeks a significant increase in exercise capacity and an increased anaerobic threshold were observed. After 6 months, however, exercise tolerance and anaerobic threshold decreased below baseline values.

Leier and coworkers [15] recently reported similar observations in a placebo-controlled study with enoximone over 16 weeks. Despite improvement of left ventricular performance, as shown by echocardiography and radionuclide angiography, exercise tolerance and aerobic capacity did not improve.

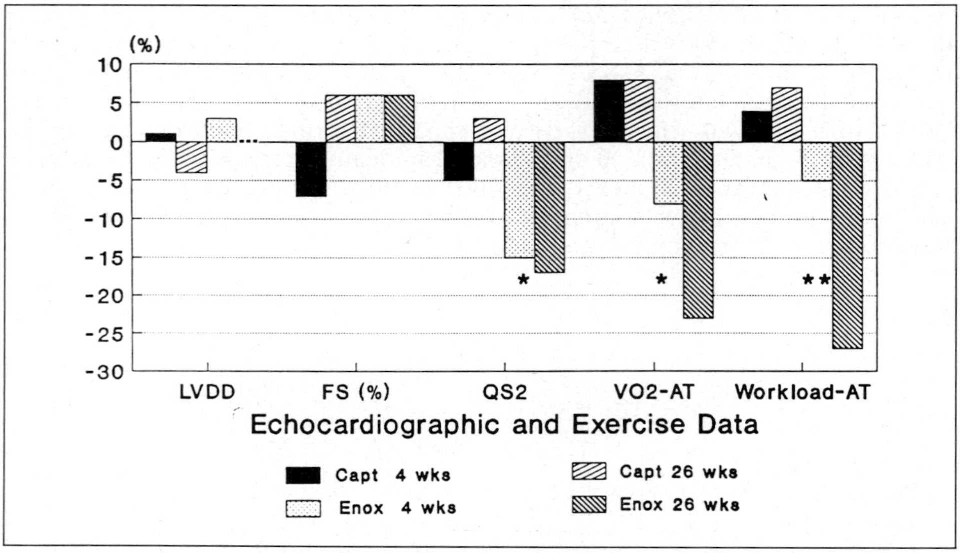

Fig. 5. Comparison of long-term treatment with enoximone and captopril in chronic heart failure. The percent-change from baseline after 4 and 26 weeks of fractional shortening (FS), total electromechanical systole (QS_2), oxygen uptake ($\dot{V}O_2$-AT), and workload (W-AT at anaerobic threshold) is shown.

Conclusion

These findings demonstrate the usefulness of cardiopulmonary exercise testing as an additional diagnostic tool to provide independent information in the assessment of drug treatment in chronic heart failure. It is of particular importance that exercise tolerance in chronic heart failure is less dependent on the degree of systolic left ventricular function, but is more related to the peripheral abnormalities that constitute the syndrome of circulatory failure. This may explain the discrepancies frequently observed between central hemodynamic changes and the functional status of the patients. Cardiopulmonary exercise testing can assess the potential long-term benefit of inotropic drugs to improve the peripheral abnormalities in chronic heart failure.

Drugs that enhance cardiac performance without improving long-term exercise capacity are less valuable in chronic heart failure and should only be used if no alternative treatment is available.

Summary

Positive inotropic drugs are useful in patients with chronic heart failure whose symptoms are not controlled by digitalis, diuretics, and vasodilators. Exercise capacity in these patients is not only limited by the inability to increase cardiac output, but also by peripheral abnormalities which result in an insufficient oxygen supply to the working muscle. Phosphodiesterase inhibitors are of particular interest as they show both positive inotropic and vasodilator properties. Improvement of cardiac performance, however, enhances exercise capacity only if the abnormalities of muscle blood flow and metabolism in chronic heart failure are reversed. Cardiopulmonary exercise testing allows the determination of the ventilatory anaerobic threshold and thus can provide some information about the peripheral abnormalities in these patients. The aerobic capacity assessed by this technique may be a valuable endpoint demonstrating potential benefits of drug treatment in chronic heart failure.

References

1. Baim DS, McDowell AV, Cheniles J, Monrad ES, Parker JA, Edelson J, Braunwald E, Grossman W (1983) Evaluation od a new bypiridine inotropic agent-milrinone- in patients with severe chronic congestive heart failure. N Engl J Med 309: 748—756
2. Benge W, Litchfield RL, Marcus ML (1980) Exercise capacity in patients with severe left ventricular dysfunction. Circulation 61: 955—959
3. Benotti JR, Grossman W, Braunwald E, Davolos DD, Alousi AA (1978) Hemodynamic assessment of amrinone: a new positive inotropic agent N Engl J med 299: 1373—1377
4. Choong CYP, Roubin GS, Shen WFm Harris PJ, Kelly DT (1985) Effects of nifedipine on systemic and regional oxygen transport and metabolism at rest and during exercise Circulation 71: 787—796
5. Choraria SK, Taylor D, Picher J (1987) Double-blind crossover comparison of enoximone and placebo in patients with congestive heart failure. Circulation 76: 1307—1311
6. Colluci WS, Wright RF, Braunwald E (1986) New positive inotropic agents in the treatment of congestive heart failure N Engl J Med 414: 290—299, 349—358
7. DiBianco R, Shabetai R, Kostuk W, Moran J, Schlant R, Wright R (1989) Oral milrinone and digoxin in patients with chronic heart failure: N Engl J Med 320: 677—673
8. Drexler H, Faude F, Hoing S, Just H (1987) Blood flow distribution within skeletal muscle during exercise in the presence of chronic heart failure: effect of milrinone. Circulation 76: 1344—52
9. Drexler H, Banhardt U, Meinertz T, Wollschläger H, Lehmann M, Just H (1989) Contrasting peripheral short-term and long-term effects of converting enzyme inhibition in patients with congestive heart failure. Circulation 79: 491—502
10. Franciosa JA, Ziesche S, Wilen M (1979) Functional capacity of patients with chronic heart left ventricular failure. Am J Med 67: 460—466
11. Franciosa JA, Park M, Levine B (1981) Lack of relation between exercise capacity and indices of resting left ventricular performance in heart failure. Am J Cardiol 47: 33—39
12. Froelicher VF (1987) Exercise and the heart: Clinical concepts 2nd ed Chicago Year Book Medical Publishers, Inc.
13. Higginbotham MB, Morris RG, Conn EH, Coleman RR, Cobb FR (1985) Determinants of variable exercise performance among patients with severe left ventricular dysfunction Am J Cardiol 51: 52—60
14. Kramer BL, Massie BM, Topic N (1983) Controlled trial of captopril in chronic congestive heart failure. Am J Cardiol 67: 807—816
15. Leier CV, Binkley PF, Starling RC, Randolph PH (1989) Disparity between improvement in left ventricular function and changes in clinical status and exercise capacity during chronic enoximone therapy. Am Heart J 117: 1089—1092
16. Likoff MJ, Weber KT, Janicki JS, Wilson et al. (1985) Milrinone in the treatment of chronic cardiac failure: A controlled trial. Am Heat J 110: 1035—1042
17. Likoff MJ, Chandler SL, Kay HR (1987) Clinical determinants of mortality in chronic congestive heart failure secondary to idiopathic dilated or to ischemic cardiomyopathy. Am J Cardiol 59: 634—638
18. Maskin CS, Forman R, Sonnenblick H, Frishman WH, LeJemtel TH (1983) Failure of dobutamine to increase exercise capacity despite hemodynamic improvement in severe congestive heart failure. Am J Cardiol 51: 177—182

19. Matsumura N, Nishijima H, Kojima S, Hashimoto F, Minami M, Yadsuda H (1983) Determination of anaerobic threshold for assessment of functional state in patients with chronic heart failure. Circulation 68: 360—367
20. Nemanich JW, Shurman AJ, Rossen JD, Kremser C, Davis F, Faifer SI (1987) Effects of longterm therapy with oral piroximone on resting hemodynamics, peak aerobic capacity and the anaerobic threshold in patients with chronic heart failure. J Cardiovasc Pharmacol 10: 580—588
21. Ribeiro JP, White HD, Arnold JMO, Artley LH, Colucci WS (1986) Exercise response before and after longterm treatment with oral milrinone in patients with severe heart failure. Am J Med 81: 759—764
22. Rubin SA, Chatterjee K, Parmley WW (1980) Metabolic assessment of exercise in chronic heart failure patients treated with short-term vasodilators. Circulation 61: 543—548
23. Scriven AJI, Lipkin DP, Sutton GC, Poole-Wilson PA (1988) Double-blind randomized cross over comparison of oral captopril and enoximone added to diuretic treatment in patients with severe chronic heart failure. J Cardiovasc Pharmacol 11: 45—50
24. Sullivan MJ, Knight JD, Higginbothan MB, Cobb FR (1989) Relation between central and peripheral hemodynamics during exercise in patients with chronic heart failure. Circulation 80: 769—781
25. Szlachic J, Massie BM, Kramer BL, Topic N, Tubau J (1985) Correlates and prognostic implication of exercise capacity in congestive heart failure Am J Cardiol 55: 1037—1042
26. Treese N, Erbel R, Rhein S, Henrichs KJ, Meyer J (1989) Additive effects of enoximone and nitroprusside in unstable chronic heart failure. Eur Heart J 10: 484—492
27. Treese N, Erbel R, Rhein S, Coutinho M, Meyer J (1990) Aerobic capacity in chronic heart failure: a randomized long-term comparison of captopril and enoximone J Am Col Cardiol 15 (2): 150A
28. Uretsky BF, Generalovich T, Reddy PS, Spangenberg RB, Follansbee WP (1983) The acute hemodynamic effects of a new agent, MDL 17.043 in the treatment of congestive heart failure. Circulation 62: 823—828
29. Wasser am K, Hansen JE, Sue DY, et al. (1987) Principles of exercise testing and interpretation. Philadelphia, Lea & Febinger
30. Weber KT, Andrews V, Janicki JS, Wison JR, Fishman AP (1981) Amrinone and exercise performance in patients with chronic heart failure. Am J Cardiol 48: 164—169
31. Weber KT, Andrews V, Janicki JS, Likoff M, Reicheck N (1982) Pirbuterol an oral beta adrenergic receptor agonist, in the treatment of chronic heart failure. Circulation 66: 1262
32. Weber KT, Janicki JS (1985) Cardiopulmonary exercise testing for evaluation of chronic cardiac failure. Am J Cardiol 55 (SupplA): 22A—31A
33. Weber KT, Janicki JS, Jain MC (1986) Enoximone (MDL 17.043) for stable chronic heart failure secondary to ischemic or idiopathic cardiomyopathy. Am J Cardiol 58: 589—595
34. Weber KZ, Janicki JS (1986) Cardiopulmonary exercise testing. Philadelphia, WB Saunders Co.
35. Weber KT, Janicki JS, Jain MC (1987) Piroximone (MDL 19.205) in the treatment of unstable and stable chronic heart failure. Am Heart J 114: 805—813
36. Wilson JR, Martin JL, Ferraro N, Weber KT (1983) Effect of hydralazine on perfusion and metabolism in the leg during upright bicycle exercise in patients with heart failure. Circulation 68: 425—432
37. Wilson JR, Martin JL, Schwartz D, Ferraro N (1984) Exercise intolerance in patients with chronic heart failure: role of impaired nutritive flow to skeletal muscle. Circulation 69: 1079—1087
38. Zelis R, Longhurst J, Capone RJ, Mason DT (1974) Comparison of regional blood flow and oxygen utilization during dynamic exercise in normal subjects and patients with congestive heart failure. Circulation 50: 137—143

Author's address:
Prof. Dr. Norbert Treese
II. Medizinische Klinik
Langenbeckstr. 1
D-6500 Mainz

Effect of a Single Oral Dose of the PDE Inhibitor Milrinone on Exercise Tolerance of Chronic Heart Failure Patients — CPX in Advanced Heart Failure

G. Mager, R. K. Klocke, U. J. Winter, A. Gitt, G. Rommert, H. W. Höpp, H. H. Hilger

Third Clinic for Internal Medicine of the University of Cologne, FRG

Introduction

In addition to improvement of the very serious mortality prognosis of patients with severe heart failure in New York Heart Association (NYHA) classes III and IV, a priority goal of therapy is to raise the exercise tolerance increasingly restricted by progressive heart failure, as well as to relieve the agonizing dyspnea in the daily life of these patients. Every treatment concept for long-term therapy of chronic heart failure must consider these two important parameters. Nitrates and diuretics offer immediate relief of the clinical symptoms of patients with severe heart failure. The beneficial influence of ACE inhibitors on the mortality prognosis and clinical symptoms in 60—80% of patients has now been established [1—3]. Yet the prognosis remains very serious once the clinical condition of patients has reached NYHA classes III and IV [4, 5]. Even an optimal therapeutic concept including digitalis, diuretics, nitrates, and ACE inhibitors can often hardly improve the significantly reduced exercise tolerance, nor can it measurably relieve the dyspnea of these patients in the advanced stage of their chronic heart failure.

The new orally administered PDE inhibitors enoximone and milrinone, with their pronounced positive inotropic and vasodilating effects, should be tested for their suitability as a supplement to the proven pharmaceutic agents in the oral long-term therapy of chronic heart failure; in particular, this should consider the two mentioned parameters, namely the influence on mortality prognosis and the improvement of exercise tolerance and, thereby, the quality of life in general.

The investigation presented here is meant to demonstrate the effect of a single oral dose of the PDE inhibitor milrinone on the exercise tolerance of advanced heart failure patients receiving long-term oral therapy with milrinone. This should produce evidence of any possible development of drug tolerance from long-term oral therapy with phosphodiesterase inhibitors.

Patients and methods

The study examined 15 chronic heart failure patients in NYHA class II (six patients) and III (nine patients) in whom the origin of the heart failure was either coronary heart disease (n = 7) or dilative cardiomyopathy (n = 8). Of the nine patients in NYHA class III, eight were designated as Weber class E. At the time of the examination all patients had received long-term oral therapy with 4 × 10 mg milrinone daily as a supplement to digitalis, diuretics, and ACE inhibitors. Excluded from the

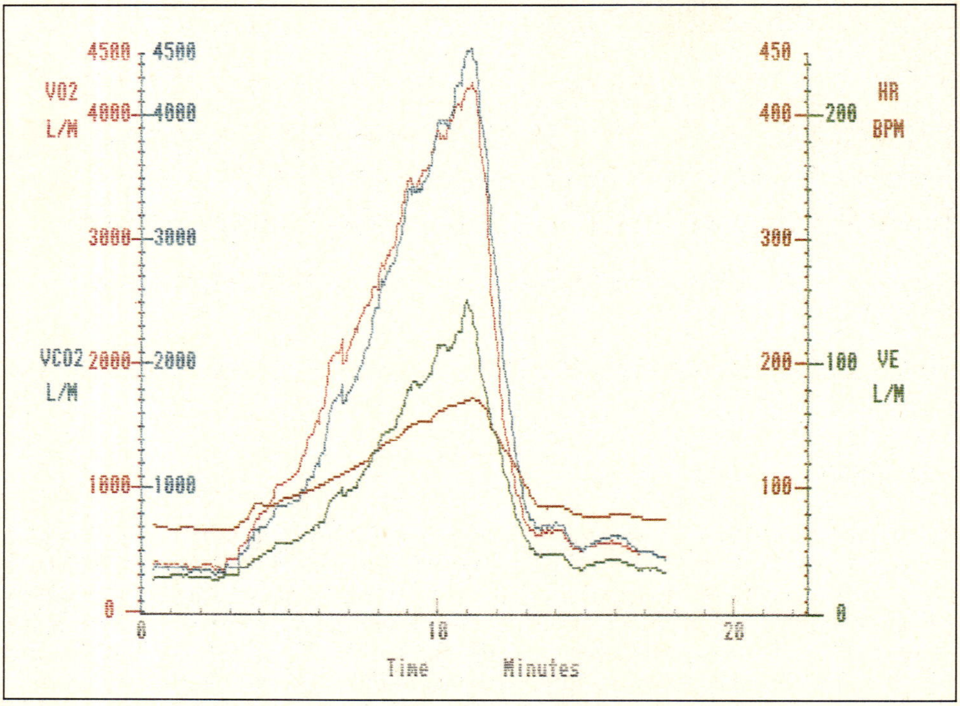

Fig. 1. O_2-uptake ($\dot{V}O_2$), CO_2-output ($\dot{V}CO_2$), respiratory minute volume ($\dot{V}E$), and heart rate (HR) of a trained subject during physical stress.

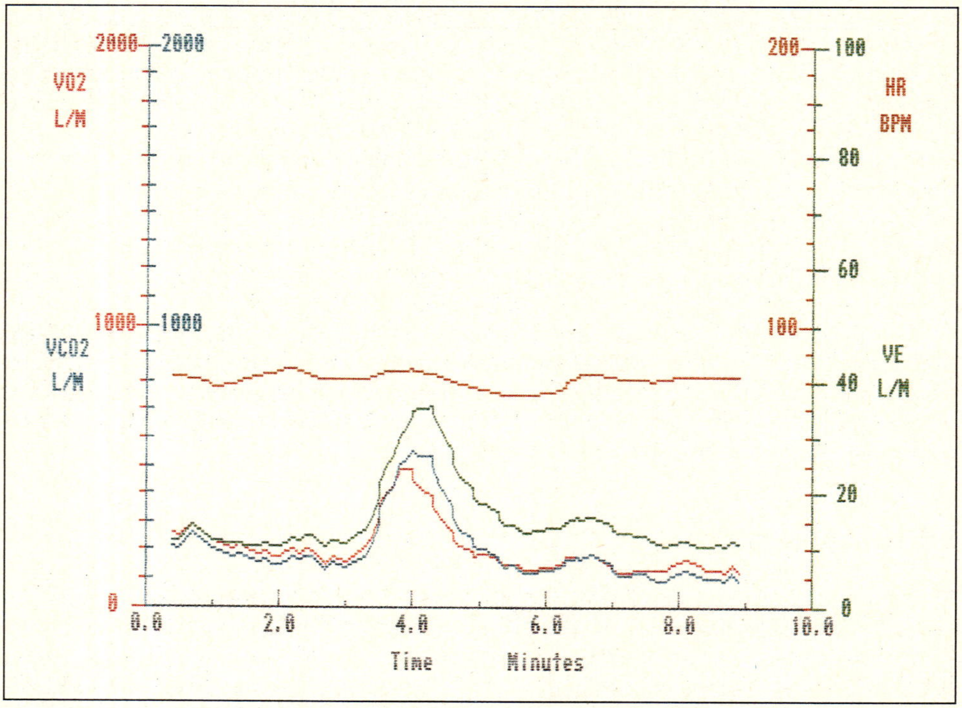

Fig. 2. O_2-uptake, CO_2-output, respiratory minute volume, and heart rate of a patient with severe heart failure under physical stress.

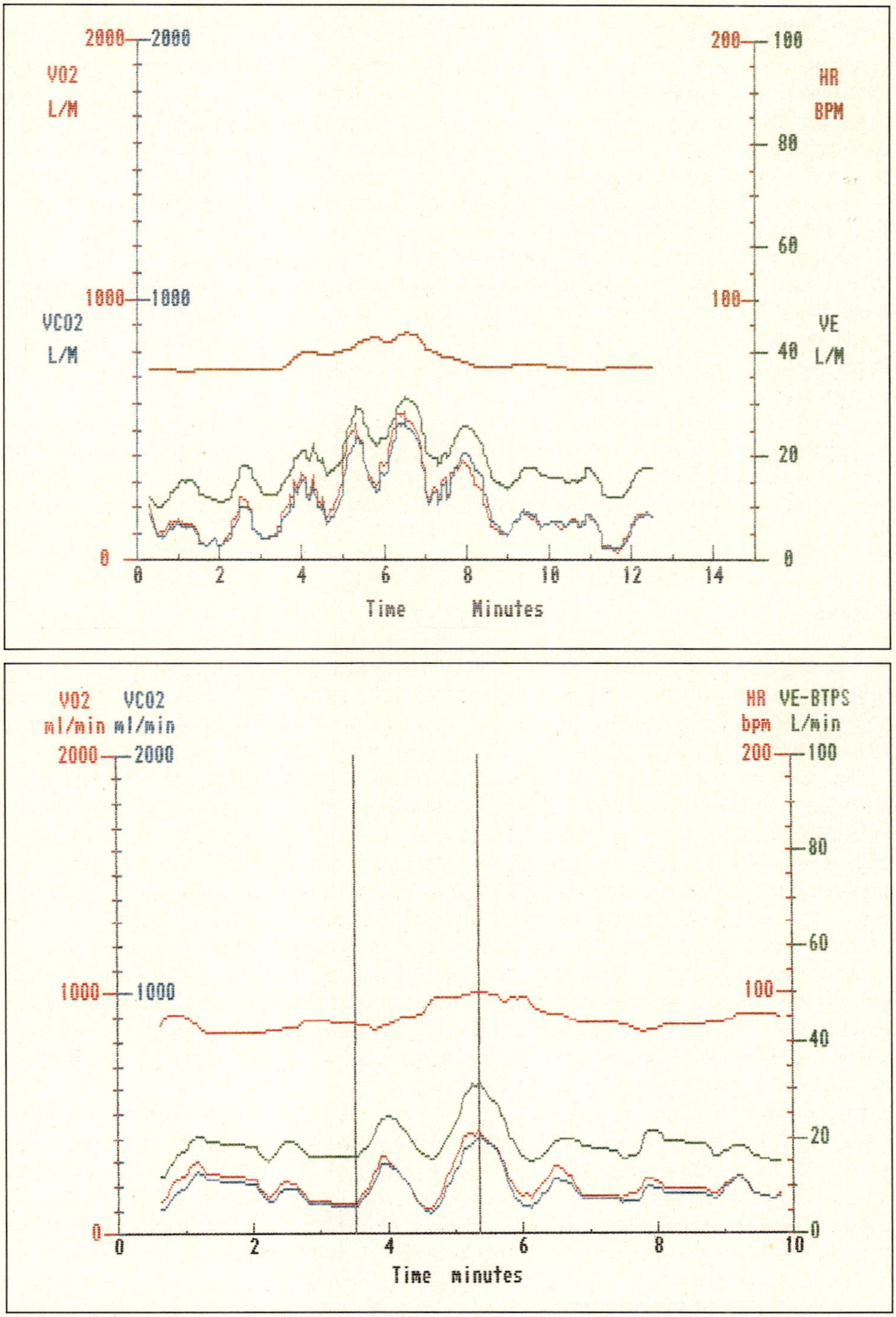

Figs. 3a, b. Cyclic fluctuations of respiratory function in patients with advanced heart failure under physical stress.

study were patients with primary lung disease and clinically pronounced right-ventricular failure, which could possibly interfere with absorption of the drug. The last meal was least 2 h before the beginning of the investigation. Before oral milrinone therapy, i.e. at least 6 months previously, all 15 patients were classified as NYHA class IV with an average cardiac index of 1.60 $l/min/m^2$ (thermodilution method).

The study design included simple blind and intraindividual placebo control. Physical stress was applied by means of computer-controlled bicycle spiroergometry (CPX), beginning at 0 watts (W) with infinitely variable continuous increase of 15 W per minute with the patient in a semisupine position. The last oral milrinone dose was administered the evening before the day of the study. On the day of the study no ACE inhibitors or delayed action nitrates were taken until the end of the investigation; diuretics and digitalis were not allowed later than 4 h prior to the beginning of the investigation.

After baseline ergometry, a 10-mg milrinone tablet was administered and spiroergometry was repeated after 90 min. One week later two exercise tolerance tests were conducted under the same conditions, the second ergometry being carried out after intake of the control medication. Statistics were determined with the paired t-test.

Results

For better comparison with the results of the heart-failure patients, Fig. 1 shows original tracings of the CPX curves for O_2-uptake ($\dot{V}O_2$), CO_2-output ($\dot{V}CO_2$), and heart rate (HR) of a healthy athlete; he reaches and O_2-uptake of 4200 ml/min at a stress of 350 watts, with his heart rate rising from 72 bpm to 178 bpm.

Figure 2 shows the respective parameters of a heart failure patient in NYHA stage III, Weber class C, under stress, before ingestion of a milrinone tablet. The O_2 uptake at the anaerobic threshold after a 7-min stress up to 105 watts was 850 ml/min, only 21% that of the healthy subject. Heart rate rose from 82 to 87/min. 90 min after intake of 10 mg milrinone this patient showed on O_2-uptake increase to 1450 ml/min at the anaerobic threshold after an 8-min stress to 120 watts; this is a 42% increase in O_2-uptake compared to the control investigation without milrinone.

Figure 3a shows an interesting wave-like course of the respiratory function of a patient with very severe heart failure whose exercise tolerance threshold was already reached at 35 W. A similar pattern is seen in Fig. 3b; this patient could only tolerate a stress of 25 W. Both of these patients with an accelerated resting heart rate showed no noticeable heart-rate increase under exercise.

In the patient group as a whole, Fig. 4 shows the development of average O_2-uptake at the anaerobic threshold; there was no significant change after placebo, but a definite increase of O_2-uptake from an average of 6.8 to 9.8 ml O_2/kg/min was observed after milrinone. This represents an average increase of 44% in cardiopulmonary performance after a single oral dose of milrinone, despite previous long-term continuous administration of the drug for at least 6 months.

The respiratory minute volume ($\dot{V}E$) also rose from 32 to 38 l/min after milrinone in comparison to the placebo test (Fig. 5). Heart rate rose after ingestion of a milrinone tablet from an average of 116 to 125 bpm under maximal stress (Fig. 6). The maximal tolerated stress rose likewise from an average of 60 to 75 W (Fig. 7). Res-

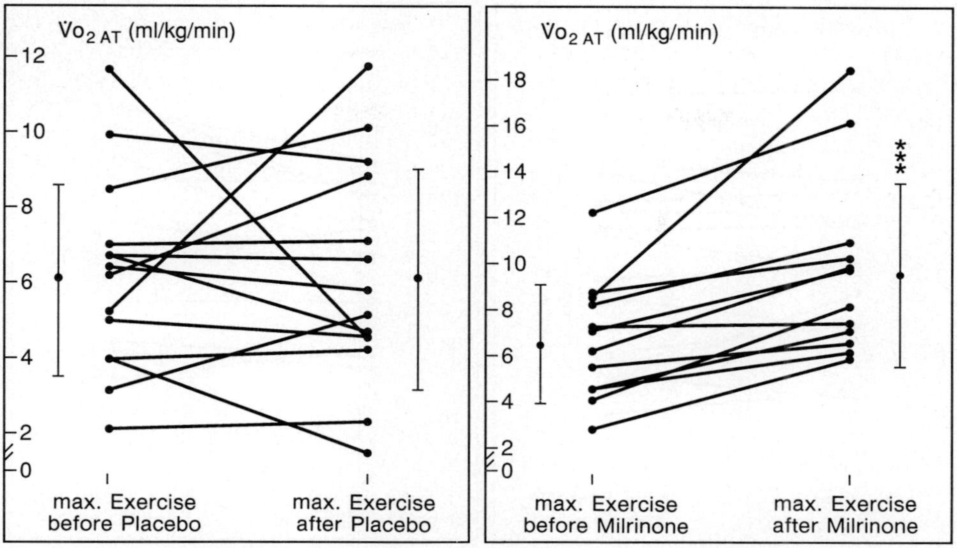

Fig. 4. Average O_2-uptake under physical stress at the anaerobic threshold ($\dot{V}O_2$-AT) after placebo and milrinone (n = 15).

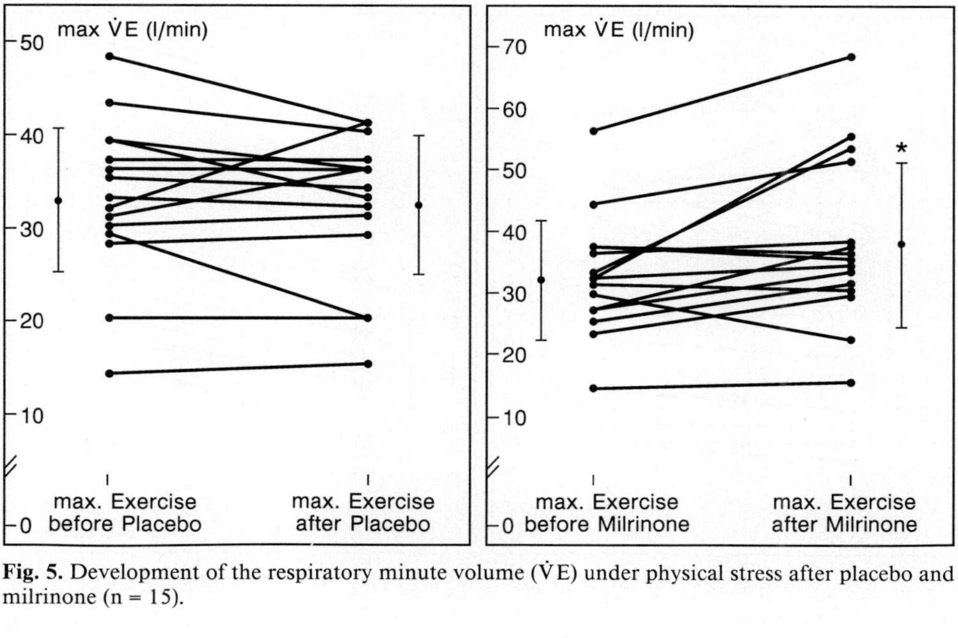

Fig. 5. Development of the respiratory minute volume ($\dot{V}E$) under physical stress after placebo and milrinone (n = 15).

piratory rate and average arterial blood pressure did not show any significant change under the influence of milrinone.

The reproducibility of investigation results expected from application of the CPX method to heart failure patients can be observed in Fig. 7. Three examinations carried out at different times on two different days with the same patients under

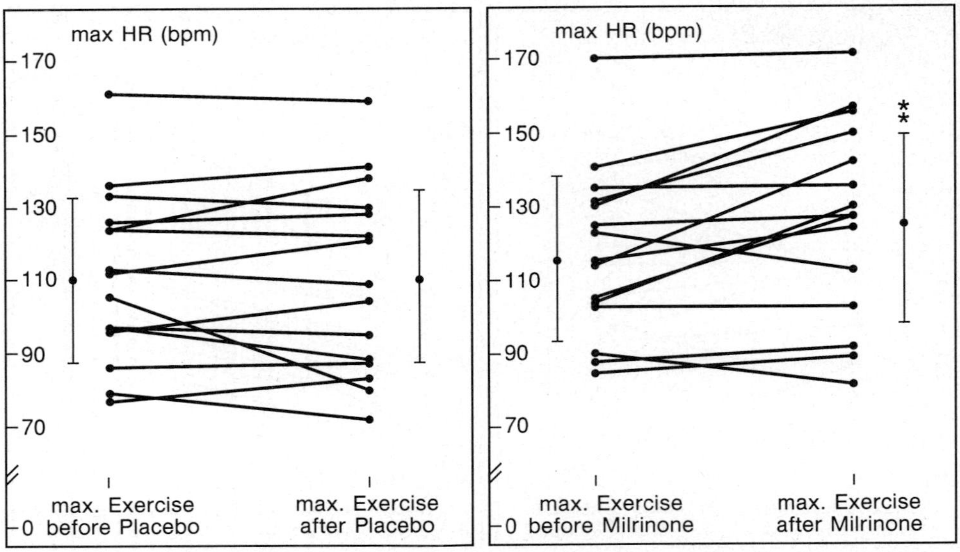

Fig. 6. Development of maximal heart rate (HR) under physical stress after placebo and milrinone (n = 15).

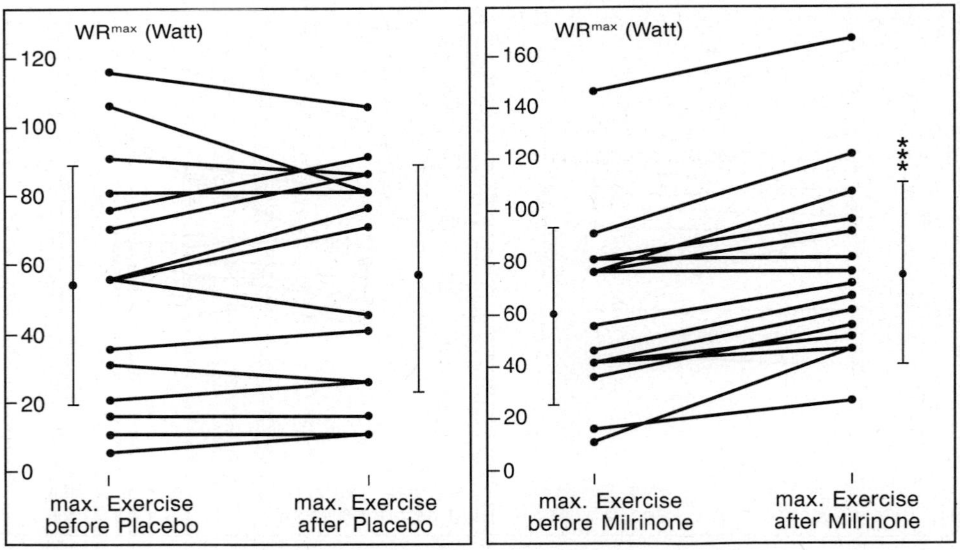

Fig. 7. Development of maximal tolerated stress max after placebo and milrinone (n = 15).

the same conditions (namely, before and after placebo, and before milrinone) gave the same results. Only the stress after milrinone showed a significant rise in the maximal tolerated stress, similar to the behavior of the O_2-uptake (Fig. 4).

Discussion

Notwithstanding the often debated influence of long-term oral therapy of heart failure patients with PDE inhibitors upon mortality prognosis, the results presented here show that oral administration of a single dose of milrinone leads to an increase in exercise tolerance, even after 6-month continuous therapy with intake of four doses per day. In this respect there was no evidence of tolerance development.

The improvement in exercise tolerance measured here, even during uninterrupted continuous therapy supports the effects of a single dose observed by other investigators [6, 7, 8] upon cardiac index (+ 51%), pulmonary capillary wedge pressure (— 48%), and systemic vascular resistance (— 40%), for which invasive measurement methods were employed.

In severe heart failure patients with an average O_2-uptake at anaerobic threshold ($\dot{V}O_2$-AT) of 6.8 ml/kg/min (normal value: > 14 ml/kg/min), the CPX method proved to be a dependable, non-invasive, and thus minimally stressful examination method for seriously ill patients, with reproducible results for the evaluation of exercise tolerance particularly for testing the influence of medications.

The wave-pattern of the respiratory function curves for the two patients with highly restricted cardiac pump function should possibly be differentiated from the oscillations described by other investigators [9]; this may be related to the Cheyne-Stokes-breathing pattern of periodically increased and decreased depth of respiration known to us in severe heart failure patients. However, further investigation is needed for clarification of these relationships.

It is noteworthy that some patients with highly restricted cardiac pumping function subjectively tolerated a stress considerably above the anaerobic threshold without an intensified feeling of exhaustion; in contrast, other patients, already physically exhausted shortly before reaching the anaerobic threshold, broke off the stress due to leg fatique in particular. These observations can only be properly interpreted after investigation of larger patient groups.

Even under continuing long-term therapy with the PDE inhibitor milrinone, administration of a single dose leads to an increase in exercise tolerance and thus to an improvement in the quality of life of patients with advanced heart failure. Possible impacts upon the mortality prognosis remain to be demonstrated.

Computer-controlled spiroergometry (CPX) is a non-invasive and minimally stressful method for the study of exercise tolerance, even in patients with highly restricted cardiac pumping function and it delivers reproducible results.

Summary

Fifteen patients with advanced heart failure (six New York Heart Association (NYHA) II; nine NYHA III, of whom eight were Weber class E) were examined by means of bicycle spiroergometry (CPX) to evaluate the influence of a single dose of milrinone on exercise tolerance. Parameters investigated were O_2-uptake ($\dot{V}O_2$-AT) at the anaerobic threshold (from 6.8 to 9.8 ml O_2/kg/min after milrinone), maximal respiratory minute volume (from 32 to 38 l/min), maximal tolerated stress (from 60 to 75 watts), heart rate under maximal physical stress (from 116 to 120/min), as well as respiratory rate and average arterial blood pressure (no change under the influence of milrinone). The investigation included intraindividual placebo control;

no change in any of the examined parameters was observed after the placebo. Results of the study were reproducible. Thus, even after long-term oral therapy, administration of a single dose of milrinone leads to an increase in exercise tolerance. There were no indications of any development of tolerance to the drug. CPX is a minimally stressful, non-invasive method for examining exercise tolerance in patients with greatly restricted cardiac pumping function, and it delivers reproducible results.

References

1. Consensus Trial Study Group (1987) Effects of Enalapril on Mortality in severe congestive heart failure. New Engl J Med (316) 1429—1435
2. Creager MA, Faxon DP, Halperin JL, Melidossian CD, McCabe CH, Schick EC, Ryan TJ (1982) Determinants of clinical response and survival in patients with congestive heart failure treated with captopril. Am Heart J (104) 1147—1154
3. Creager MA, Massie BM, Faxon DP, Friedmann SD, Kramer BL, Weiner DA, Ryan TJ, Topic N, Melidossian CD (1985) Acute and Long-Term Effects of Enalapril on the Cardiovascular Response to Exercise and Exercise Tolerance in Patients With Congestive Heart Failure. J Am Coll Cardiol (6, No 1) 163—170
4. Wilson JR, Schwartz JS, Sutton M, Ferraro N, Horowitz LN, Reichert N, Josephson ME (1983) Prognosis in Severe Heart Failure. J Am Cardiol (2) 403—410
5. Gorilin R (1983) Incidence, Etiology and Prognosis of Heart Failure Cardiovasc Rev Rep (4) 765—770
6. Costanzo-Nordin MR, O'Connell JB, Engelmeier RS, Moran JF, Scanlon PJ (1985) Dilated Cardiomyopathy: Functional Status, Hemodynamics, Arrhythmias, and Prognosis. Cath Cardiovasc Diagn (11) 445—453
7. Colucci WS, Wright RF, Braunwald (1986) New Positive Inotropic Agents in The Treatment of Congestive Heart Failure. New Engl J med (314, No 6) 349—458
8. Fitzpatrick PG, Cinquegrani MP, Vakiener AR, Baggs JG, Biddle TL, Liang C, Hood WB (1987) Hemodynamic and regional blood flow response to milrinone in patients with severe congestive heart failure: A dose-ranging study. Am Heart J (114) 97—105
9. Packer M (1989) Effect of phosphodiesterase inhibitors on survival of patients with chronic congestive heart failure. Am J Cardiol (63, No 2) 41—45
10. Wood MA, Hess ML (1989) Review: Long term oral therapy of congestive heart failure with phosphodiesterase inhibitors. Am J Med Sci (297, No 2) 105—113
11. Cohen-Solal A for the VO2 French Study Group (1989) Improving exercise tolerance in patients with chronic heart failure: should we treat the heart or the periphery? Eur Heart J (10), 866—871
12. Cody RJ (1988) Do positive Inotropic Agents Adversely Affect the Survival of Patients With Chronic Congestive Heart Failure? J Am Coll Cardiol (12) 559—569
13. Wassermann K (1990) Cardiopulmonary Exercise (CPX) Testing in Heart and Lung Disease. Circulation (81, No 1) II—26

Author's address:

Priv.-Doz. Dr. G. Mager
Klinik III für Innere Medizin der Universität zu Köln
Joseph-Stelzmann-Str. 9
5000 Köln 41, FRG

Spiroergometry in Post Myocardial Infarction Patients with Compromised Left Ventricular Function

F. X. Kleber, L. Niemöller, F. Weißthanner, and W. Doering

Division of Cardiology, Teaching Hospital München-Schwabing, Ludwig-Maximilians-University, Munich, FRG

Introduction

Coronary artery disease is by far the most common cause of congestive heart failure in the industrialized world [1, 2] and bears a major risk for the development of congestive heart failure [11]. Exercise capacity in patients after myocardial infarction is dependent on reduction of left-ventricular function and peripheral, neurohormonal, and cardiac adaptations. Usually, exercise capacity is estimated by applying the NYHA-classification. This classification is rather insensitive for milder degrees of impairment and also for evaluation of therapeutic influences [4]. Other measures of left-ventricular performance in congestive heart failure do not correlate well with exercise capacity [6]. Measurement of exercise duration on the other hand is very much dependent on motivation.

Afterload reducing agents such as ACE-inhibitors can favorably influence left-ventricular remodeling after myocardial infarction [10, 15]; they can also improve exercise capacity [13] and favorably influence survival in congestive heart failure (CHF) [1, 17]. On the other hand, even temporarily increased afterload [12] and training programs in high-risk patients [9] have been shown to promote ventricular dilatation and thus unfavorably influence long-term left ventricular function.

Cardiopulmonary exercise testing has gained widespread acceptance and is a cornerstone in assesing exercise capacity in patients with congestive heart failure [19]. We therefore used cardiopulmonary exercise testing as the major endpoint in a trial evaluating the efficacy of ACE-inhibition in early myocardial infarction over a period of 3 months.

Methods

Forty patients were entered into a pilot trial of ACE-inhibition in myocardial infarction. All patients had survived acute myocardial infarction (proven by electrocardiograms) and typically had increased serum enzymes. Patients older than 75 years, those with pulmonary and/or peripheral vascular disease were excluded. Cardiopulmonary exercise tests were performed 4 and 12 weeks after myocardial infarction. The 12-week-test was done after the test-drug was withheld for 12 to 24 hours.

A medical graphics system for breath-by-breath analysis of O_2-uptake and CO_2-output was used during treadmill exercise tests. Exercise time was recorded as well. Exercise tests were performed using a modified Naughton-protocol with stages of 2 min, starting with a speed of 1.6 km/h and a slope of 0% and reaching a speed of 5.5 km/h and a slope of 14% at 18 min. In this setup with treadmill exercise tests using a modified Naughton-protocol it has been emphasized that the plateau phase of O_2-uptake can be demonstrated by researchers at least in patients with chronic congestive heart failure [19], while many researchers have not been able to demonstrate a plateau phase in the majority of their patients using bicycle ergometry.

Patients performed a symptom-limited maximal exercise test while online O_2-uptake and CO_2-delivery were measured. Maximal O_2-uptake ($\dot{V}O_2$ max) was defined as the highest O_2-uptake reached and the plateau phase was defined as a failure of O_2-uptake to increase over a period of more than 2 min, i.e. failure to increase O_2-uptake in the presence of increased speed or slope. Anaerobic threshold ($\dot{V}O_2$-AT) was defined according to Wasserman [18] as the sudden slope increase of CO_2-delivery or sudden slope increase of ventilation, while a steady increase of $\dot{V}O_2$ is observed. Usually, this was evaluated by plotting $\dot{V}O_2$ on the X-axis and $\dot{V}CO_2$ and $\dot{V}O_2$ on the Y-axis. Thus, the slope deviation of $\dot{V}CO_2$ from the slope of $\dot{V}O_2$ could easily be detected.

Left-ventricular enddiastolic and endsystolic volumes as well as ejection fraction were determined by echocardiography using a single plane method from the four-chamber view at baseline and at 3 months. Echocardiography has been shown to reliably detect left-ventricular volumes compared to cineangiography in our laboratory [11] as well as by other investigators [5, 7]. Enddiastolic and/or endsystolic volume increased over 10% was defined as left-ventricular dilatation. Patients with and without left-ventricular dilatation were compared with respect to exercise capacity.

Another 31 consecutive controls and patients with CHF served to correlate exercise capacity with NYHA-classification, with left-ventricular ejection fraction (n = 24), and to established normal values.

Twenty patients with acute myocardial infarction were treated with captopril (target dose 50 mg b.i.d) from day 2 to 3 months in addition to standard therapy; 20 patients received placebo. Of the 40 patients, comparisons were made between patients with and without left-ventricular dilatation, irrespective of therapy (see above), and between the two groups assigned to treatment with or without ACE-inhibition.

Descriptive statistical analysis was performed using Chi-square test, Fisher's exact-test, or the two-sided t-test. Only data of patients on randomized therapy were used for the comparison of treatment efficacy. A p-value of 0.05 was judged as significant.

Results

Description of patients with acute myocardial infarction and of the 31 controls with or without CHF is given in Tables 1 and 2. In the patients with acute myocardial infarction there were no differences between the captopril- and the placebo-group with respect to age, height, weight, sex, test-drug dose at hospital discharge, serum creatin kinase, and measures of ventricular function at baseline.

In the control patients there was only a modest interrelationship between NYHA functional class and aerobic and maximal exercise capacity as measured by $\dot{V}O_2$ AT

Table 1. Description of controls and patients with CHF of varying degrees according to NYHA-classification.

		n	Age Years (m ± SE)	m/f	DCM/CAD	LV-EF
Healthy controls		5	33 ± 6	5 / 0	0 / 0	—
CHF NYHA	I	7	55 ± 5	7 / 0	1 / 6	46 ± 4
	II	7	50 ± 6	6 / 1	3 / 4	34 ± 5
	III	10	53 ± 3	6 / 4	4 / 6	27 ± 4
	IV	2	28 / 47	1 / 1	1 / 0*	15 / 67*
Total	Σ	31	50 / 3	25 / 6	9 / 16	35 ± 3

* cor pulmonale; DCM = dilative cardiomyopathy; CAD = coronary artery disease; LV-EF left-ventricular ejection fraction; NYHA = New York Heart Association class; CHF = congestive heart failure.

Table 2. Description of patients with myocardial infarction.

	n	Sufficient Echo follow-up (n)	exercise tests 3 months (n)	Age (years) mean ± SE	m/f	EF Baseline mean ± SE	CK-max mean ± SE
Captopril	20	15	12	59 ± 3	17 / 3	46 / 3	1021 ± 114
Placebo	20	13	14	55 ± 2	16 / 4	43 ± 4	1073 ± 107
Σ	40	28	26	57 ± 2	33 ± 7	44 ± 2	1047 ± 111

CK = creatine kinase
EF = ejection fraction (echo)

Table 3. Anaerobic threshold and maximal oxygen uptake in normal controls and patients with congestive heart failure NYHA I, II, III, and IV.

	$\dot{V}O_2AT$ ml/min/kg	$\dot{V}O_2$ max ml/min/kg	Age years
Healthy controls	17—30	34—54	17—52
NYHA I	13.1—24.1	19.7—44.7	38—75
NYHA II	11.9—19.3	17.7—24.9	28—65
NYHA III	8.0—15.6	13.8—16.6	41—70
NYHA IV	5.3— 6.5	8.2— 8.4	28—47

NYHA = New York Heart Association classification.

or $\dot{V}O_2$ max. As is shown in Table 3, normal controls have a maximal oxygen uptake over 30 ml/kg/min. In contrast, oxygen uptake was usually diminished in patients with heart failure of any etiology in NYHA Classes I—IV.

However, there was a considerable overlap in oxygen uptake between the NYHA functional groups, suggesting that the NYHA classes cannot easily be translated into oxygen uptake data.

The correlation between exercise capacity and ejection fraction was weak as well, as demonstrated in Fig. 1.

Exercise time in the patients after acute myocardial infarction was in the range that is considered to be "normal" in congestive heart failure trials. Nevertheless, oxygen uptake showed a slight to moderate impairment of functional capacity, as compared to normal controls (Table 3).

Furthermore, the patients with ventricular dilatation (11 of 28 patients with echo-studies of sufficient quality), although most of them were not in clinical overt heart failure, had a significantly smaller oxygen uptake than patients without ventricular dilatation (see Fig. 2).

Effects of Captopril

In the patients after acute myocardial infarction a 3-months' therapeutic effect of ACE-inhibition on ventricular remodeling and exercise performance was tested in comparison to placebo.

Patients on captopril had a higher anaerobic threshold and maximal oxygen uptake in comparison to patients on placebo, which, however, was not significant in

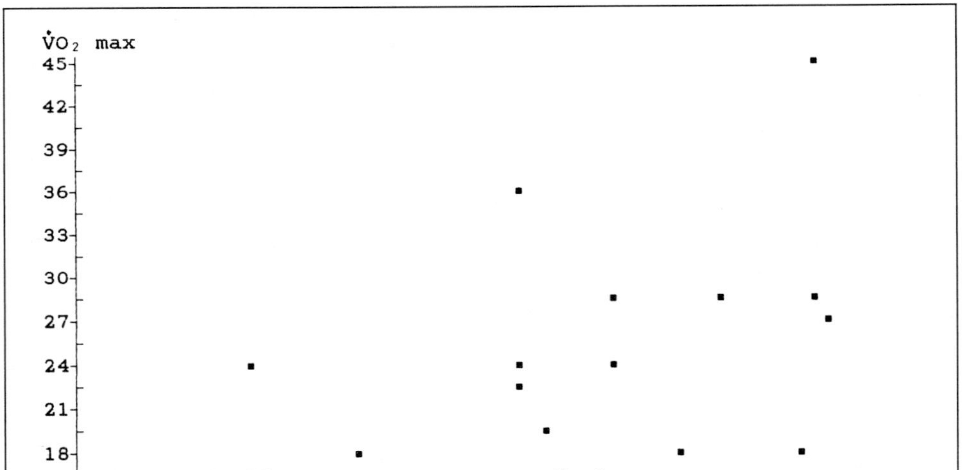

Fig. 1. Correlation between maximal oxygen uptake and left-ventricular function. EF = 14.56 ± 0.91 $\dot{V}O_2$ max. Regression coefficient r = 0.49.

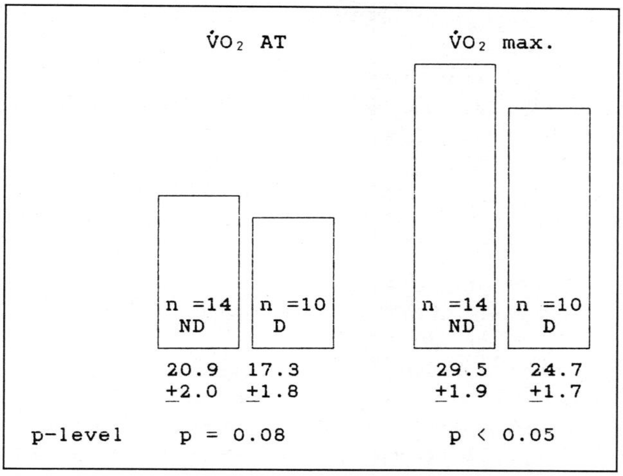

Fig. 2. Anaerobic threshold and maximal oxygen uptake in patients with and without progressive left-ventricular dilatation.

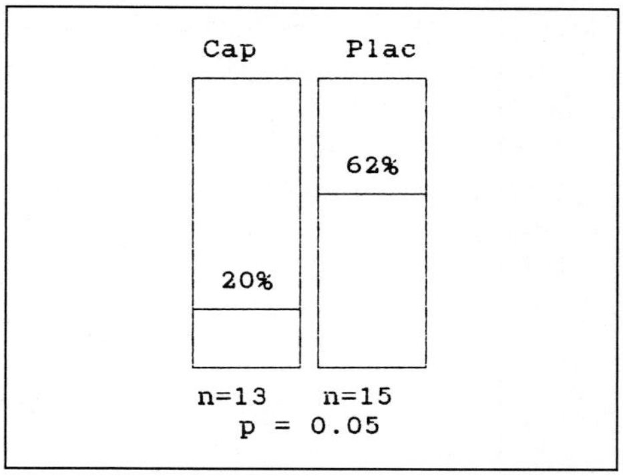

Fig. 3. Percentage of patients with progressive ventricular dilatation 3 months after acute myocardial infarction in patients treated with captopril vs. patients treated with placebo in addition to standard therapy.

Table 4. Anaerobic threshold and maximal oxygen uptake and exercise capacity in patients 4 and 12 weeks after myocardial infarction.

	4 weeks	3 months
		$\dot{V}O_2$ max ml/min/kg
Captopril	17.0 ± 1.8	19.6 ± 2.6
Placebo	14.9 ± 1.1	18.6 ± 1.1
		$\dot{V}O_2$ max ml/min/kg
Captopril	24.5 ± 2.0	27.9 ± 2.3
Placebo	23.2 ± 2.1	26.5 ± 1.4
		Exercise time s
Captopril	887 ± 60	976 ± 79
Placebo	813 ± 76	911 ± 60

this relatively small sample (see Table 4). The effect on exercise capacity was more pronounced at 4 weeks than at 3 months.

The group of patients on captopril had only insignificantly smaller volumes (Fig. 3) at 3 months. However, marked left-ventricular dilatation occurred significantly less often in patients treated with captopril (see Fig. 3).

Discussion

At hospital discharge after acute myocardial infarction usually only a submaximal exercise test is performed for safety reasons. In this trial we showed that a symptom-limited maximal exercise test can be achieved safely in otherwise stable patients 3 to 4 weeks after acute myocardial infarction. After 12 weeks exercise capacity was moderately improved. As did Weber et al. [19], we were able to demonstrate a plateau of $\dot{V}O_2$ uptake in most instances of congestive heart failure, while we were unable to show this plateau in patients with basically normal O_2-uptake ($\dot{V}O_2$ max. over 30 ml/min/kg).

After acute myocardial infarction our patients had moderately impaired left-ventricular function. Left-ventricular function, however, is not an indicator of impairment of exercise capacity [6]. This lack of correlation is explained by the interactions of peripheral adaptations and central hemodynamics in congestive heart failure [3]. Most investigators therefore rely on exercise time as major endpoint in congestive heart failure trials. The exercise time in our set-up correlates nicely with maximal O_2-uptake, however, an exercise time with online measurements of gas exchange analysis might not be the equivalent to that achieved without cardiopulmonary testing. Therefore, the exercise time is not a good predictor of maximal $\dot{V}O_2$-uptake. Anaerobic threshold was found to be equally sensitive for impairment of exercise capacity.

Cardiopulmonary exercise testing was helpful in distinguishing patients with CHF from normal controls. Most patients, even with NYHA functional class I, had a compromised exercise capacity as measured by maximal oxygen uptake. There was some overlap between the groups according to NYHA-classification, as has been shown by others as well. This is largely due to the subjective judgement in assigning patients to the NYHA functional classes. This scale is mainly based on the compromise of the individuel lifestyle, i.e. patients with a sedentary life style tend to be assigned to a better functional class, since they are asymptomatic in their daily activities during a long period in the course of their disease. On the contrary, patients who are used to an active lifestyle will recognize a compromise in their daily activity long before they have a severely compromised exercise capacity. The measurement of anaerobic and maximal oxygen uptake will therefore give a more objective view of their exercise capacity.

This report focuses on our experiences with cardiopulmonary exercise testing in the evaluation of patients with congestive heart failure and within the first 3 months after myocardial infarction, i.e. the most common etiology of congestive heart failure.

Acute myocardial infarction is the leading underlying cardiac disease for development of congestive heart failure. During pharmacologic intervention or training programs in the time-course of healing after myocardial infarction, i.e. in the first 3 months after myocardial infarction, patients' exercise performance should be monitored carefully. While some groups show improvement in exercise capacity after training programs [14, 16], others have shown worsening of symptomatology and left-ventricular dilatation [8, 9], while therapy with ACE-inhibitors has been shown to blunt progressive ventricular dilatation [15] and increase exercise capacity [13] after 1 year of treatment.

One of the major pathophysiologic mechanisms leading to progression of CHF is left-ventricular dilatation [11, 13]. However, it is very difficult to clinically separate patients with this condition based on history and compromise in daily activities. Usually, these patients are judged to have either "no heart failure" or are assigned to NYHA functional class I. As is demonstrated in this study, patients with NYHA functional class I usually have a compromised oxygen uptake. Furthermore, even patients with left-ventricular dilatation in the very early stages of development of congestive heart failure after myocardial infarction have a compromised oxygen uptake. Therefore, measurement of oxygen uptake in patients either with very mild congestive heart failure or in the developmental stage from left-ventricular dysfunction to congestive heart failure is helpful in depicting patients with already compromised exercise capacity, who can be assumed to be at higher risk for progressive deterioration of pump dysfunction.

The effects of captopril in the group with myocardial infarction

Overall, there was only a tendency towards smaller left-ventricular volumes and better exercise capacity in this group of patients. However, marked left-ventricular dilatation occurred significantly less often in patients on captopril than in patients on placebo (Fig. 3, $p = 0.05$). Furthermore, exercise capacity showed a good correlation with a measure of progressive ventricular dysfunction: the ventricular volumes. Ventricular volume enlargement has been shown to be a good predictor of evolving CHF [11] and of prognosis [20]. Therefore, avoiding ventricular dilatation after myocardial infarction results in better functional capacity and can be expected to improve prognosis.

Conclusions

Cardiopulmonary exercise testing in post myocardial infarction patients with determination of maximal oxygen consumption is usually possible without complications. It shows compromised functional capacity even in patients with normal exercise time and in patients with NYHA functional class I. It is safe and provides information for interventional studies. Even in patients after only moderate degree myocardial infarctions without major compromise of left-ventricular function, impairment of exercise capacity is possible. ACE-inhibitors administered early after myocardial infarction positively influence left-ventricular remodeling by lessening the increase in systolic and diastolic volumes. The increase in volumes is associated with impairment of exercise capacity, as shown in this study. ACE-inhibitors have significant effects on remodeling while effects on exercise capacity failed conventional statistical levels in this small subset of patients. Since left-ventricular dilatation has been shown to carry substantial prognostic risks, an impaired exercise capacity after acute myocardial infarction may thus be associated with a poor prognosis as well.

Summary: Cardiopulmonary exercise tests were performed in 71 patients. Thirty-one patients were evaluated to establish normal values and to correlate oxygen consumption with New York Heart Association (NYHA) classification. NYHA classification correlated only weakly with oxygen uptake.

Forty patients were treated in a double-blind randomized trial evaluating the efficacy of captopril on exercise performance in myocardial infarction patients. Captopril was administered within 2—3 days after acute myocardial infarction. Captopril blunted left-ventricular (LV)-volume increase, which was associated with impaired exercise tolerance.

We conclude that ACE-inhibition administered early after myocardial infarction might have favorable effects and large-scale trials with this therapeutic regimen are encouraged.

References

1. Cannon PF, et al (1983) A placebo-controlled trial of captopril in refractory chronic congestive heart failure. J Am Coll Cardiol 2: 755—763
2. Cohn JN, Archibald DG, Ziesche S, Franciosa JA, Harston WE, Tristani FE, Dunkman WB, Jacobs W, Francis GS, Flohr KH, Goldman S, Cobb FR, Shah PM, Saunders R, Fletcher RD, Loeb HS, Hughes VD, Baker B (1988) Effects of Vasodilator therapy on mortality in chronic congestive heart failure. Results of a Veterans Administration Cooperative Study. N Engl J Med 314: 1547—1552
3. Drexler H, Banhardt U, Meinertz T, Wollschläger H, Lehmann M, Just HJ (1989) Contrasting peripheral short-term and long-term effects of converting-enzyme inhibition in patients with congestive heart failure. Circulation 79: 491—502
4. Dunselmann PH, Kuntze EE, Bruggen A, Beekhuis H, Piers B, Scaf AH, Wesseling H, Lie KI (1988) Value of New York Heart Association Classification, radionuclid-ventriculography, and cardiopulmonary exercise tests for selection of patients for congestive heart failure studies. Am Heart J 116: 1475—1482
5. Erbel R, Schweizer P, Lambertz H, Henn G, Meyer J, Krebs W, Effert R (1983) Echoventriculography — A Simultaneous Analysis of Two-dimensionel Echocardiography and Cinventriculography. Circulation 67: 205—215
6. Franciosa JA, Park M, Levine TB (1981) Lack of correlation between exercise capacity and indexes of resting left ventricular performance. Am J Cardiol 47: 33—39
7. Gordon EP, Schnittger J, Fitzgerald PJ, Williams P, Popp RL (1983) Reproducibility of Left Ventricular Volumes by Two-Dimensional Echocardiography. J Am Coll Card 2: 506—513
8. Iskandrian ASJ (1988) Exercise Training after Anterior Q-Wave Myocardial Infarction, Harmful or Beneficial? J Am Coll Cardiol 12: 373—374
9. Jugdutt BI, Michorowski BL, Kappagoda CT (1988) Exercise Training After Anterior Q Wave Myocardial Infarction: Importance of Regional Left Ventricular Function and Topography. J Am Coll Cardiol 12: 362—372
10. Jugdutt BI (1988) Improved left ventricular geometry and function during healing after anterior and inferior myocardial infarction in the dog. Circulation 78 (suppl II): 643
11. Kleber FX, Einwang HP, Kronski D, Ohly A, Osterkorn K, Doering WJ (1990) Progrediente linksventrikuläre Dilatation nach Vorderwandinfarkt als Determinante für die Entwicklung einer Herzinsuffizienz. Z Kardiol 79: 1—7
12. Nolan SE, Mannisi JA, Bush DE, Healy N, Weisman HF (1988) Increased afterload aggravates infarct expansion after acute myocardial infarction. J Am Coll Cardiol 12: 1318—1325

13. Pfeffer MA, Lamas GA, Vaughan DE, Parisi AF, Braunwald E (1988) Effect of captopril on progressive ventricular dilatation after anterior myocardial infarction. N Engl J Med 319: 8—86
14. Shabetai R (1988) Beneficial effects of exercise training in compensated heart failure. Circulation 78: 775—776
15. Sharpe N, Smith H, Murphy J, Hannan S (1988) Treatment of patients with symptomless left ventricular dysfunction after myocardial infarction. Lancet 1: 255—259
16. Sullivan MJ, Higginbotham MB, Cobb FR (1988) Exercise Training in Patients with Severe Left Ventricular Dysfunction. Hemodynamic and Metabolic Effects. Circulation 78: 506—515
17. The Consensus Trial Study Group (1987) Effects of Enalapril on mortality in severe congestive heart failure. N Engl J Med 316: 1429—1435
18. Wassermann K (1988) New Concepts in assessing cardiovascular function. Circulation 78: 1060—70
19. Weber KT, Kinasewitz GT, Janicki JS, Fishman AP (1982) Oxygen Utilization and Ventilation During Exercise in Patients with Chronic Cardiac Failure. Circulation, 65: 1213—1223
20. White HD, Norris RM, Brown MA, Brandt PWT, Whitlock RML, Wild CJ (1987) Left ventricular end-systolic volume as the major determinant of survival after recovery from myocardial infarction. Circulation 76: 44—51

Author's address:

F. X. Kleber, M.D.,
II. Med. Krankenhaus München-Schwabing
— Kardiologie und Pneumologie —
Akademisches Lehrkrankenhaus
der Ludwig-Maximilians-Universität,
Kölner Platz 1,
8000 München 40

3. Clinical Value in Pacemaker Therapy

Evaluation of Algorithms for Rate Adaptive Pacing by Gas Exchange Measurements

D. J. MacCarter and J. Millerhagen

Telectronics/Köln, FRG

Algorithms or mathematical formulas for the modulation of heart rate in pacemaker patients with chronotropic incompetence, based upon mechanical or biological sensor input, have been in clinical use for the past 10 years. It is well known that the basis for the use of such algorithms is to increase heart rate, the major contributing parameter to an elevation in cardiac output during isotonic exercise [3, 12, 13]. Concomitant with the elevation in cardiac output during exercise, an increase in oxygen uptake occurs, thus resulting in an improved exercise tolerance or functional capacity of the patient.

It is the primary objective of a rate-adaptive algorithm to restore normal chronotropic function or heart-rate reserve in accordance with the patients metabolic demand and functional class. Normal chronotropic function will, in turn, contribute to an improvement in functional capacity or the ability of the pacemaker patient to perform daily activities. Also of importance is that the restoration of the heart rate response to activity be achieved in a physiologic way, i.e. in a way simulating the changes in heart rate observed in subjects with intact intracardiac conduction and normal neural and hormonal regulation during rest, exercise, and recovery. The increase in heart rate during exercise should be relatively linear with increasing work rate or metabolic demand.

For review purposes, one must keep in mind that cardiac output (C.O.) is directly related to oxygen uptake ($\dot{V}O_2$) [1] and can be expressed by the following equation: C.O. = $\dot{V}O_2$/A-VO_2 difference. Cardiac output in L/min is equal to oxygen uptake in ml/min divided by the arterial mixed venous oxygen content difference in volumes percent times 10. According to Fick's theorem above, at maximal exercise when cardiac output and the extraction of oxygen in the peripheral, active muscle tissue is maximal, cardiac output is directly correlated to $\dot{V}O_2$ max [9]. Since cardiac output is linearly related to oxygen uptake, changes in oxygen uptake in response to increasing work rate level is an important parameter to assess, not only in terms of a measurement of functional capacity, but also as a correlate to the more frequently measured variable, cardiac output. The invasive measurement of cardiac output by dye- or thermal-dilution techniques served as one of the most frequently used methods of assessing cardiac output, other than the "gold standard" technique using the direct Fick method with oxygen uptake measurements. Most cardiologists preferred the use of dye- or thermal-dilution techniques. However, due to significantly improved data processing, computer graphics, and rapidly responding analyzers for measuring expired carbon dioxide and oxygen during exercise, the use of noninvasive breath-by-breath oxygen uptake measurements have become increasingly useful to the cardiologist as a clinically diagnostic and prognostic tool [4, 5, 7, 8, 14]. The noninvasive, direct assessment of oxygen uptake has been recognized as the most accurate and acceptable means of evaluating the functional capacity of subjects with cardiovascular or pulmonary disease.

McElroy, Janicki, and Weber have previously described the relationship between heart rate and oxygen uptake, minute ventilation, and mixed venous oxygen saturation [10]. Table 1 shows the relationship between heart rate and oxygen uptake with various patient functional classes, as reported by Weber et al. Note that the lower the functional class, i.e. class A vs. B or C, the greater the linear slope. The average linear regression analysis slope of HR to $\dot{V}O_2$ in normals is approximately 3.0 and increases to a slope of 4.6 in functional class D patients who have a significantly lower peak oxygen uptake or $\dot{V}O_2$ at anaerobic threshold. Focusing upon changes in the minute ventilation ($\dot{V}E$) during exercise, McElroy and colleagues have, in contrast to $\dot{V}O_2$, noted a rather consistent relationship between HR and $\dot{V}E$, i.e. an average linear regression slope of approximately 1.5, which is independent of the subject's functional classification as shown in Table 2.

Additional investigation using breath-by-breath gas exchange and computerized "best fit" regression analysis have disclosed, in many patients, a more logarithmic relationship between HR and VE, as shown in Fig. 3. In subjects who are relatively fit, the HR to $\dot{V}O_2$ relationship is more curvelinear in form, as shown in Fig. 1. However, in some patients with cardiac disease or subjects who are markedly deconditioned, the HR to $\dot{V}O_2$ curve appears to follow a curvelinear slope or derivation from linearity [1] beyond the anaerobic threshold, as shown in Fig. 2. If two linear slopes or tangents to the regression curves in Figs. 1 and 3 are constructed via selective computerized regression analysis, one would observe that the slope from rest or the onset of exercise to the anaerobic threshold (AT) is always greater

Table 1. Heart rate to oxygen uptake slope (beats/ml/kg). Note that as the subject's functional class decreases from normal to class C, the HR to $\dot{V}O_2$ regression analysis slope increases.

	Functional class			
	Normals	A	B	C
HR to $\dot{V}O_2$ slope	2.91 ± 0.51	3.43 ± 0.81	3.67 ± 1.13	4.66 ± 1.35
Sample Size	26	15	16	38

Note: N = 6; 0.9 $<r>$ 0.8 (r = correlation coefficient) (Used with permission from McElroy (10).)

Table 2. Heart rate to minute ventilation slope (beats/liter). In contrast to the HR to $\dot{V}O_2$ linear regression slopes listed in Table 1, the HR to $\dot{V}E$ slope remains relatively independent of the patient's functional class.

	Functional class			
	Normals	A	B	C
HR to $\dot{V}E$ Slope	1.49 ± 0.49	1.55 ± 0.61	1.43 ± 0.69	1.52 ± 0.67
Sample Size	26	15	17	31

Note: N = 8; 0.9 $<r>$ 0.8 (r = correlation coefficient) (9).)

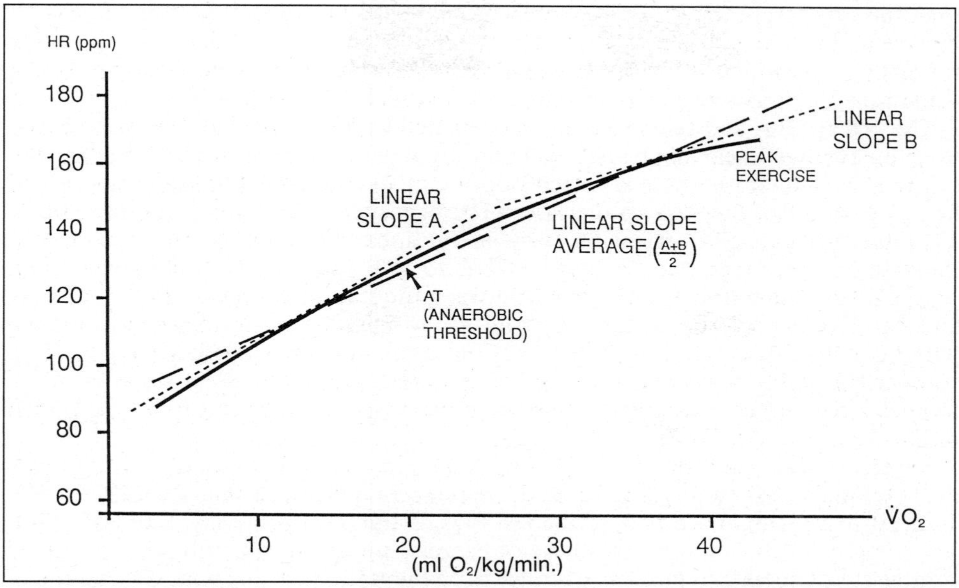

Fig. 1. The heart rate to $\dot{V}O_2$ regression analysis curve (solid line) observed in most normal or fit subjects is curvelinear in nature. Individual linear slopes A and B can be constructed from rest to the AT, and AT to peak exercise, respectively. Note that linear slope A is slightly greater than linear slope B.

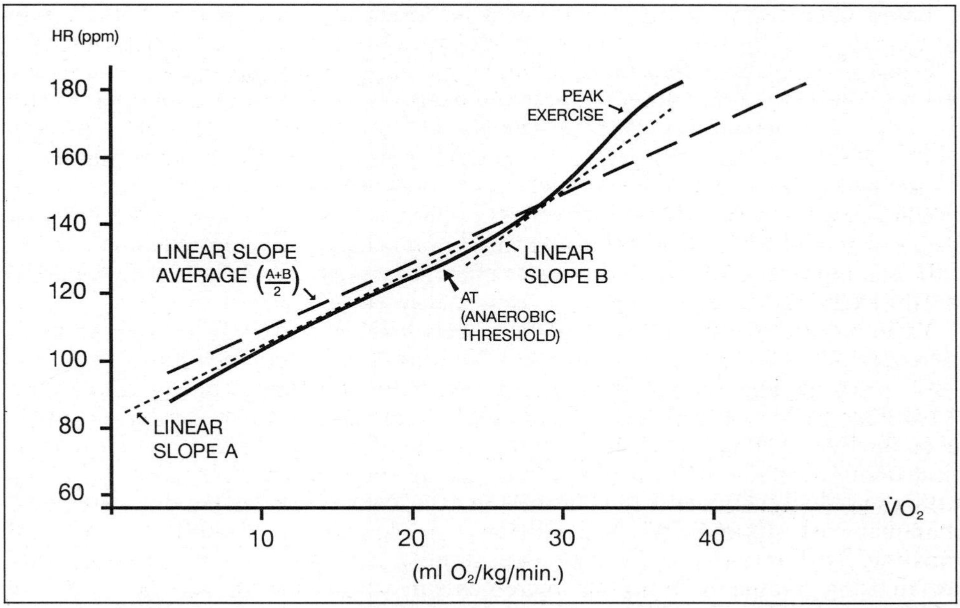

Fig. 2. The heart rate to $\dot{V}O_2$ regression analysis curve is also curvelinear in nature; however, linear slope B can be greater that linear slope A, demonstrating a deviation from linearity near the anaerobic threshold.

than the slope from the anaerobic threshold to peak exercise or $\dot{V}O_2$ max. In Fig. 2, however, linear regression analysis of the second phase of the HR to $\dot{V}O_2$ curve reveals a slope which is greater than the first from rest to AT. This increase in the slope was previously reported by Wasserman et al. [18].

The HR to $\dot{V}O_2$ and HR to $\dot{V}E$ slopes reported by McElroy et al. [10] were based upon an average linear slope analysis throughout exercise from its onset to the peak of exercise. Therefore, these reported slopes may be lower than the slopes observed from the onset of exercise to the AT point, especially when analyzing the HR to $\dot{V}E$ slope, since its true regression curve is not linear, but logarithmic in nature. In the case of linear regression analysis of HR to $\dot{V}O_2$ in normal or fit subjects (Fig. 1), the linear regression analysis slope between the start of exercise and the AT may also be greater than the later slope from AT to peak exercise. However, in some patients with cardiac disease, when $\dot{V}O_2$ increases at a slower rate after the AT in comparison to the observed rate of increase in heart rate, the linear slope from AT to peak exercise becomes greater than the slope observed from rest to AT, as shown in Fig. 2.

Recent studies by Treese et al. [15] with 44 deconditioned patients without cardiopulmonary disease (average age: 53 years), demonstrated that the HR to $\dot{V}O_2$ and HR to $\dot{V}E$ slopes are as described in Figs. 2 and 3, respectively. The HR to $\dot{V}E$ slope is greater during the first phase of exercise up to the anaerobic threshold, as compared to the second phase of exercise from the AT to peak exercise. For example, in 26 men, the first phase of exercise for the HR to VE slope was 2.03 ± 0.89 vs 1.22 ± 0.44 for the second phase of exercise.

The HR to $\dot{V}O_2$ slope, however, showed an increase in the second phase of exercise, as compared to the first phase: for men from 2.6 ± 0.69 to 3.2 ± 0.09 from 3.71 ± 1.27 to 4.34 ± 1.42 for women.

Based upon the previously mentioned information, it seems logical that, with increasing work during exercise, the modulation in heart rate to be achieved by a rate adaptive paceaker algorithm should be accomplished by means which simulate the normal relationship observed between heart rate and various cardiopulmonary parameters, as shown in Figs. 1—3. The HR to $\dot{V}O_2$ and HR to $\dot{V}E$ slopes for both phases of exercise, i.e. from rest to AT, and AT to peak exercise should be simulated by the pacemaker's rate-adaptive algorithm, in accordance with the patients' functional class. Likewise, during the recovery phase following exercise or activity, the decay or rate of decrease of heart rate should represent a slope proportionate to the subjects' physical condition in order to effectively repay the oxygen debt incurred during exercise.

Various exercise tests or protocols have been developed to evaluate the rate-adaptive pacemaker algorithm, such as stair-climbing, steady-state ergometer protocols with relatively large increments in work rate, outdoor walking courses, and Holter recordings during various, logged patient activities: however, few tests have actually been devised to study the entire work-rate range of the patient in a relatively short time period. Wasserman et al. have developed an ergometer ramping protocol which utilizes gradual increments in work rate in accordance with the patient's predicted maximal work rate and physical condition [17]. For example, if a patient's predicted maximal work rate is 150 Watts (W) per minute, a 10-min exercise protocol is selected using gradual or "ramping" increments in a work rate of 15 W per min. The advantage of such a protocol is that the test is subsequently short and the patient does not percieve the smaller work rate increments, as is experienced with other protocols such as the Bruce protocol. In addition, the exercise test spans the entire

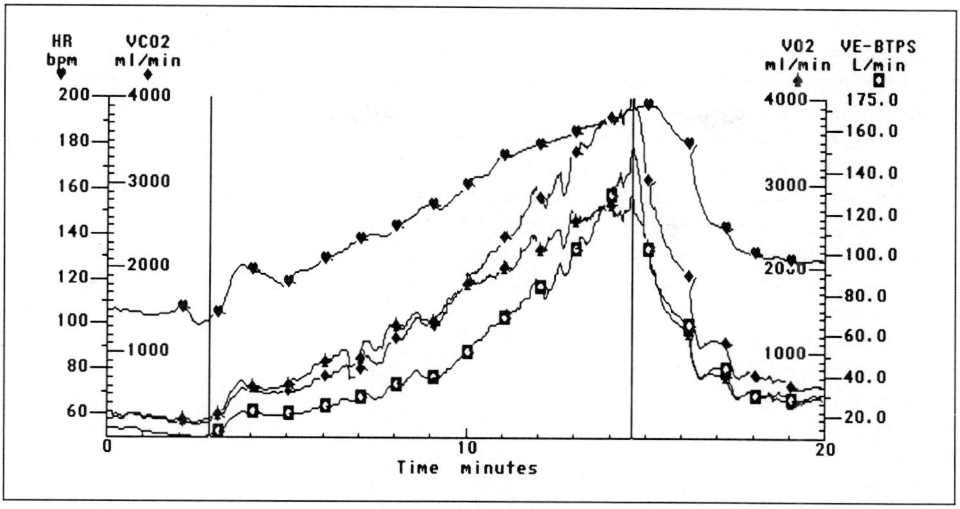

Fig. 3. The graph shows the changes in heart rate, oxygen uptake, carbon dioxide output, and minute ventilation with a linear increase in the work rate (ramp protocol of 25 Watts/minute). Note the initial rise in HR and $\dot{V}O_2$ with the onset of exercise marked by the first vertical line. The HR decreases gradually after the cessation of exercise (second vertical line on the right at about 14.5 min), in order to repay the oxygen debt incurred during exercise.

	AT VO2	P VO2
Time Min	9:34	14:38
VO2	1633	2888
VCO2	1571	4147
R	0.96	1.44
HR	155	196
VE	43	153
Watts	160	281

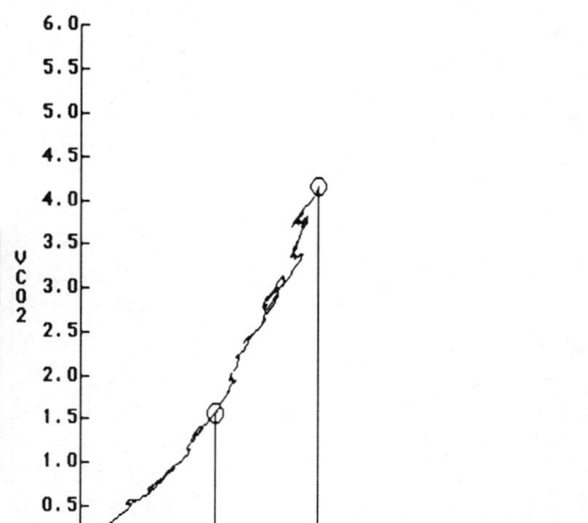

Fig. 4. The graph demonstrates the V-slope technique of determining the anaerobic threshold. Carbon dioxide output is plotted against oxygen uptake on the X-axis. The first vertical line with the small circle at its top end marks the anaerobic threshold, whereby an acceleration in $\dot{V}CO_2$ is observed relative to $\dot{V}O_2$. The corresponding values for other cardiopulmonary parameters are displayed in the table to the left of the graph. The peak exercise point is denoted by P $\dot{V}O_2$.

work-rate range of the patient, so that all intensities of activity can be evaluated. The use of "real time" breath-by-breath gas-exchange measurement obviates the need for steady-state levels of exercise to evaluate submaximal exercise points, such as the anaerobic threshold.

During the exercise protocol, gas-exchange parameters such as oxygen uptake ($\dot{V}O_2$), carbon dioxide output ($\dot{V}CO_2$), end tidal oxygen and carbon dioxide (ET O_2 and ET CO_2, respectively), the respiratory exchange ratio ($\dot{V}CO_2/\dot{V}O_2$) or RER, ventilatory equivalents of O_2 and CO_2 ($\dot{V}E/\dot{V}O_2$ and $\dot{V}E/\dot{V}CO_2$), respiratory rate, and tidal volume are all monitored on a breath-by-breath basis to provide an adequate number of data points for easy assessment of the most clinically relevant information, such as the anaerobic threshold (AT), peak $\dot{V}O_2$ or $\dot{V}O_2$ max, and the HR to $\dot{V}O_2$ or $\dot{V}E$ regression analysis slopes.

By definition, a patient has reached his $\dot{V}O_2$ max during exercise if there is less than 1 ml/min/kg increase in $\dot{V}O_2$, despite an increase in work load [9]. If the subject does not demonstrate a true $\dot{V}O_2$ max, then the greatest $\dot{V}O_2$ point attained is defined as the peak $\dot{V}O_2$. However, since a majority of patients do not demonstrate a $\dot{V}O_2$ max, and a peak $\dot{V}O_2$ is often dependent on the patient's level of motivation or stamina and the physician's subjective judgment of the patient's endperformance, a more submaximal point called the anaerobic threshold can be determined which is more reproducible and independent of patient motivation. Despite discrepancy in the literature concerning the term "anaerobic" for this threshold, one can envision this reference point during submaximal exercise as an operational threshold whereby, beyond this point, the subject cannot comfortably sustain or continue exercise for any great length of time. The anaerobic threshold is defined from a biochemical standpoint as the level of oxygen uptake attained during exercise above which energy production by aerobic means (tricarboxylic acid cycle) is supplemented by anaerobic metabolic pathways, thus creating an increase in lactate production in accordance with the rate of glycolysis [16]. Due to the sustained increase in blood lactate and the lactate/pyruvate ratio above the AT, metabolic acidosis occurs. Lactic acid is buffered by bicarbonate, resulting in an increase in $\dot{V}CO_2$ in addition to the CO_2 produced by aerobic metabolism. This increase in $\dot{V}CO_2$ results in an acceleration in $\dot{V}CO_2$ relative to $\dot{V}O_2$. Minute ventilation accelerates in parallel with $\dot{V}CO_2$ above the AT, causing an increase in the ventilatory equivalent of O_2 and ET O_2, but relatively no change in the ventilatory equivalents of CO_2 or the ET CO_2. This phase, termed the isocapnic buffering phase, represents an initial hyperventilation with respect to oxygen, not CO_2, and normally lasts several minutes.

The gas-exchange method to measure the anaerobic threshold is based upon the V-slope method, as described by Beaver et al. [2]. The technique determines the onset of the anaerobic threshold at stage I or the cellular level of respiration, and is independent of the sensitivity of the respiratory chemoreceptors. Stage-II criteria for assessing the anaerobic threshold are based upon changes in the ventilatory equivalents of O_2 and CO_2, ET O_2 and ET CO_2 and the RER value; however, these changes may serve more reliably as supportive criteria for confirming the V-slope method. The most recent computerized method for determination of the AT by location of the acceleration point in $\dot{V}CO_2$ production relative to O_2 uptake has been reported by Dickstein and coworkers [6].

The anaerobic threshold is most appropriately expressed in terms of ml O_2 per kg body weight per minute and represents a submaximal exercise performance point relative to the patient's daily exercise capacity. In other words, the greater the $\dot{V}O_2$

at AT, the greater the patient's capacity for higher intensity daily activities. The AT has been shown to improve significantly in comparison to SSI or single-chamber, fixed-rate pacing in pacemaker patients with appropriately programmed rate algorithm slopes [4, 7, 8, 14].

The clinically relevant point to remember concerning the anaerobic threshold is that pacemaker algorithms which can significantly increase the heart rate at AT, as compared to that observed with chronotropic insufficiency, will, in most cases, demonstrate an increase in the patient's $\dot{V}O_2$ at this point, thus indicating a greater submaximal exercise tolerance or aerobic exercise capacity. The important issues remaining are 1) whether the rise in heart rate attained was achieved in a physiologic way with respect to the patient's oxygen uptake or minute ventilation, and 2) whether the heart rate increase was sufficient enough to aleviate the initial condition of chronotropic incompetence. In other words, based upon the definition of chronotropic incompetence, is the heart rate achieved at the AT with rate-adaptive pacing greater than 60% of the patient's predicted, age-adjusted heart rate max?

In conjunction with the appropriate rate-adaptive slope is the programming of the most suitable maximal or upper paced rate. If too low of an upper rate is programmed, the heart rate at AT may be inadequate to improve the oxygen uptake at AT and correct for the patient's chronotropic impairment at submaximal levels of activity. On the contrary, if the maximal upper rate is too high, perhaps the heart rate is inappropriately greater than necessary for improvement of the patient's submaximal exercise capacity. In addition, especially in the patient with ischemic heart disease, too high of a heart rate may induce an imbalance in the myocardial oxygen supply and demand, predisposing the patient to ischemia or symptomatic chest pain.

If the rate-adaptive algorithm has been designed appropriately, with the correct mathematical expression for correlation to sensed changes in a specific biologic parameter which closely correlates to the patient's true metabolic demand, the clinician need not be concerned about programming the patient's age-adjusted heart rate max for exercise, other than perhaps for cases of valvular disease or myocardial ischemia, as discussed above. For example, if the paced heart rate is appropriately correlated with the indirect monitoring of minute ventilation, it will follow the true relationship between heart rate and minute ventilation during exercise, as shown in Fig. 3. The heart rate will not exceed any specifically monitored minute ventilation value relative to changes in metabolic demand during exercise, by virtue of the employed logarithm's regression analysis curve of the algorithm.

Clinical centers active in pacemaker follow-up that have access to and the expertise available for the employment of non-invasive gas-exchange measurements can benefit from the technology by being able to accurately adjust the individual pacemaker patient's rate-adaptive algorithm.

In summary, non-invasive breath-by-breath gas-exchange measurements provide an easy and accurate clinical means to evaluate the efficacy of a rate-adaptive pacemaker algorithm, whether intended for single-chamber or dual-chamber stimulation. Direct measurement of the oxygen uptake at anaerobic threshold can be used to determine whether the rate-adaptive algorithm results in an improvement in functional capacity and hence, daily exercise ability of the patient. In addition, measurement of the heart rate to oxygen uptake and minute ventilation slopes is useful to 1) evaluate whether chronotropic function of the pacemaker patient is restored in a physiologic way simulating the normal heart-rate response, and 2) to select, via programming, the rate-adaptive slope most suitable for the patient.

References

1. Astrand PO, Rodahl K (1986) Body and fluids, blood and circulation (Chapter 4). Textbook of Work Physiology; Physiological Bases of Exercise
2. Beaver WL, Wasserman K, Whipp BJ (1986) A new method for detecting the anaerobic threshold by gas exchange. J Appl Physiol 39: 354
3. Benchimol A, Ligget MS (1966) Cardiac hemodynamics, right ventricle and left ventricle in normal and abnormal hearts. Circulation 33: 933—944
4. Brachmann J, MacCarter DJ, Frees U, Millerhagen J, Kübler W (1989) Cardiopulmonary evaluation during submaximal exercise with a ventilation based VVIR pacemaker. PACE Vol 12/7: 1159
5. Cohn JN (1987) Quantitative exercise testing for the cardiac patient: The value of monitoring gas exchange. Circulation Suppl (Part II, 76) no 6): VI-I — VI-58
6. Dickstein K, Millerhagen J, Barwick S, Aarsland T, Andersen D, Snapinn S (1989) Validation of a computerized technique for determining the anaerobic threshold. Circulation (Suppl II) 80 (4): II—246
7. Frees U, Aubele R, Brachman J, MacCarter DJ, Kübler W (1990) Kardiopulmonale Leistungsfähigkeit bei Patienten mit Aktivitäts-, Atemfrequenz- und Atemminutenvolumen-gesteuerten VVIR/AAIR Schrittmachern bei submaximaler Belastung. Zeitschrift für Kardiologie 79 (Suppl 1): 55
8. MacCarter DJ, Brachmann J, Frees U, Aubelle R, Grunze M, Kübler W (1989) The use of oxygen uptake measurements to optimize the rate response pacemaker. PACE Vol 12/9: 1568
9. McElroy PA, Janicki JS, Weber KT (1988) Cardiopulmonary exercise testing in congestive heart failure. Am J Cardiol 1 62: 35A—40A
10. McElroy PA, Janicki JS, Weber KT (1988). Physiologic Correlation of the Heart Rate Response to Upright Isotonic Exercise: Relevance to Rate Responsive Pacemakers. J Am Coll Cardiol II: 94—99
11. Neuberg K (1988) Cardiopulmonary exercise testing. An Idea whose time has almost come. Chest 97: (2), 257—267
12. Rushmer RF (1970) Cardiovascular responses during exertion, chapter 7. Cardiovascular Dynamics, WB Saunders Co p 239
13. Rushmer RF, Smith DA (1959) Cardiac control physiology review 39: 41—68
14. Treese N, Coutinho, Stegmaier A, Meyer J (1990) Optimierung frequenzvariabler Schrittmachersysteme durch Spiroergometrie. Herzschrittmachertherapie & Elektrophysiologie 1: 13—17
15. Treese N, MacCarter D, Abkulut O, Werneyer A und Meyer J (1991) Atmung und Herzfrequenz unter Belastung: Bedeutung für frequenzvariable Stimulation. Herzschrittmachertherapie & Elektrophysiologie 2: 90
16. Wasserman K (1987) Determination and detection of anaerobic threshold and consequences of exercise above it. Circulation 76 (Suppl VI): VI-29
17. Wasserman K (1988) New Concepts in Assessing Cardiovascular Function. Circulation 78: 1060—1071
18. Wasserman K (1987) Measurement of physiologic response to exercise. Principles of exercise testing and interpretation. Lea and Fabiger.

Authors' address:

Dean J. MacCarter, PH.D.
Emil-Hoffmann-Str. 1
5000 Köln 50

Influence of Rate Responsive Pacing on Aerobic Capacity in Patients with Chronotropic Incompetence

N. Treese, M. Coutinho, A. Stegmeier, S. Jungfleisch, A. Werneyer, U. Nixdorf, N. Ophoff, and J. Meyer

II. Medizinische Klinik Joh. Gutenberg-Universität Mainz, FRG

Chronotropic incompetence

In most subjects maximal exercise capacity is defined by maximal oxygen uptake ($\dot{V}O_2$ max). According to Fick's principle maximal oxygen consumption is the product of heart rate, arteriovenous oxygen difference, and stroke volume at maximal exercise. At lower workload stroke volume increases by the Frank-Starling-mechanism. At higher workload exercise tachycardia is more important [1] and despite increasing filling pressure, systolic and diastolic volume may decrease [11].

Exercise capacity in normals and moreover in patients with chronic heart failure is very much dependent on the ability to increase heart rate. An abnormal heart rate response to exercise therefore appears to be related to reduced exercise performance and low aerobic capacity [13, 17]. The patient's disability to provide an appropriate heart rate response to exercise defined as 70% of normal age-adjusted peak exercise rate has been considered as chronotropic incompetence. An abnormal heart rate behaviour, however, may also be found in patients despite a normal peak rate with a too-slow heart rate increase at the beginning, an unstable heart rate during prolonged exercise, or a too-slow decrease at the end of exercise.

Rate-responsive pacing

The traditional goal of pacemaker therapy is to prevent symptoms associated with excessive bradycardia. Modern cardiac pacing has, in addition, attempted to not only maintain atrioventricular synchrony but also to provide an appropriate heart rate response to exercise. In the absence of normal sinus node function, patients may benefit from pacing systems that simulate physiologic heart-rate changes during exercise using sensors to provide heart-rate variability independent of atrial activity. It has been proposed that rate-responsive pacing should normalize the heart-rate response to exercise in proportion to oxygen uptake [16]. Therefore, the analysis of respiratory gas exchange during exercise may be of particular interest in patients with sensor triggered rate-responsive pacing.

The usefulness of such pacing systems in selected patients is established. Many studies have demonstrated that single-chamber rate-responsive pacing is superior to fixed-rate atrial or ventricular pacing [1, 5, 6, 8, 9, 15, 18—22, 30]. In a crossover study, Smedgard et al. [22] demonstrated a 7% increase of exercise capacity on the bicycle and a 19% increase during treadmill exercise when activity-triggered pacing was compared with fixed-rate ventricular pacing. Benditt and coworkers [6] found a consistently lower level of perceived exertion during activity-triggered rate-variable single-chamber pacing compared to fixed-rate stimulation. In addition, these authors assessed exercise capacity during both pacing modalities using cardiopulmonary exercise testing. During treadmill exercise rate-responsive pacing provided a 42% increase of heart rate which was related to a 22% increase of aerobic capacity [5].

Cardiopulmonary exercise testing

Rossi et al. [19, 20, 21] were the first to assess respiratory-controlled pacemaker systems employing the principles of cardiopulmonary exercise testing. According to their findings, rate-responsive pacing is of particular value in patients with chronotropic incompetence and heart failure [20]. To achieve a sufficient level of exercise, these patients appear to be dependent on an appropriate increase in heart rate as the myocardial contractile reserve and stroke volume capacity are limited. More recently, Kay and coworkers [14] showed that respiratory-controlled pacing improved maximal oxygen uptake by 22% from 13.4 to 16.3 ml/kg/min, as compared to fixed-rate pacing. We used respiratory gas exchange analysis to assess exercise capacity in 17 patients with rate-responsive pacing systems. In 13 patients an activity-triggered single-chamber system (7 × Sensolog, 6 × Activitrax), in two patients a temperature-controlled (NOVA MR), and in two more patients a respiratory-controlled system (META MV) was implanted. Chronotropic incompetence was present in all patients, due to His-bundle ablation in four, high grade AV-block after open-heart surgery in five, and acquired third degree AV-block in another eight patients who required battery exchange.

All patients were exercised sequentially either in a fixed-rate (VVI-70 bpm) or in the sensor-triggered pacing mode (VVIR) 4 to 6 months after pacemaker implantation.

Exercise testing was performed on a bicycle in a semisupine position using a ramp protocol with 10 to 20 watts increments of workload [8]. Respiratory gas exchange was analyzed using a computerized breath-by-breath technique (Medical Graphics Corporation, St. Paul, Min., USA). Anaerobic threshold was assessed according to the V-slope method proposed by the Wasserman group [4, 29] and the determination of the respiratory compensation point (RQ = 1 method). Both methods did not deviate much in the present study population; therefore, only the data of the RQ=1 determination are presented. In Table 1 cardiopulmonary exercise data during fixed-rate pacing and rate-responsive pacing are compared. Our findings demonstrate that the observed heart-rate increase during rate-responsive pacing was associated with a 40% increase in aerobic capacity [23].

The observed change of anaerobic threshold is of particular clinical importance. 1) Anaerobic threshold is not influenced by the motivation of the patient and the medical supervisor. 2) The anaerobic threshold determines a submaximal exercise level below which work can be performed for a longer period of time without fatigue. 3) Anaerobic threshold describes a critical point in the interaction between central hemodynamics and performance of skeletal muscle during exercise [25]. The delayed onset of the anaerobic glycolysis that is due to a normalized heart-rate response in patients with sensor-triggered pacemakers demonstrates the close coupling of cardiac and muscular function. These findings have been recently extended by

Hatano et al. [23] who showed that rate-responsive pacing at a given workload lowered the venous lactate production when compared to fixed-rate pacing, indicating an increase of aerobic capacity.

Oxygen uptake and work rate

Oxygen uptake during exercise is closely related to the level of work that can be performed. Hansen and coworkers [10] showed that the ratio between increase in oxygen uptake and increase in performed work ($\dot{V}O_2$/WR) is constant over a wide range of workloads. During incremental exercise this ratio appears to be predictable for normal men and a reduction in this ratio may indicate cardiovascular dysfunction.

In 64 patients with different degrees of heart failure, we performed analysis of respiratory gas exchange during bicycle exercise using a ramp protocol with uniform work increments of 10 or 20 watts/min. In these patients, we could confirm that the oxygen uptake relative to work rate is dependent on the degree of cardiac impairment [7]. When the patients were classified according to their peak oxygen consumption [27, 28] it appeared that the lower functional class had a lower $\dot{V}O_2$/work-rate ratio compared to normals or patients with lesser degree of heart failure (Fig. 1).

Rate-responsive pacing in patients with chronic heart failure and chronotropic incompetence might also influence the $\dot{V}O_2$/work-rate ratio. Figure 2 shows a typical example in a patient with advanced chronic heart failure and third degree AV Block in whom a respiratory-controlled ventricular pacing system (META MV) was implanted. The $\dot{V}O_2$ work-rate ratio was 9.2 during fixed-rate pacing and increased to 12.5 during exercise with the pacemaker programmed to rate-response pacing. This observation suggests that the $\dot{V}O_2$/work rate ratio might be an additional parameter to assess the potential benefit of rate-response pacing in selected patients. This para-

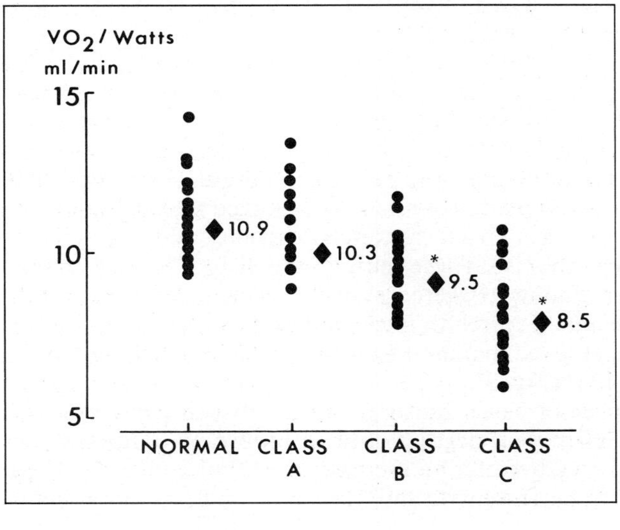

Fig. 1. Oxygen uptake work-rate ratio ($\dot{V}O_2$/WR) in 28 normal subjects and 64 patients with different degrees of heart failure classified according to the Weber functional classes [26, 27]. With increasing impairment of left ventricular function the $\dot{V}O_2$ work-rate ratio decreases.

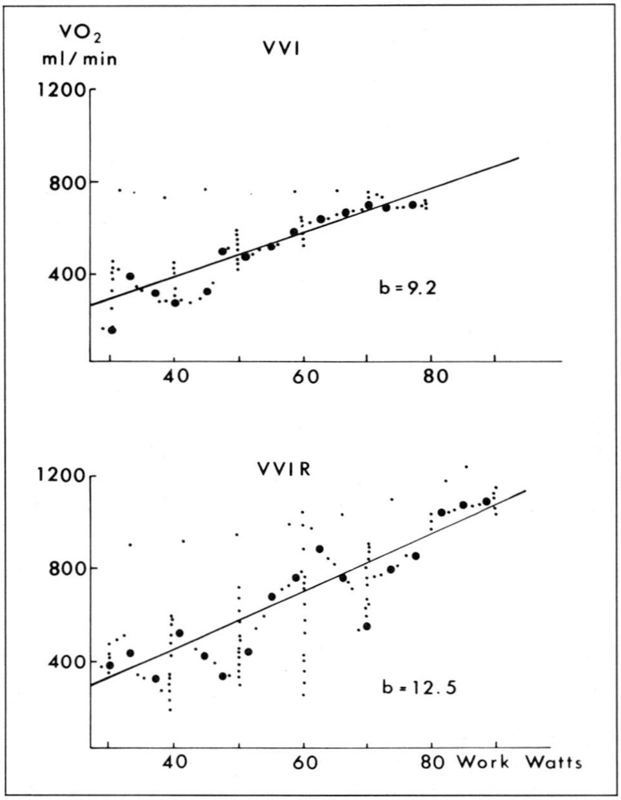

Fig. 2. Influence of rate-response pacing on the oxygen uptake/work-rate ratio ($\dot{V}O_2$/WR) in a patient with advanced heart failure and chronotropic incompetence. The upper panel shows the $\dot{V}O_2$/WR ratio during fixed-rate pacing and the lower panel demonstrates this ratio during rate-responsive pacing (META MV). The exercise settings were identical during both tests. It is shown that the oxygen uptake work-rate ratio is a sensitive measurement to confirm the beneficial effect of rate-response pacing in this patient.

meter is not influenced by age or sex and is independent of the work increments. The method is best used for rapid, short exercise tests on the bicycle, which allows for constant work increments [26].

Heart rate and oxygen uptake

The heart rate/oxygen uptake relation appears to be the most useful tool to optimize rate-responsive pacing systems. Alt and coworkers [29] observed that temperature-controlled pacing provided a greater increase in exercise capacity than the activity-triggered systems during bicycle exercise. These findings are due to the fact that the bicycle test is less suitable for activity-triggered systems, because peak heart rate cannot be attained. In our patients a correlation was found between the individual increase in heart rate and the achieved maximal oxygen uptake, independent of the implanted pacemaker system [23] (Fig. 3).

McElroy and coworkers [6] described a linear relation between heart rate and oxygen uptake in patients with different degrees of heart failure. Individual slopes of this response ranged from 2 to 6 bpm for an increase in $\dot{V}O_2$ of 1 ml/min. These findings may also be applied to patients with rate-responsive pacemaker systems.

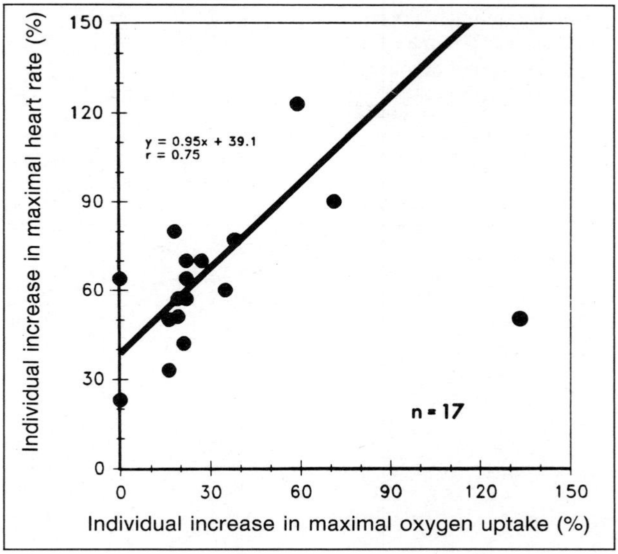

Fig. 3. Individual maximal heart rate increase (%) in relation to the improvement of maximal oxygen uptake (%) from fixed-rate to rate-responsive pacing. The increase in aerobic capacity is a direct function of the degree of heart-rate increase during rate-responsive pacing, independent of the implanted pacemaker system.

An optimal programmed rate-variable pacemaker should increase the heart rate according to this relationship.

In our patients, we examined the heart rate/oxygen uptake ratio of different rate-response pacing systems [24]. The mean slope of this ratio was 4.2 ± 1.8 beats/ml/kg (Table 2). Figure 4 shows a typical example in a patient with a respiratory-controlled system (META MV). The rate response to exercise was programmed according to the criteria proposed by the pacemaker company. The observed slope of 6 beats/ml/kg appears to be at the upper end of the normal physiological range.

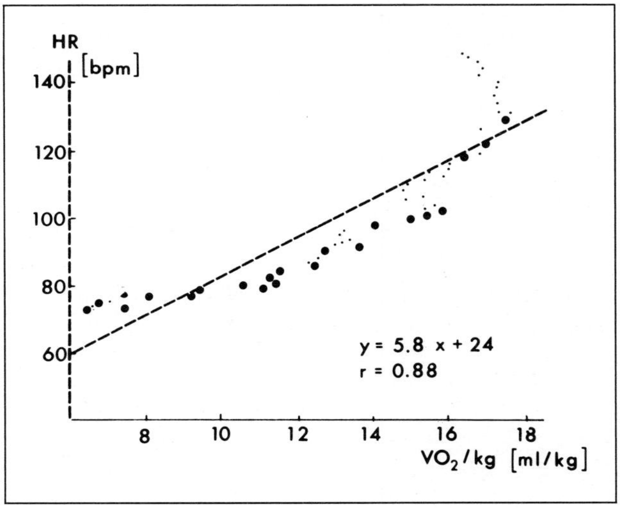

Fig. 4. Correlation of heart rate (HR: bpm) and oxygen uptake ($\dot{V}O_2$: ml/kg/min) during CPX in a patient with a respiratory-controlled rate-responsive ventricular pacing system (META MV). The close relationship between heart rate and oxygen uptake is demonstrated. To increase oxygen uptake by 1 ml/min/kg a heart rate increase of about 6 beats/min was needed.

Table 1. Findings of cardiopulmonary exercise testing (CPX) in the fixed-rate (VVI-70) and the rate-responsive (VVIR) pacing mode. Abbreviations: HR max (bpm), $\dot{V}O_2$max (ml/kg/min) and Watt max: heart rate, oxygen uptake, work load at maximal exercise. HR-AT (bpm), $\dot{V}O_2$-AT (ml/kg/min), Watt-AT: heart rate, oxygen uptake, and work load at anaerobic threshold. m: mean value, sd: standard deviation. Exercise time (min).

No	HR max		HR-AT		VO_2 max		VO_2-AT		Watt max		Watt-AT		exercise time	
	VVI	VVIR	VVI	VVIR	VVI	VVIR	VVI	VVIR	VVI	VVIR	VVI	VVIR	VVI	VVIR
1	70	110	70	92	18.3	21.7	14.3	15.7	120	150	90	105	8.5	10.5
2	62	88	60	88	14.5	17.5	14.5	16.6	65	85	65	85	5	7.5
3	72	96	70	90	21.4	24.8	16.5	20.8	150	175	105	135	11	12
4	70	112	70	102	17.1	23	15.2	22	150	170	110	150	7	8
5	70	124	70	124	15.3	21.1	15.3	21.1	60	80	60	80	3	4.5
6	70	106	70	70	19.8	23.6	13.1	13.8	90	110	50	50	4.5	5.5
7	70	110	70	110	9	11	7	10.3	69	81	63	81	8	11
8	70	115	79	115	14	14	12	12	91	98	85	93	11	12
9	80	98	80	98	9	9	5	7	52	63	10	30	6	6
10	60	90	60	76	16	18.5	14.5	16.1	90	110	70	90	4	5.5
11	80	118	80	100	7.2	16.8	6.5	15.8	90	110	50	70	3.5	5.5
12	70	133	70	121	7	12	3	8	70	67	45	45	7	7
13	70	115	70	101	9	11	7	8	60	75	32	55	6.1	7.5
14	70	126	70	104	11	13	7	10	75	75	72	72	5.5	6.3
15	98	167	80	160	23	28	15	18	120	140	80	90	6.4	7.3
16	70	156	70	136	17	27	9	18	95	105	50	80	6.5	7.4
17	100	140	91	117	15	19	6	15	100	125	75	100	7	8
m	74	118	72	106	14.3	18.3	10.6	14.6	91	107	65	83	6.5	7.7
sd	11	22	8	22	4.9	5.9	4.5	4.7	30	35	25	30	2.3	2.3

Table 2. Correlation between pacing rate (HR) and instantaneous oxygen uptake ($\dot{V}O_2$) during exercise testing of seven patients in the rate-responsive pacing mode (VVIR). The slope varied between 2.83 and 7.10 beats/ml/kg.

No	age sex	pacemaker system	HF/$\dot{V}O_2$ slope	correlation coefficient
1	51 W	Sensolog	2.31	0.84
2	67 m	Nova MR	2.73	0.93
3	23 w	Meta MV	3.07	0.98
4	25 w	Meta MV	4.27	0.95
5	51 w	Nova MR	2.83	0.91
6	70 w	Meta MV	5.80	0.95
7	18 w	Meta MV	4.92	0.98

In clinical practice different pacemaker settings may be examined according to this relationship and an individual optimal heart rate increase may be established.

Conclusion

Cardiopulmonary exercise testing is of particular value in patients with rate-responsive pacemaker systems. The ramp protocol allows maximal workload to be attained in a short period of time. Therefore this technique is well tolerated by most patients. The physiologic heart rate/$\dot{V}O_2$ ratio can predict the appropriate heart rate response to exercise and may be useful to optimize the pacemaker programming according to the individual metabolic demands.

Summary:

Cardiopulmonary exercise testing appears to be of particular value in patients with rate responsive pacing. The influence of an appropriate sensor-triggered heart-rate response to exercise on the patient's aerobic capacity can be assessed by continuous monitoring of respiratory gas exchange. In a group of 17 patients with chronotropic incompetence rate-responsive pacing was associated with a 40% increase of aerobic capacity as compared to fixed-rate pacing. Changes of the anaerobic threshold as an objective measure of a submaximal exercise level are most useful to demonstrate the overall benefit of rate-responsive pacing in these patients. The oxygen-uptake work-rate ratio appears to provide additional information. Finally, the close relationship between heart rate and oxygen uptake can be used to optimize the individual programming of the pacemaker system according to variables of metabolic demand.

References

1. Alt E, Hirgstetter C, Heinz M, Blömer H (1986) Rate control of physiologic pacemakers by central venous blood temperature. Circulation 73: 1206
2. Astrand PO, Cuddy TE, Saltin B, Stenberg J (1964) Cardiac output during submaximal and maximal work. J appl Physiol 19: 268—274
3. Alt E, Völker R, Högl B, McCarter D (1988) Kardiopulmonale Belastungstests unter frequenzvariabler Stimulation: Ein Vergleich von Activitrax und nova-MR Schrittmachern zu VVI-/AAI-Stimulation. Z Kardiol 77: 456
4. Beaver WL, Wasserman K, Whipp BJ (1986) A new method for detecting the anaerobic threshold by gas exchange. J Appl Physiol 60: 2020
5. Benditt DG, Mianulli M, Fetter J, Benson DW, Dunningan A, Molina E, Gornick CC, Almquist A: (1987) Single-chamber cardiac activity-initiated chronotropic response: evaluation by cardiopulmonary exercise testing. Circulation 75: 184
6. Benditt DG, Milstein S, Buetikoffer J, Gornick CC, Mianulli M, Fetter J (1987) Sensor triggered, rate-variable cardiac pacing: current technologies and clinical implications. Ann Intern Med 107: 714
7. Coutino M (1990) Spiroergometrische Untersuchungen bei chronischer Herzinsuffizienz. Inauguraldissertation, Main 1990
8. Davis JA, Whipp BJ, Lamarra N, Huntsman DJ, Frank MH, Wasserman K (1982) Effect of ramp slope on measurements of aerobic parameters from the ramp exercise test. Med Sci Sports Exerc 14: 339
9. Den Dulk K, Bouwels L, Lindemans F, Rankin I, Brugada P, Wellens H (1988) The activitrax rate response pacemaker system. Am J Cardiol 61: 107
10. Hansen JE, Sue DY, Oren A, Wasserman K (1987) Relation of oxygen uptake to work rate in normal men and men with circulatory disorders. Am J Cardiol 59: 669—674
11. Higginbothan MB, Morris KG, Williams RS, McHale PA, Coleman RE, Cobb FR (1986) Regulation of stroke volume during submaximal and maximal upright exercise in normal man. Circ res 58: 281—291
12. Hatano K, Kato R, Hayashi H, Noda S, Sotobata I, Murase M (1989) Usefulness of rate response pacing in patients with sick sinus syndrome. Pace 12: 16—24

13. Ikkos D, Hanson JS (1960) Response to exercise in congenital complete atriventricular block. Circulation 22: 583
14. Kay GN, Bubien RS, Epstein AE, Plumb VJ (1989) Rate-modulated cardiac pacing based on transthoracic impedance measurements of minute ventilation: correlation with exercise gas exchange. J Am Coll Cardiol 14: 1283
15. Lindemans FW, Rankin IR, Murtaugh R, Chevalier PA (1986) Clinical experience with an activity sensing pacemaker. Pace 9: 978
16. McElroy P, Janicki JS, Weber KT (1988) Physiologic correlates of the heart rate response to upright isotonic exercise: relevance to rate-responsive pacemakers. J Am Coll Cardiol 11: 94
17. Reybrouck T, Eynde BV, Dumoulin M, Van der Hauwaert LC (1989) Cardiorespiratory response to exercise in congenital completre atriventricular block. Am J Cardiol 64: 896—899
18. Rickards AF, Donaldson RM, Thalen HJTh (1983) The use of QT interval to determine pacing rate: early clinical experience. Pace 10: 650
19. Rossi P, Rognoni G, Occhetta E, Aina F, Prando MD, Plicchi G, Minella M (1985) Respiration-dependent ventricular pacing compared with fixed ventricular and atrial-ventricular synchronous pacing: aerobic and hemodynamic variables. J Am Coll Cardiol 6: 646
20. Rossi P, Prando MD, Occhetta E, Aina F, Rognoni G, Magnami A (1986) Influence of heart rate on anaerobic threshold. Adv Cardiol 35: 108
21. Rossi P, Prando MD, Ochezza E, Rognoni G, Aina F (1986) Rate-responsive pacing in patients with left ventricular failure. Adv Cardiol 34: 115—123
22. Smedgard P, Kristensson BE, Kruse I, Ryden L (1987) Rate-response pacing by means activity sensing versus single rate ventricular pacing: a double-blind cross-over study. Pace 10: 902—915
23. Treese N, Coutinho M, Ophoff N, Rhein S, Pop T, Meyer J (1990) Kardiopulmonale Belastung: Funktionskontrolle für frequenzvariable Schrittmachersysteme. Z Kardiol 79 (6): 396—402
24. Treese N, Coutinho M, Stegmaier A, Meyer J (1990) Optimierung frequenz-variabler Schrittmachersysteme durch Spiroergometrie. Herschr Elektrophys 1: 13—17
25. Wasserman K (1987) Determinants and detection of anaerobic threshold and consequences of exercise above it. Circulation 76: (suppl VI) 29
26. Wassermann K (1990) New concepts in assessing cardiovascular function. Circulation 81 (Suppl II): 59
27. Weber KT, Kinasewitz GT, Janicki JS, Fishman AP (1982) Oxygen utilization and ventilation during exercise in patients with chronic cardiac failure. Circulation 65: 1213
28. Weber KT, Janicki JS (1985) Cardiopulmonary exercise testing for evaluation of chronic heart failure. Am J Cardiol 55: 22A
29. Whipp BJ, Davis JA, Torres F, Wasserman K. A test to determine parameters of aerobic function during exercise. J appl Physiol 191; 50: 217
30. Wirtzfeld A, Goedel-Meinen L, Bock Th, Heinze R, Liess HD, Munteanu J (1982) Central venous oxygen saturation for the control of automatic rate response pacing. PACE 5: 829

Authors' address:
Prof. Dr. Norbert Treese
II. Medizinische Klinik
Langenbeckstraße 1
D-6500 Mainz

Cardiopulmonary Exercise Testing in Rate-Modulated Cardiac Pacing Based on Minute Ventilation and QT-Interval

F. van Erckelens, M. Sigmund, Ch. Reupcke, B. Heiermann, P. Hanrath

Medical Clinic I, RWTH Aachen, FRG

Introduction

In pacemaker patients, both atrio-ventricular (AV)-synchronity and an appropriate rate response to exercise are desirable. Given primary atrial arrhythmias or an abnormal sinoatrial conduction, atrial tracking devices (VDD or DDD) cannot be utilized for adequate rate-adaptive pacing. Therefore, the development of pacemaker devices that provide exercise-related rate-adaption independent of atrial function has gained special interest [23]. Several sensors have been tested for rate-responsive pacing as for their suitability to effect an exercise-induced increase of stimulation rate [1, 4, 10, 12, 14, 18, 19, 23, 25, 28, 40].

The use of changes in the evoked QT-interval as a sensor to regulate stimulation rate is based on the exercise-induced shortening of the QT-interval mediated by catecholamine release [5, 7, 8, 14, 15, 22, 25—27]. By measuring the QT-shortening or, to be precise, the shortening of the stimulus-T-interval with exercise the pacemaker's algorithm provides a modulation of pacing rate (Quintech, Vitatron). After the delivery of a stimulus, the system measures the interval from the stimulus to the backslope of the evoked T-wave. The subsequent stimulus escape interval is then set as a function of the preceeding stimulus-T-interval. Shortening causes an increase of pacing rate and vice versa. The programmable parameter determining the extent of rate response to a given change of stimulus-T-interval is the so-called slope.

As respiratory flow is linearly related to oxygen consumption and normal sinus nodal rate during aerobic exercise (16, 17, 20, 34), pacing systems that measure minute ventilation (e.g. Meta MV, Telectronics) — quantified by means of respiratory changes of transthoracic impedance — provide an adequate rate response. Impedance is calculated by emitting an impulse of known current from the proximal ring electrode of the bipolar pacing lead and measuring the resultant voltage between the distal up tip electrode and the pulse generator case. The product of the frequency and the amplitude of changes in transthoracic impedance is an estimate of minute ventilation [1, 16—18, 28]. The slope of the relation between the change in pacing rate for a given change in the impedance signal is a programmable parameter which determines the rate response to exercise.

This comparative study uses graded bicycle exercise with combined spiroergometry to assess the benefits of these two aforementioned single-chamber ventricular rate-responsive pacing devices. Cardiopulmonary exercise testing involves measurement of respiratory oxygen uptake, carbon dioxide outflow, tidal volume, respiratory rate, and derived parameters during a symptom-limited exercise tolerance test [24, 36, 37, 39]. Rate adaption by determination of QT-interval (Quintech) and

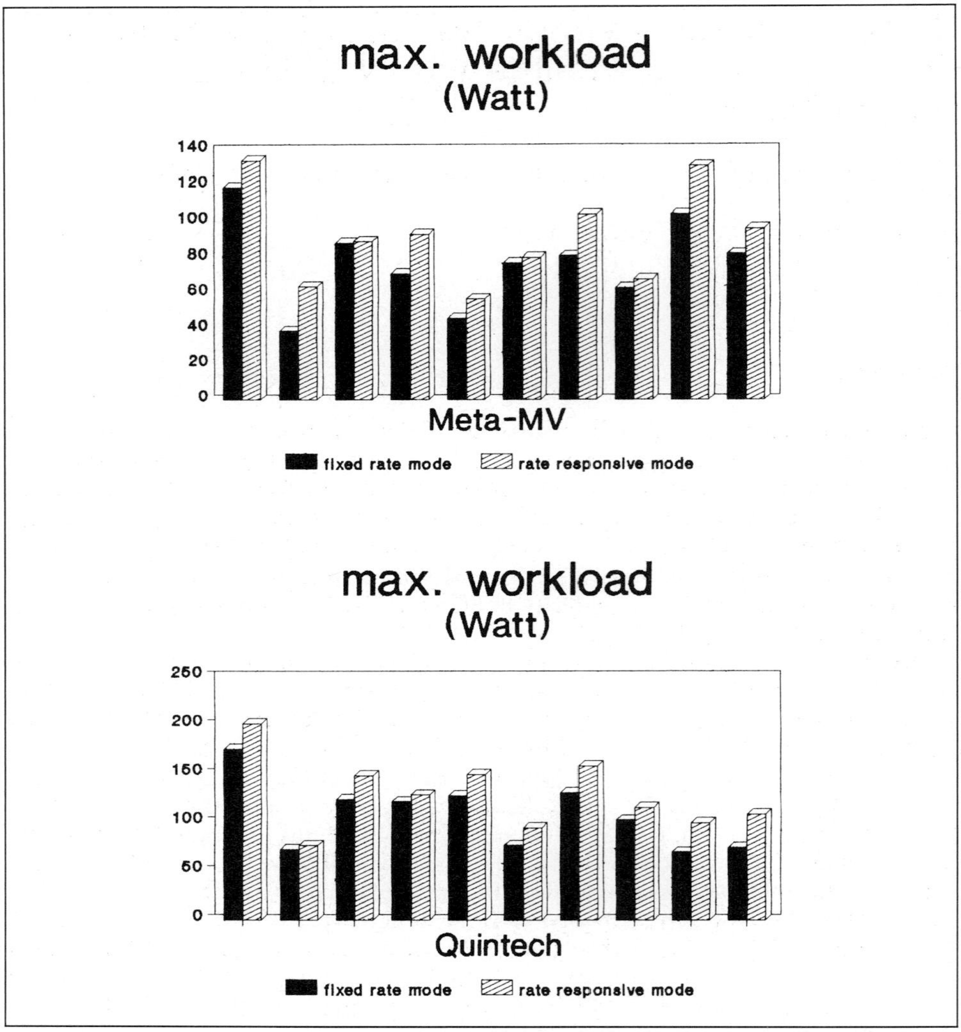

Fig. 1. Maximal work load achieved by each member of both groups (fixed rate VVI / rate variable VVIR pacing).

minute ventilation (Meta-MV) are compared as to their effects on cardiopulmonary work capacity.

Methods

Cardiopulmonary exercise testing (CPX) comprised two sequential tests with the pulse generator programmed initially to either the fixed-rate (VVI) or rate-variable (VVIR) pacing mode and the alternate pacing mode for the second test.

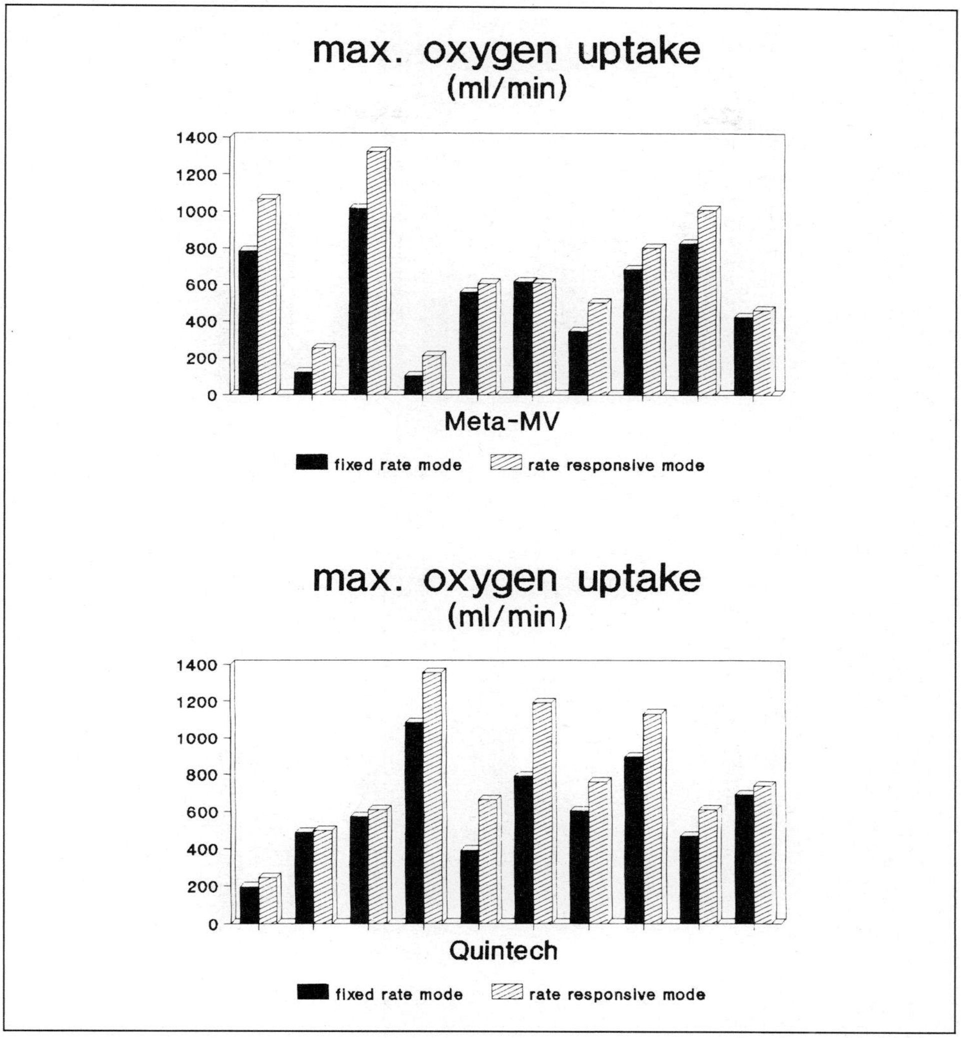

Fig. 2. Maximal oxygen uptake achieved by each member of both groups (fixed rate VVI / rate variable VVIR pacing).

Patients

Two groups of 10 patients each were studied (group 1: 10 patients; three female, seven male, mean age 67 years, with a Meta-MV-pacemaker; rate modulation by measurement of minute ventilation; 6—36 months after implantation for AV-block [3], sick sinus syndrome [5], bradyarrhythmia [2]; group 2: 10 patients, four female, six male, mean age 69 years, with a QT-interval driven Quintech-pacemaker; 12—60 months after implantation for AV-block [2], sick sinus syndrome [5], bradyarrhythmia [3]). In all patients both upper and lower rate limit as well as the slope

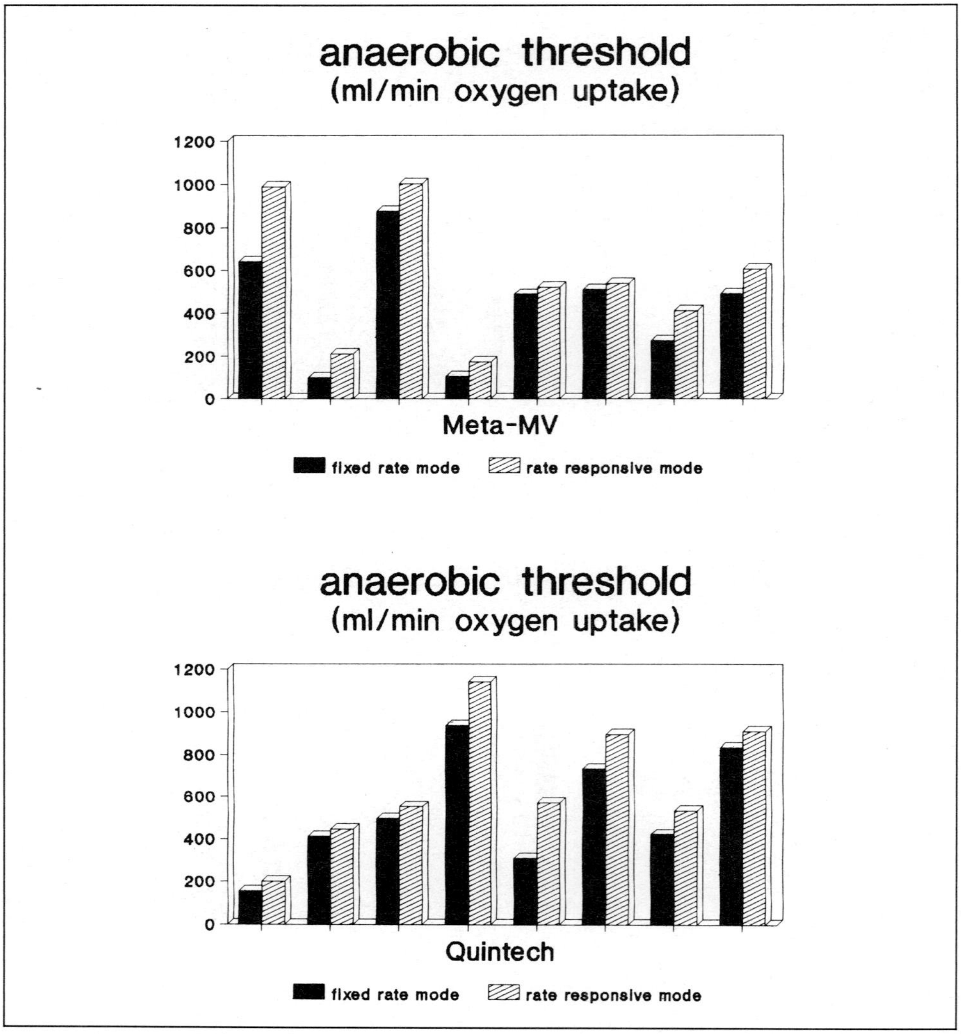

Fig. 3. Oxygen uptake at the anaerobic threshold achieved by each member of both groups (fixed rate VVI / rate variable VVIR pacing).

had been established and controlled by several exercise tests comprising standardized daily activities [35]. Rate response had been found adequate in all patients.

Exercise protocol

A symptom-limited bicycle exercise-test was performed starting at 25 watts (W) with gradeless increments of 15 W every minute.

The effects of exercise on cardiopulmonary function were assessed with a computerized breath-by-breath spiroergometric system (Medical Graphics Corp.,

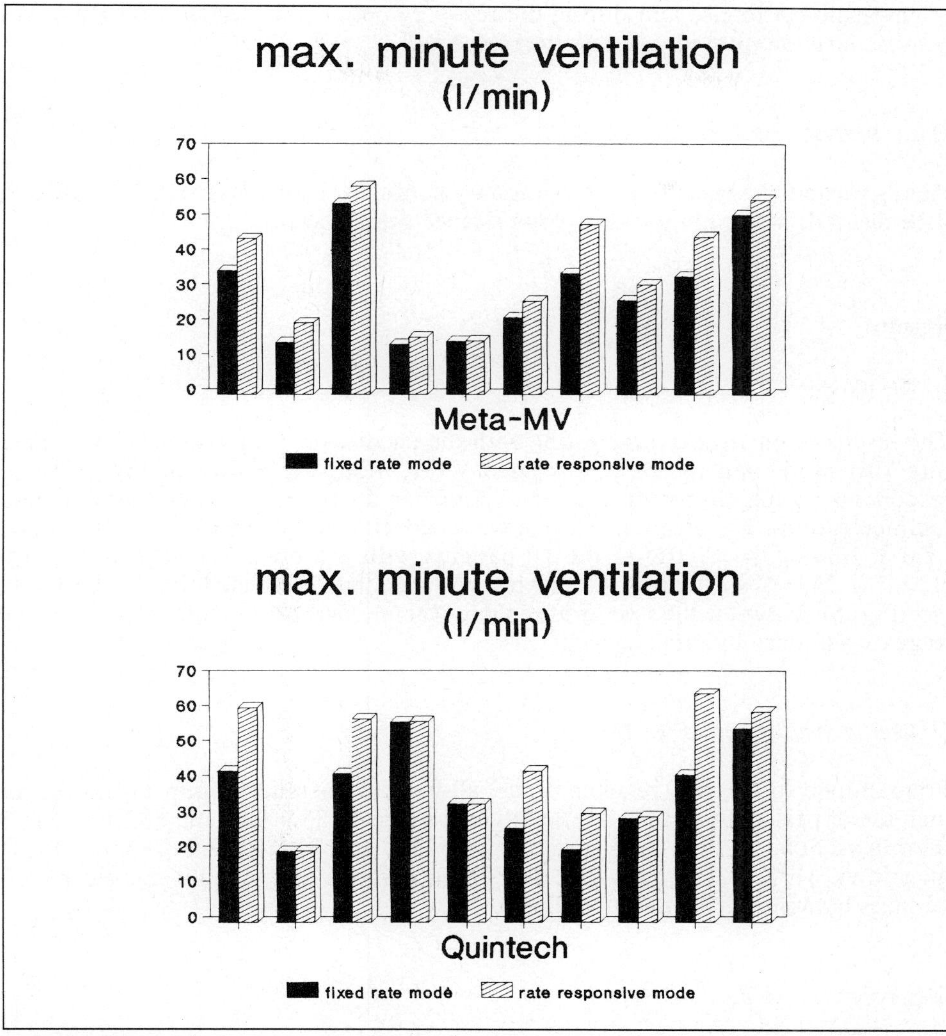

Fig. 4. Maximal minute ventilation achieved by each member of both groups (fixed rate VVI / rate variable VVIR pacing).

St. Paul, Minnesota, USA) employing an infrared CO_2-analyzer, a zirkonium cell O_2-analyzer, and a pneumotachometer. Minute ventilation ($\dot{V}E$), oxygen uptake ($\dot{V}O_2$), and carbon dioxide output ($\dot{V}CO_2$) were determined by analysis of expired air for each breath.

Anaerobic threshold (AT) was estimated by the plotting of $\dot{V}CO_2$ as a function of $\dot{V}O_2$ with AT being the point of departure from linearity of this relation. This parameter defines the level of exercise above which a sustained lactic acidosis occurs as anaerobic metabolism is neccessary to supplement aerobic energy production during exhausting exercise (6, 21, 31, 36—39).

Throughout exercise and during the recovery period the electrocardiogram was continuously monitored to assess rate response.

Data analysis

Pacing related changes of cardiopulmonary parameters were statistically evaluated with the Wilcoxon rank sum test. Significance was set at $p < 0.05$.

Results

Exercise tolerance

The results of paired exercise testing with the pacemaker programmed in the fixed rate VVI mode and the rate-modulated VVIR mode are shown in Fig. 1. Rate-responsive pacing improved exercise tolerance in all patients of both the Meta and Quintech group. The mean increase of work capacity was 22.6% (91.6 ± 21.7 W vs. 77.0 ± 18.4 W, $p < 0.05$) in the 10 patients with a Meta-pacemaker and 31.1% (112.7 ± 26.4 W vs. 84.0 ± 16.8 W, $p < 0.01$) in the Quintech group, respectively (see Fig. 5). Between the two groups there was no significant difference as to the increase achieved by rate adaption.

Oxygen consumption (Fig. 2)

Programmed to the rate variable mode, all but one member (group 1) showed an increase of peak-$\dot{V}O_2$ (= max $\dot{V}O_2$) with an average of 35.6% (Meta, 685.1 ± 131.7 ml/min vs. 505.6 ± 153.8 ml/min, $p < 0.05$) and 27.1% (Quintech, 783.0 ± 176.4 ml/min vs. 617.0 ± 111.6 ml/min, $p < 0.05$), respectively, without significant differences between the two groups (Fig. 5).

Anaerobic threshold

With both VVI and VVIR pacing, $\dot{V}O_2$-AT was achieved in 8/10 Meta- and 8/10 Quintech-patients (Fig. 3). Compared with findings during exercise with VVI pacing, exercise in the VVIR mode was associated with a mean increase in $\dot{V}O_2$-AT of 28.6% (Meta, 576.7 ± 123.4 ml/min vs. 448.9 ± 98.6 ml/min, $p < 0.05$) and 24.2% (Quintech, 647.8 ± 107.9 ml/min vs. 521.0 ± 116.4 ml/min, $p < 0.05$), respectively. Statistics revealed no significant difference between the two groups (Fig. 5).

Minute ventilation

Figure 4 presents the effect of rate-adaptive pacing with both systems on peak minute ventilation. According to the improved work tolerance with the VVIR-mode,

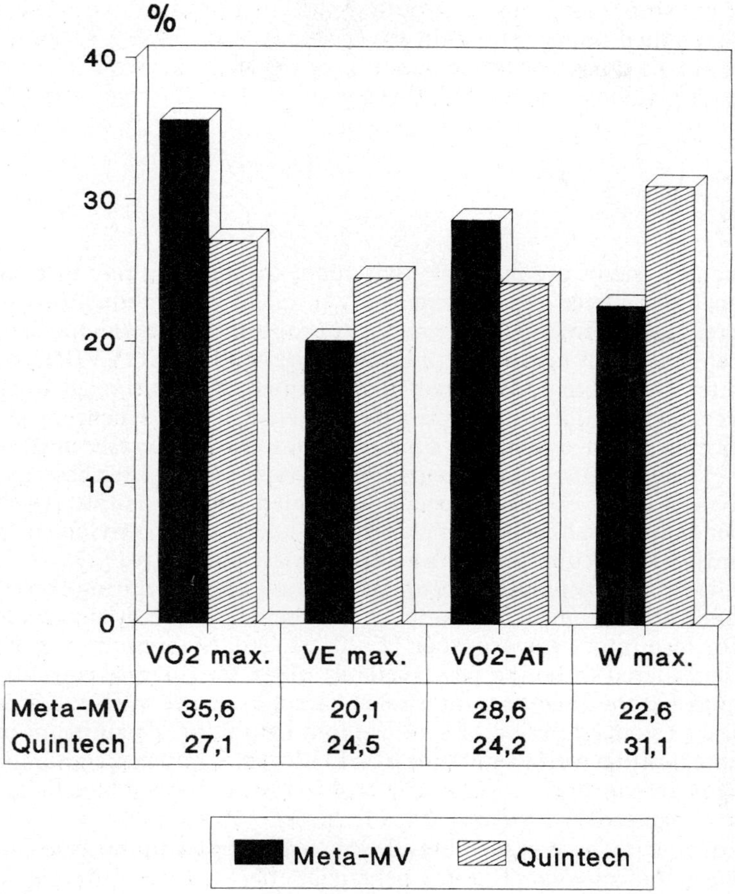

	VO2 max.	VE max.	VO2-AT	W max.
Meta-MV	35,6	20,1	28,6	22,6
Quintech	27,1	24,5	24,2	31,1

Fig. 5. Average percental increase of maximal oxygen uptake ($\dot{V}O_{2max}$), maximal minute ventilation ($VE_{max.}$), anaerobic threshold ($\dot{V}O_2$-AT), and maximal workload ($W_{max.}$) by rate-responsive pacing compared to fixed-rate VVI pacing. For each parameter there is no statistically significant difference between the minute ventilation (black) and the QT (dashed) principle.

minute ventilation was increased as well (Meta group: 20.1%, 36.4 ± 6.9 l/min vs. 30.3 ± 8.4 l/min, $p < 0.05$; Quintech group: 24.5%, 45.7 ± 10.8 l/min vs. 36.7 ± 9.6 l/min, $p < 0.05$). The achieved effect was comparable in both pacemaker groups without significant difference (Fig. 5).

Heart rate

Analyzing the heart-rate response after the onset of exercise, the QT-interval driven increase of the pacing rate was found to be less immediate and less steep, due to being dependent on sympathetic tone and circulating catecholamine levels. Modification of the stimulation rate by minute ventilation produces an earlier reaction.

The programmed upper rate limit was reached by 8/10 Meta patients and 9/10 Quintech patients during or immediately after maximal exertion. The rate decline during recovery period was regulated within a comparable range with both principles.

Discussion

Several pacing systems are available that adapt their pacing rate in response to a physiological parameter during exercise. An ideal rate-modulating pacemaker should increase the stimulation rate in direct proportion to metabolic demand [23]. The clinical benefits of ventricular-inhibited, rate-modulated (VVIR) as compared to fixed-rate VVI pacing have been demonstrated [23]. Although dual-chamber (DDD)-pacemakers additionally provide atrioventricular synchronization, rate-adaptive pacing produces a nearly similar cardiac output increase and exercise capacity [3, 9]. In (DDD)-paced patients, Fananazapir [9] reported that the approximate 40% increase in exercise capacity associated with heart-rate responsiveness was independent of whether AV-synchrony was additionally provided or not. Thus, rate-responsive ventricular pacing is an appropriate alternative [23].

The quality of rate response is documented by monitoring during exercise testing; the effect on work tolerance, however, can only be quantified by simultaneous measurement of respiratory gas exchange [2, 20, 32, 33]. Maximum oxygen uptake is generally considered to be the best available index for exercise capacity [24, 36]. Oxygen uptake at the anaerobic threshold characterizes the workload a patient can sustain for a prolonged period of time without exhibiting a significant increase in serum lactate limiting work endurance [6, 21, 37—39]. Thus, cardiopulmonary exercise testing is an appropriate diagnostic tool in estimating the beneficial effects of rate-adaptive pacemaker systems [2, 4, 11, 20, 32, 33].

This present study used graded bicycle exercise testing with measurement of cardiopulmonary indices to analyze the beneficial effects of two different sensors for rate-responsive pacing: QT-interval (Quintech) and respiratory minute ventilation (Meta MV). Parameters were determined during rate-responsive VVIR pacing and compared with those achieved during conventional fixed-rate ventricular pacing.

Our results indicate that both principles consistently extend exercise tolerance and increase maximum oxygen uptake. Peak oxygen uptake mirrors improved cardiac output [36] as the most important consequence of chronotropic competence. Controlled by the QT-interval, rate increase at the onset of exercise is delayed and is dependent on sympathetic tone and circulating catecholamines [29]. Nevertheless, an adequate exercise-induced rate response is produced [30]. With our patients, rate reaction at peak exercise was satisfactory and exhibited no difference compared with that achieved by the minute ventilation principle.

To a comparable degree, rate-responsive pacing with both sensors, QT-interval and minute ventilation, delayed the achievement of anaerobic threshold to a higher level of oxygen consumption. The profit gained by rate-responsive pacing compared to mere VVI stimulation is evident. Both the QT-interval and minute ventilation for rate adaption produce a marked improvement of long-term submaximal exercise capacity. Our patients attained the anaerobic threshold in 80% of paired tests. We conclude that this parameter, easily and non-invasively assessed by breath-to-breath analysis of gas exchange, serves as an objective means to quantify the beneficial effects of rate-responsive pacing. A chronotropic reaction proportional to metabolic requirements increases oxygen uptake and extends the time to attain the anaerobic threshold.

Conclusions

The results of this study suggest that both sensors, the QT interval as well as minute ventilation, provide an adequate rate adaption to graded exercise. Cardiopulmonary exercise testing points out the benefit of both QT- and respiratory-driven rate-response pacing.

Abbreviatons

VVI pacing: fixed rate ventricular pacing
VVIR pacing: rate responsive ventricular pacing
DDD pacing: dual chamber pacing
W: workload
$\dot{V}O_2$: oxygen uptake
peak $\dot{V}O_2$ = max. $\dot{V}O_2$
$\dot{V}CO_2$: carbon dioxide output
$\dot{V}E$: minute ventilation
AT: anaerobic threshold
$\dot{V}O_2$-AT: oxygen uptake at the anaerobic threshold
$\dot{V}O_2$-max: maximal oxygen uptake

Summary: This study used graded cardiopulmonary exercise testing with quantification of gas exchange parameters to analyze the beneficial effects of two different sensors for rate-responsive pacing: QT-interval (Quintech; Vitatron) and minute ventilation (Meta MV; Telectronics). Bicycle exercise testing was performed with the pacemaker programmed to both the fixed-rate ventricular pacing (VVI) and rate-modulating ventricular, pacing (VVIR) modes in random sequence. The mean increase of exercise tolerance achieved by rate adaption was 22.6% ($p < 0.05$) in the Meta and 31.1% ($p < 0.01$) in the Quintech group. With both systems maximal oxygen uptake increased ($p < 0.05$) by 35.6% (Meta) and 27.1% (Quintech), respectively. Oxygen consumption at the anaerobic threshold was improved ($p < 0.05$) in the VVIR mode by 28.6% in the Meta group and by 24.2% in the Quintech group. According to the improved work tolerance, minute ventilation was increased as well (Meta group: + 20.1%; Quintech group: + 24.5%; $p < 0.05$). Despite the initially delayed rate increase at the onset of exercise mediated by the QT-interval regulation, the programmed upper rate limit was satisfactorily attained by both principles.

Thus, both sensors, minute ventilation and QT-interval, provide an adequate rate-modulation in response to exercise and a marked improvement of cardiopulmonary work capacity.

References

1. Alt E, Heinz M, Hirgstetter C (1987) Control of pacemaker rate by impedance based on respiratory minute ventilation. Chest 92: 247
2. Alt E, Völker R, Högl B, McCarter D (1988) Kardiopulmonale Belastungstests unter frequenzvariabler Stimulation: Ein Vergleich von Nova MR Schrittmachern zu VVI-/AAI-Stimulation. Z Kardiol 77: 456
3. Ausubel K, Steingart RM, Shishmi M; Klementowicz P, Furman S (1985) Maintenance of exercise stroke volume during ventricular versus atrial synchronous pacing. Circulation 72: 1037
4. Benditt DG, Mianulli M, Fetter J, Benson DW, Dunnigan A, Molina E, Gornick CC, Almquist A (1987) Single-chamber cardiac activity-initiated chronotropic response: evaluation by cardiopulmonary exercise testing. Circulation 75: 184
5. Browne KF, Prystowsky E, Heger JJ, Zipes DP (1983) Modulation of the QT interval by the autonomic nervous system. PACE 6/II: 1050
6. Dickstein K, Barvik S, Aarsland T, Snappin S, Karlsson J (1990) A comparison of methodologies in detection of the anaerobic threshold. Circulation 81: III—38
7. Donaldson RM, Rickards AF (1982) Evaluation of drug-induced changes in myocardial repolarisation using the paced evoked response. Br Heart J 48: 381
8. Donaldson RM, Rickards AF (1983) Rate responsive pacing using the evoked QT principle. A physiological alternative to atrial synchronous pacemakers. PACE 5: 1344
9. Fananapazier L, Bennet DH, Monks P (1983) Atrial synchronized ventricular pacing: contribution of the chronotropic response to improved exercise performance. PACE 6: 601
10. Foerestrand S (1989) Comparison among different biosensors. 4th Europ Symp Cardiac Pacing 79
11. Fujiki A, Tani M, Mizumaki K, Asoni H, Sasayama S (1990) Pacemaker syndrome evaluated by cardiopulmonary exercise testing. PACE 13: 1236
12. Gilette P (1984) Critical analysis of sensors for physiological responsive pacing. PACE 4: 1263
13. Hedman A, Nordlander R, Kenneth Pehrsson S, Astrom H (1986) Clinical experience with rate responsive pacing by the evoked QT. Stimucoeur 14: 22
14. Hedman A, Nordlander R (1988) Changes in QT and Q-aT intervals induced by mental and physical stress with fixed rate and atrial triggered ventricular inhibited cardiac pacing. PACE 11: 1426
15. Hedmann A, Nordlander R (1988) QT-sensing rate responsive pacing versus fixed-rate ventricular pacing. A controlled clinical study. PACE 11: 506
16. Jordaens L, Bergmans L, van Wasserhove E, Clement DL (1989) Behaviour of a respiratory driven pacemaker and direct respiratory measurements. PACE 12: 1600
17. Kay GN, Bubien RS, Epstein AE, Plumb VJ (1989) Rate-modulated cardiac pacing based on transthoracid impedance measurements of minute ventilation: correlation with exercise gas exchange. J Am Coll Cardiol 14: 1283
18. Lau CP, Leigh-Jones M, Kingwell S (1988) Comparative evaluation of two respiratory sensing rate responsive pacemakers. PACE 11: 487
19. Maisch B, Langenfeld H (1986) Rate adaptive pacing — clinical experience with three different pacing systems. PACE 9: 997
20. McElroy P, Janicki JS, Weber KT (1988) Physiologic correlates of the heart rate response to upright isotonic exercise: relevance to rate-responsive pacemakers. J Am Coll Cardiol 11: 94
21. Myers J, Buchanan N, Shimizu M, Walsh D, Kraewmer M, McAuley P, Froehlicher V (1990) The ventilatory threshold (ATge) Method, protocol and evaluator agreement. Circulation 82: III—240
22. Milne JR, Ward DE, Spurell RAJ, Camm AJ (1982) The ventricular paced QT interval — The effect of rate and exercise. PACE 5: 352
23. Mond HG (1989) Rate responsive cardiac pacing — A perspective. PACE 12: 1309
24. Neuberg GW (1990) Cardiopulmonary exercise testing. Chest 97—2: 257
25. Rickards AF, Norman J (1981) Relation between QT interval and heart rate — New design of physiologically adaptive cardiac pacemaker. Br Heart J 43: 56
26. Rickards AF, Donaldson RM, Thalen AM (1983) The use of QT interval to determine pacing rate: early clinical experience. PACE 10: 650

27. Rickards AF (1986) Rate responsive pacing using QT sensing. Clin Progr Electrophysiol and Pacing 4: 7
28. Rossi P, Plicchi G, Canducci G (1984) Respiration as a reliable physiological sensor for controlling cardiac pacing rate. Br Heart J 51: 7
29. Rouwen T, Krulls J, Wagner J (1986) Sensitivity of the Stim-T time to different workloads. Clin Prog Electrophysiol Pacing 4: 9
30. Sigmund M, Uebis R, Recker S, Effert S (1987) Frequency adaptation of QT controlled pacemakers. Pacing and Clinical Electrophysiology 10: 742
31. Sullivan M, Cobb F (1990) The anaerobic threshold in chronic heart failure. Circulation 81: III-47
32. Treese N, Coutinho M, Stegmaier A, Meyer J (1990) Optimierung frequenzvariabler Schrittmachersysteme durch Spiroergometrie. Herzschr Elektrophysiol 1: 13
33. Treese N, Coutinho M, Ophoff N, Rhein S, Pop T, Meyer J (1990) Kardiopulmonale Belastung: Funktionskontrolle für frequenzvariable Schrittmachersysteme. Z Kardiol 79: 396
34. Vai F, Bonnet JL, Ritter Ph, Pioger G (1988) Relationship between heart rate and minute ventilation, tidal volume and respiratory rate during brief and low level exercise. PACE 11: 1860
35. Van Erckelens F, Sigmund M, Firnich G, Speckamp F, Pesches U, Hanrath P (1990) Belastungsinduzierte Frequenzantwort unter QT-gesteuerter Stimulation: automatische Slope-Einstellung versus individuelle Programmierung. Z f Kardiol 79: 54
36. Wasserman K (1987) Determinants and detection of anaerobic threshold and consequences of exercise about it. Circulation 76, VI: 29
37. Wasserman K, Hansen JE, Sue DY, Whipp BJ (1987) Principles of exercise testing and interpretation. Philadelphia. Lea & Febiger
38. Wasserman K, Beaver WL, Whip BJ (1990) Gas exchange theory and the lactic acidosis (anaerobic) threshold. Circulation 81: II—16
39. Weber KT, Janicki JS (1986) Cardiopulmonary exercise testing. Philadelphia. WB Saunders
40. Wirtzfeld A, Stangl K, Maubach P (1989) Biological sensors: different types and combinations. 4th Europ Symp cardiac Pacing 15

Author's address:

Franz van Erckelens, M.D.
Medical Clinic I
RWTH Aachen
Pauwelsstr. 30
5100 Aachen, FRG

Evaluation of Temperature- and Activity-Controlled Rate-Adaptive Cardiac Pacemakers by Spiroergometry

E. Alt, H. Theres, M. Heinz

I. Medical Clinic, Technical University of Munich, FRG

Introduction

The indication for pacemaker therapy has clearly changed in the almost 30 years of its existence. While the primary purpose in the first two decades was to prevent life-threatening bradycardia or Stokes-Adams seizures, implantation is performed nowadays mainly for patients with sick sinus syndrome (18), the purpose being primarily to improve their quality of life (1). At the same time, rate-adaptive pacemaker systems are being used more and more since an exercise-adequate increase in the pacing rate can increase the patient's physical capability and thus improve his quality of life.

Various parameters have been proposed for controlling the pacing rate and some have already been realized: activity (12), respiratory rate (20), QT interval (19), temperature (2), oxygen saturation (26) and pH value (7).

In the present study, we concerned ourselves with two rate-adaptive pacemaker systems. The first was the Activitrax (Medtronic Inc., Minneapolis, Minnesota, USA), a single-chamber pacemaker with a piezocrystal integrated into the can for converting mechanical vibrations into electrical signals. If these signals exceed a threshold with a programmable level (low, medium, high) the pacing rate is affected, with the steepness of the rate increase also being adjustable telemetrically (level 1 = slight increase to level 10 = steep increase). The second was the Nova MR (Intermedics Inc., Freeport, Texas, USA), also a single-chamber pacemaker which varies its pacing rate analogously to the change in central venous blood temperature which is measured by means of a small thermistor near the distal end of the pacing electrode. The rate change per degree of temperature change can be fixed telemetrically; the algorithm also distinguishes between brief, steeper temperature changes during exercise etc., and long-term slower fluctuations, e.g. during the 24-h circadian rhythm.

The aim of our study was to examine the influence of increasing isotonic exercise on cardiopulmonary parameters with different types of pacing: both with conventional VVI or AAI pacing at 70/min and with rate adaptive pacing using the two above-mentioned systems: activity-controlled with the Activitrax and temperature-guided with the Nova MR.

Patients

We examined seven patients (three male, four female) with an average age of 69.1 ± 10.8 years in whom the Nova MR pacemaker had been implanted, after informed written consent, in the course of the clinical testing of this pacemaker in our hospital*. The indication was sick sinus syndrome in three patients, a binodal disease in two patients and a third-degree AV block and a bradyarrhythmia in the other patients.

Methods

Three exercise tests of each patient were conducted. In one, the pacemaker was set to the VVI or AAI mode at 70/min (referred to in the following as SSI 70); in the second, the pacemaker worked in the temperature-controlled rate-adaptive mode; and in the third, the pacemaker was set to the VVT or AAT mode, being triggered via skin electrodes by an Actrivitrax taped externally to the upper left thorax region. The Activitrax was programmed to "low", i.e. high sensitivity, and "7", i.e. strong rate increase. In all patients the Nova MR was unchanged compared to the settings already used before for the daily routine. The basic rate was set at 65/min at an average basic temperature of 36.64 °C. The steepness of the exercise characteristic was 5.6 on the average (1 = very slow to 10 = very fast), the steepness of the basic characteristic (slow temperature fluctuations) was 18 beats/min per °C of change. The sensitivity of the initial dip detection was set to level 6 (1 = very insensitive to 10 = very sensitive), the steepness of heart rate drop after exercise was 6.3 on the average (1 = very slow to 10 = very fast). The order of the three exercise tests was randomized and neither the patient nor the doctor supervising the ergospirometry knew in what mode the pacemaker was working. Between each two tests was an adequate recovery phase of at least 30 min.

For the exercise tests we used the computer-supported ergospirometry unit Medical Graphics System 2001 (Medical Graphics Corp., St. Paul, Minnesota, USA) with an attached bicycle ergometer. Due to a fast gas analyzer this device can analyze all cardiopulmonary parameters (heart rate, oxygen uptake, carbon dioxide output, respiratory minute volume, tidal volume, etc.) breath-by-breath. This makes it possible to select a continuously increasing form of exercise (ramp protocol) so that the test persons can be maximally exercised within a few minutes before muscular exhaustion limits exercise in the normal case. The ergospirometry system increases the exercise on the ergometer at intervals of 1 s, giving rise to the subjective impression of gradually increasing exercise, as when going up a ramp. In our tests the increase was 10 W/min. Besides the above-mentioned parameters, the current blood temperature and pacing rate were also measured telemetrically and recorded with the aid of the Datalog (Intermedics Inc., Freeport, Texas, USA) every 6 s. Also, the ECG was monitored continuously and written out every minute, and the blood pressure was measured every 2 min.

For the first 3 min of a test the patient sat at rest on the bicycle to get used to the test structure (in particular the mouthpiece and breathing through the tube), thus ensuring stable value detection. Then the gradually increasing exercise began with the above-mentioned increase of 10 W/min. The patient was asked to exercise to the point of maximum exhaustion in each test; the respiratory ratio at the end of exercise signalled a comparable degree of exhaustion in each test. In no case did an exercise test have to be broken off by the doctor beforehand. All tests could be

* According to the protocol approved by the IRB of the Rechts der Isar Medical Center.

conducted without any complications. In addition, the lung function was determined for each patient at the beginning of the test series, whereby essential restrictive or obstructive ventilation disorders could be ruled out.

The statistical calculations were performed with the aid of the paired t-test (8). The significance level was at least $p < 0.05$. The statistical calculations and graphic evaluations were conducted with the aid of the programs StatView and Cricket Graph on an Apple Macintosh Plus computer.

Results

Physical capability

The maximum performance obtained could be improved with both rate adaptive pacing modes, but clearly more with Nova MR than with Activitrax. The maximum exercise tolerance was 67 ± 25 W with SSI 70, 71 ± 27 W with Activitrax, and 91 ± 29 W with Nova MR. The increase with Nova MR was significant with 36% ($p < 0.001$) compared to SSI 70, and 28% ($p < 0.01$) compared to Activitrax, while the improvement by 6% from SSI 70 to Activitrax was not significant (Fig. 1, top).

Due to the linking of performance and oxygen uptake, the latter showed similar behavior in the different pacing modes. The maximum oxygen absorption ($\dot{V}O_2$ max) was 17.6 ± 3.5 ml/min/kg with SSI 70, was raised with Activitrax to 19.5 ± 4.1 ml/min/kg ($p < 0.05$), and could be increased with Nova MR to 21.5 ± 5.6 ml/min/kg ($p < 0.01$) (Fig. 1, bottom).

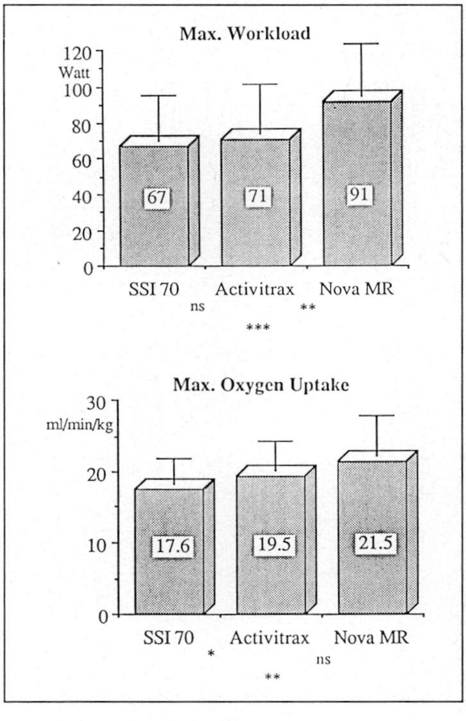

Fig. 1. Maximum performance (top) and maximum oxygen uptake (bottom) with the three pacing modes. Significances in this and the following figures: ns = not significant; * = $p < 0.05$; ** = $p < 0.01$; *** = $p < 0.001$.

Heart rate

While the maximum heart rate reached with SSI 70 was 81 ± 17/min, it could again be clearly increased with both rate adaptive modes: With Activitrax to 98 ± 19/min and with Nova MR to 118 ± 20/min. The increase with Nova MR by 46 % compared with SSI 70 ($p < 0.001$) or by 20 % compared with Activitrax ($p < 0.05$) was significant, as well as the increase with Activitrax by 21 % compared with SSI 70 ($p < 0.05$).

Figure 2 upper left shows the different heart rate curves with increasing exercise for the three types of pacing. Both rate-adaptive modes led, at each level of exercise, to a heart rate higher than that reached with SSI 70, and both also showed a clear rate increase even at low exercise (10 W). Whereas at lower levels of exercise the rate response with Activitrax was more pronounced compared to Nova MR, at higher levels this behavior was vice versa with the Nova MR showing a more marked rate increase than the Activitrax.

The other diagrams of Fig. 2 indicate the close heart rate increase and the standard deviations ($\bar{x}$ ± SD) with increasing exercise for each pacing mode. As can be clearly seen, the rate increase with Nova MR was relatively homogeneous, while larger fluctations occurred with SSI 70 at higher exercise and with Activitrax — even from the very beginning. The possible cause for this variance will be dealt with below.

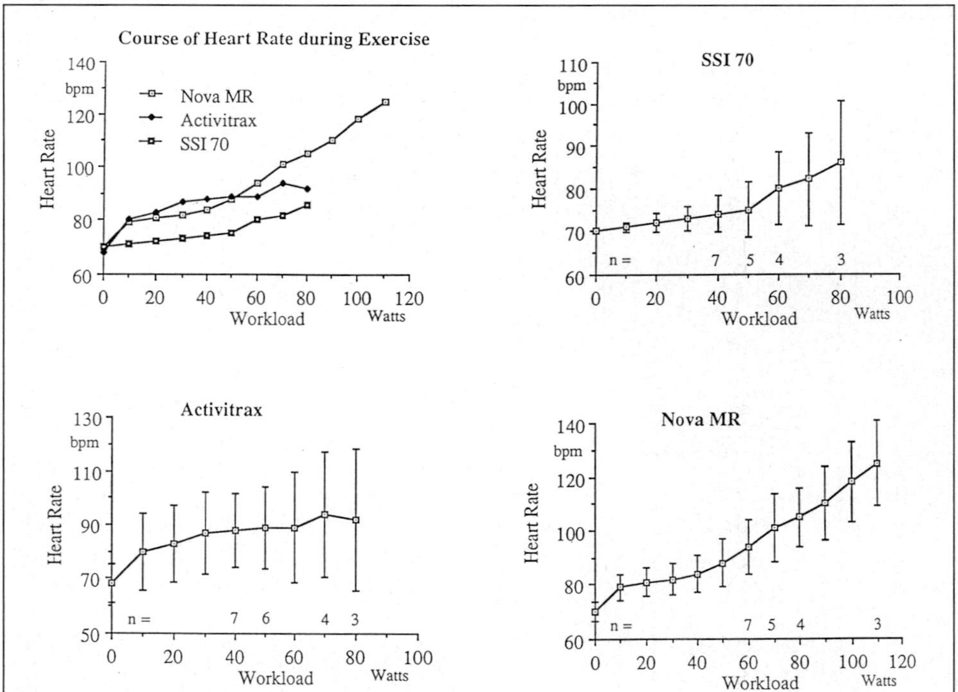

Fig. 2. Heart-rate curve with increasing exercise for the three types of pacing, altogether (upper left) and separately including the standard deviations ($\bar{x}$ ± SD) stated for each heart rate reached.

Figure 3 shows the absolute maximum heart rate (above) and the heart rate increase above resting values (below) for the three types of pacing. The increase was 11 ± 17 beats/min for SSI 70; 29 ± 15 beats/min for Activitrax; and 47 ± 18 beats/min for Nova MR. The differences were significant: SSI 70 — Activitrax: $p < 0.01$; SSI 70 — Nova MR: $p < 0.001$; Activitrax — Nova MR: $p < 0.05$.

Respiration

In accordance with the varying maximum oxygen uptake ($\dot{V}O_2$ max), which is due to the varying cardiovascular oxygen transport capacity, respiration also differed (Fig. 4). The maximum respiratory minute volume in the three types of pacing was 42 ± 11 l/min with SSI 70, 50 ± 10 l/min with Activitrax, and 58 ± 14 l/min with Nova MR. The differences were all significant (SSI 70 — Activitrax: $p > 0.01$; SSI 70 — Nova MR: $p < 0.01$; Activitrax — Nova MR: $p < 0.05$).

The maximum tidal volume was 1440 ± 456 ml with SSI 70; 1530 ± 412 ml with Activitrax; and 1610 ± 494 ml with Nova MR. The differences were not significant.

The maximum respiratory rate reached was 33 ± 8/min with SSI 7, 35 ± 9/min with Activitrax, and 38 ± 8/min with Nova MR. Here, only the differences Activitrax — Nova MR ($p < 0.01$) and SSI 70 — Nova MR ($p < 0.05$) were significant.

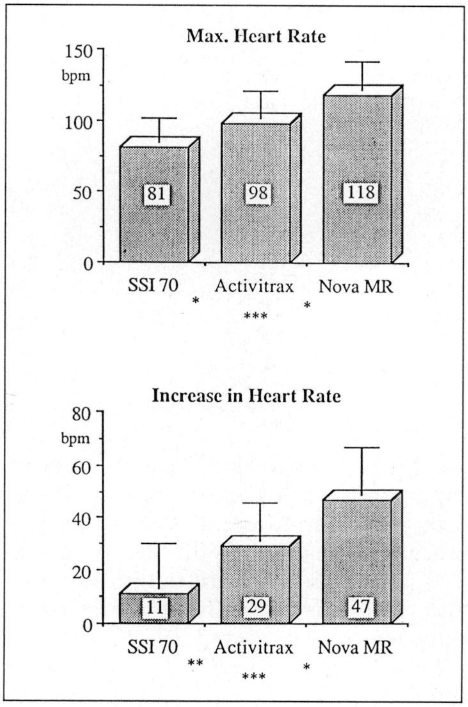

Fig. 3. Absolute maximum heart rate attained (top) and relative heart rate increase from the resting values to the maximum values (bottom) for the three different types of pacing.

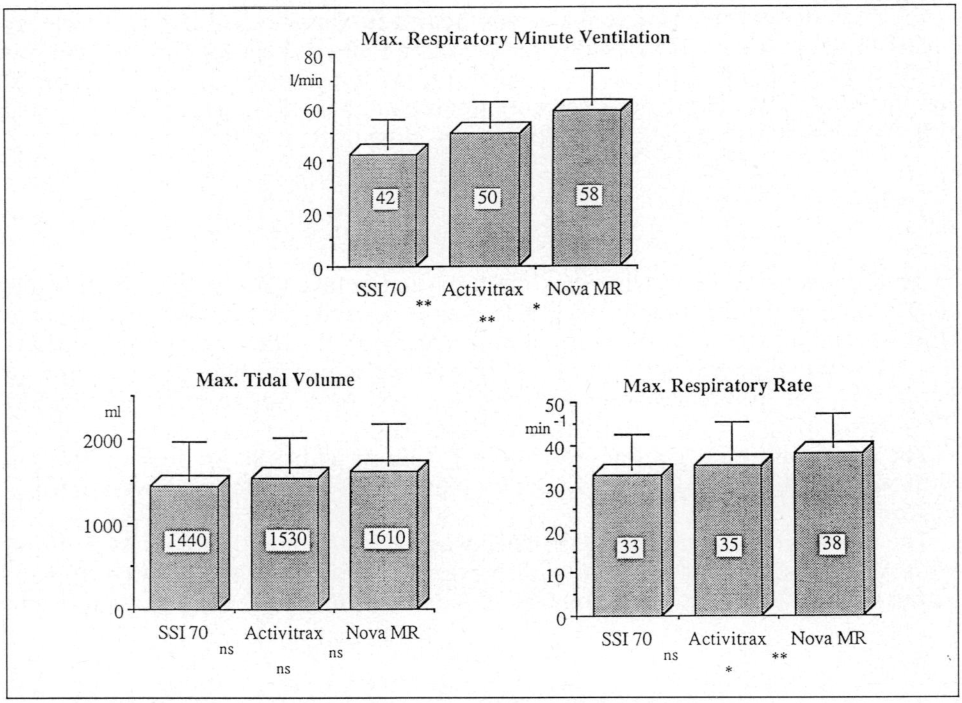

Fig. 4. Maximum ventilatory parameters with different pacing modes.

Table 1. Data of the patients.

Patient	Age	Indication	Mode
E. Wo.	57	AV-block III	VVI
E. Wa.	57	Sick sinus syndrome	AAI
R. N.	73	Bradyarrhythmia	VVI
O. R.	60	Sick sinus syndrome	AAI
H. R.	80	Binodal disease	VVI
G. R.	81	Binodal disease	VVI
R. R.	76	Sick sinus syndrome	AAI

Central venous blood temperature

In accordance with the varying maximum performance and thus with the varying heat production (about 75% of the total energy are transformed to heat and only about 25% are transformed to muscular work) with the different types of pacing, the increase in central venous blood temperature also varied. With SSI 70, it was 0.28 ± 0.15 °C, with Activitrax 0.32 ± 0.18 °C, and with Nova MR 0.44 ± 0.19 °C. The differences between Nova MR and both SSI 70 ($p < 0.001$) and Activitrax ($p < 0.001$) were significant, whereas that between Activitrax and SSI 70 was not.

A summary of all test results is given in Table 2 with the individual values for each patient, the mean values, and the standard deviations.

Table 2. Test results of the patients with individual values, mean values, and standard deviations: Δ = increase from rest to maximum values; Resp. minute vent. = respiratory minute ventilation; SD = standard deviation.

Patient	Test Sequence			Max. Heart Rate bpm			Δ Heart Rate bpm		
	SSI 70	Activ.	Nova MR	SSI 70	Activ.	Nova MR	SSI 70	Activ.	Nova MR
O. R.	2	3	1	88	112	146	18	42	74
R. N.	1	2	3	73	87	102	3	27	35
E. Wo.	3	2	1	70	62	114	0	2	49
E. Wa.	1	3	2	115	112	141	45	42	68
H. R.	2	1	3	78	95	117	8	30	47
G. R.	3	1	2	70	100	110	0	20	35
R. R.	2	1	3	70	115	39	0	43	23
$\bar{x}$				81	98	118	11	29	47
± SD				17	19	20	17	15	18

Patient	Max. Oxygen Uptake ml/min/kg			Max. Resp. Minute Vent. l/min			Δ Temperature °C		
	SSI 70	Activ.	Nova MR	SSI 70	Activ.	Nova MR	SSI 70	Activ.	Nova MR
O. R.	21.1	24.5	26.5	56	66	81	0.36	0.49	0.65
R. N.	13.3	14.1	15.3	31	36	45	0.20	0.24	0.35
E. Wo.	17.1	18.3	24.6	39	47	56	0.41	0.38	0.56
E. Wa.	22.8	25.3	29.2	33	46	64	0.52	0.61	0.70
H. R.	15.4	16.4	14.7	30	44	36	0.17	0.11	0.32
G. R.	18.9	18.3	22.0	52	52	64	0.14	0.20	0.30
R. R.	14.9	19.8	18.4	52	61	58	0.19	0.19	0.23
$\bar{x}$	17.6	19.5	21.5	42	50	58	0.28	0.32	0.44
± SD	3.5	4.1	5.6	11	10	14	0.15	0.18	0.19

Discussion

The development of rate-adaptive pacemaker systems is without doubt an important advance in pacemaker therapy. By allowing for an increase in heart rate with exercise, its hemodynamic gain comes close to that of dual chamber pacemakers (9, 14). In our study, we could confirm this gain for both rate-adaptive systems examined. Both with the activity-controlled Activitrax and with the temperature controlled Nova MR, an increase in maximum heart rate, maximum work rate, and maximum oxygen uptake could be obtained in the short-term exercise test on bicycle ergometer. However, the improvement of these parameters was much more clearly marked with the Nova MR than with the Activitrax.

The higher maximum oxygen uptake reached with Nova MR is related to the higher cardiovascular maximum oxygen transport capacity and a higher maximum respiratory minute ventilation. The increase in oxygen uptake is reached physiologically, mainly by a rise in respiratory minute ventilation and only to a lesser degree by an increase in oxygen utilization, as is shown by our data.

In accordance with the varying maximum exercise performed the rise in blood temperature also differed; the relation of the body's heat production to the exercise level is about 3 : 1 if the thyroid function is normal (2).

For the Activitrax, several studies (13, 21, 17, 24) have already demonstrated an improvement in exercise tolerance compared to VVI pacing, but largely for exercise on the treadmill. Smedgard (24) observed an increase in performance of 10 % during exercise on the bicycle ergometer (from 89 to 98 W) compared to VVI pacing and a pacing rate during maximum exercise of 96/min. This corresponds approximately with the values observed by us: increase in performance of 6% (measured in W) and a maximum heart rate of 98/min.

Since the temperature-controlled pacemaker system Nova MR came into the clinical testing stage just recently, only a few comparative studies exist. Seger (23) also compared the two systems examined by us and found similar results, although the difference between Nova MR and Activitrax was even more clearly marked. In particular, the rate increase during maximum exercise on the bicycle ergometer was more marked with Nova MR than with Activitrax (130/min as opposed to 75/min).

Looking now at the rate increase during exercise with the various rate-adaptive systems, the question arises what increase is physiologically reasonable. There is

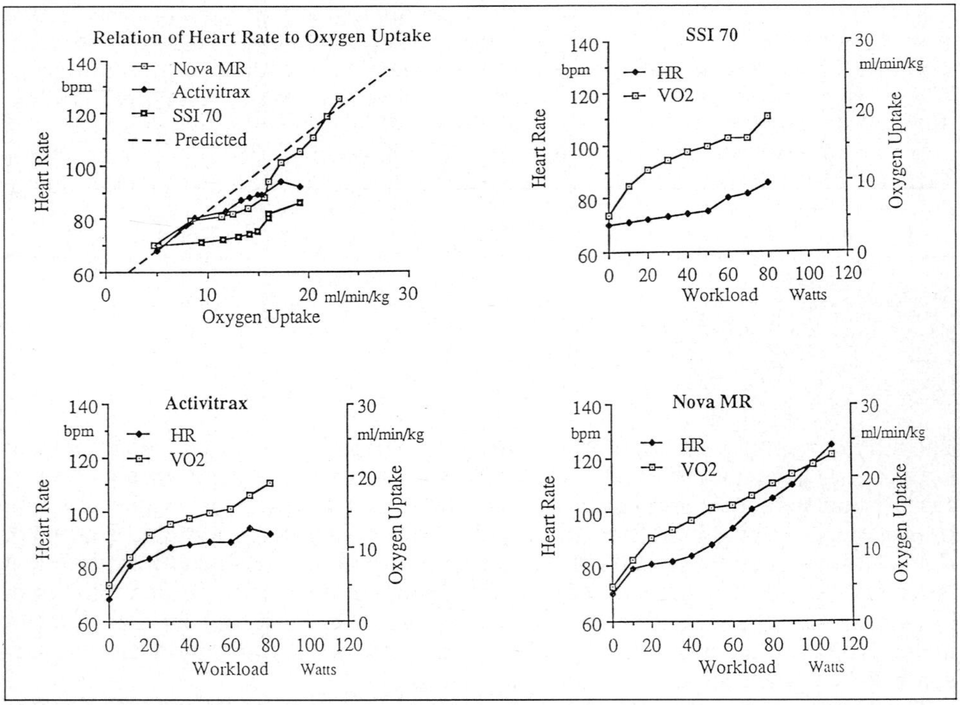

Fig. 5. Upper left: Heart rate curve in relation to oxygen uptake for the three types of pacing. Shown in dotted lines are the maximum oxygen uptake calculated according to age, sex, weight, and size for normal persons and the corresponding heart rates at given oxygen uptake (see text). Upper right and lower left and right: Heart rate curve and oxygen uptake curve during exercise for the three types of pacing.

known to be a largely linear relation between oxygen uptake (as a measure of physical exercise) and heart rate, this relation varying individually, depending on fitness etc. We therefore calculated the corresponding relation of heart rate and oxygen uptake for our patients according to a few formulae stated for this purpose (5, 10, 15) and contrasted it as the normal value with the values actually observed for the various types of pacing (Fig. 5, upper left). The assumption is made that a corresponding optimum rate value can be associated with each level of exercise. Heart-rate values that are below the calculated normal line constitute a rate too slow for the given exercise, while rates above it are considered too fast for the given exercise. One accordingly sees that the heart rates obtained with the Nova MR come closest to this normal curve, while the heart rate increase with the activity-controlled pacemaker is too low for higher exercise levels, and the increase in intrinsic heart rate (SSI 70) relative to the particular exercise level is always too low. Finally, if one separately compares the oxygen uptake and the corresponding heart rate at each exercise level for each type of pacing (other diagrams of Fig. 5), it appears that the individual curves for oxygen uptake are naturally almost identical, while the rate response is of varying adequacy, being least adequate with SSI 70, more adequate with Activitrax, and most adequate with Nova MR.

The reason for this is presumably that the central venous blood temperature is a biological parameter which varies in accordance with the metabolic conditions of the organism (3, 11) and allows, by means of an intelligent algorithm (4), for a pacing rate response which is largely adequate in terms of the metabolism and in terms of exercise. Mechanical vibrations, on the other hand, which are used to control the Activitrax, are only an indirect parameter for physical exercise in general, without any direct correlation to the level of exercise (25). This also becomes clear when one looks at the standard deviations in the particular pacing rates (Fig. 2). While the variance of the intrinsic heart rate increase with SSI 70 (which is marked during

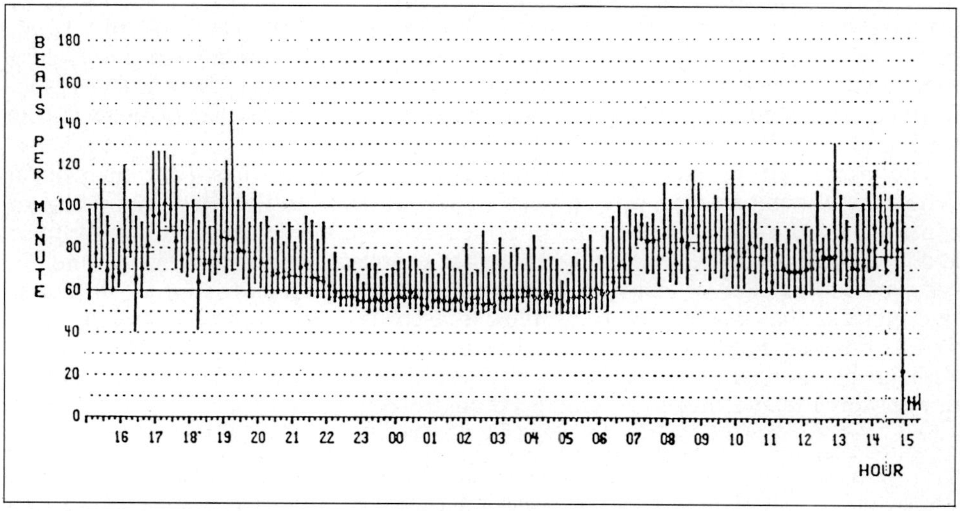

Fig. 6. Print-out of a 24-h Holter monitoring of a patient with a Nova MR pacemaker.

higher exercise) was a sign of our patients' basic diseases, the fluctuation clearly present with Activitrax from the beginning is a sign that the pacing rate obtained on an exercise level is not a direct correlate of the metabolism in accordance with the different movements of the patient on the bicycle, regardless of the genuine exercise-level. With Nova MR, however, the rate response is clearly more homogeneous and corresponds to the linearly increasing oxygen uptake (Fig. 5, lower right) and thus to the metabolism.

It is known that the Activitrax shows a more marked rate response with treadmill exercise than with bicycle exercise, since in the former case the mechanical shocks in general (16) and the movements in the thoracic region are more marked. However, since it is possible to perform maximum circulatory exercise within a short time with the bicycle ergometer by means of the above-mentioned ramp protocol and before muscular exhaustion normally occurs, exercise tests with measurement of the oxygen uptake on the bicycle are better suited for determining the maximum cardiopulmonary functional parameters. Furthermore, holding the mouthpiece for treadmill exercise makes additional considerable demands on the mechanical coordination of the older patients. In order to compensate the disadvantage of lower mechanical shocks on the bicycle ergometer for the Activitrax, we therefore set it to steep angle (level 7) and the highest sensitivity level ("low"), which is normally less suitable for daily life since it already leads to a rate increase due to minimal shock (24).

The central venous blood temperature allows not only an adequate rate increase with exercise, but also a rate decrease at night, according to the well-known circadian rhythm. Figure 6 shows a print-out of a 24-h Holter monitoring of a patient with a Nova MR pacemaker under constant pacing rhythm. As can be clearly seen, the heart rate goes back to about 50 to 60 bpm at night, while it rises during the day according to the various exercises, thus showing a nearly normal rate behavior.

Table 3 shows that the rate increase results in an objectively and subjectively improved physical capability. It shows the rate increase of a patient with a Nova MR pacemaker during an increasing treadmill exercise. Besides the heart rate, this table also demonstrates the corresponding value of the Borg scale for each stage of exercise that is a measure of the subjectively perceived exercise level (6) and ranges in extremes from 6 = very easy to 20 = very strenuous. As can be seen, the highest exercise stage reached with the temperature-controlled rate-adaptive mode was subjectively perceived as less strenuous than the maximum exercise performed with the VVI mode.

The present study shows that in spite of all doubts in the past (22), the central venous blood temperature, when processed adequately with the aid of an intelligent control algorithm (4) as used in the Intermedics Nova MR, can ensure a more marked heart-rate increase, especially at higher exercise intensities (Figs. 2 and 5), compared to the activity-controlled system. Furthermore it allows for a continuous rate increase that is adequate to exercise in accordance with the metabolism (Fig. 5). Further studies should be done to determine if the improved physical capability with bicycle exercise in the laboratory also results in an improved physical capability in everyday life and thus in an enhanced quality of life.

Summary

We examined in seven patients with implanted Intermedics Nova MR pacemakers the cardiopulmonary effects of maximum bicycle ergometer exercise for three types of pacing: VVI or AAI at 70/min (SSI 70), rate-adaptive temperature-controlled with the implanted Nova MR, and rate-adaptive activity-controlled by means of a Medtronic Activitrax pacemaker taped to the chest wall, which triggered, via skin electrodes, the implanted Nova MR in the VVT or AAT mode.

The maximum exercise tolerance was 67 Watts (W) with SSI 70, 71 W with Activitrax, and 91 W with the Nova MR; the maximum oxygen uptake was accordingly 17.6 ml/min/kg with SSI 70, 19.5 ml/min/kg with Activitrax, and 21.5 ml/min/kg with Nova MR. The highest heart rate reached was 81/min with SSI 70, 98/min with Activitrax and 118/min with Nova MR. The rate increase from rest to maximum exercise was 11 beats/min with SSI 70, 29/min with Activitrax, and 47/min with Nova MR.

With both rate-adaptive types of pacing, an increase in exercise tolerance and maximum heart rate could be achieved, but heart rate increased significantly more clearly with the temperature-controlled Nova MR than with the activity-controlled Activitrax. However, with a different form of exercise, e.g. treadmill ergometry, the rate response of the Activitrax would presumably have been somewhat clearer.

References

1. Alt ER, Völker R, Wirtzfeld A, et al (1985) Survival and Follow-up After Pacemaker Implantation: A Comparison of Patients with Sick Sinus Syndrome, Complete Heart Block, and Atrial Fibrillation. Pace 8, 849
2. Alt E, Hirgstetter C, Heinz M, et al (1986) Rate control of physiologic pacemakers by central venous blood temperature. Circulation 73, 1206
3. Alt E, Hirgstetter C, Heinz M, et al (1986) Measurement of Right Ventricular Blood Temperature During Exercise as a Means of Rate Control in Physiological Pacemakers. Pace 9, 970
4. Alt E, Theres H, Völker R, et al (1987, in press) Temperature-Controlled Rate Responsive Pacing with the Aid of an Optimized Algorithm. J Electrophysiol
5. Astrand PO, Ryhming I (1954) A Nomogram for Calculation of Aerobic Capacity (Physical Fitness) from Pulse Rate during Submaximal Work. Acta Med Scand 7, 218
6. Borg G, Noble BJ (1974) Perceived exertion. In: Exercise and Sports Sciences Review. Ed. by J. H. Wilmore. Academic Press, London, 2, 1974, p. 131
7. Cammilli L, Alcidi L, Papeschi G, et al (1978) Preliminary experience with the pH-triggered pacemaker. PACE 1, 448
8. Cavalli-Sforza (1972) Biomathematik. Gustav Fischer Verlag, Stuttgart
9. Fananapazier L, Bennert DH, Monks P (1983) Atrial synchronized pacing: contribution of the chronotropic response to improved exercise performance. PACE 6, 601
10. Givoni B, Goldman R-F (1971) Predicting metabolic energy cost. J Appl Physiol 30, 429
11. Griffin JC (1985) Central Venous Temperature: An Indicator of Exercise. In: Cardiac Pacing. Electrophysiology — Tachyarrhythmias. Ed. by F. P. Gómez. Editorial Grouz, Madrid, p 792
12. Humen DP, Anderson K, Brumwell D, et al (1983) A pacemaker which automatically increases its rate with physical activity. World Symposium of Cardiac Pacing: Proceedings. Steinkopff Verlag, Darmstadt, p 259
13. Humen DP, Kostuk WJ, Klein GJ (1985) Activity-sensing, rate-responsive pacing: Improvement in myocardial performance with exercise. PACE 8, 52
14. Karlöff J (1975) Hemodynamic effect of atrial triggering versus fixed rate pacing at rest and during exercise in complete heart block. Acta Med Scand 197, 195
15. Löllgen H (1983) Kardiopulmonale Funktionsdiagnostik. Ciba-Geigy GmbH, Wehr/Baden

16. Matula M, Alt E, Theres H (1987) Rate Responsive Pacing Based on a New Activity Sensing Principle. PACE 10, 1220
17. Moura PJ, Gessmann LJ, Lai T, et al (1987) Chronotropic Response of an Activity Detecting Pacemaker Compared with the Normal Sinus Node. PACE 10, 78
18. Rickards AF, Donaldson RM (1983) Rate Responsive Pacing. Clin Prog Pacing Electrophysiol 1, 12
19. Rickards AF, Donaldson RM, Thalen HJTh (1983) The use of QT interval to determine pacing rate: early clinical experience. PACE 6, 346
20. Rossi P, Plicchi G, Canducci GC, et al (1983) Respiratory rate as a determinant of optimal pacing rate. PACE 6, 326
21. Ryden L, Smedgard R, Kurse I, et al (1984) Rate-responsive pacing by means of activity sensing. Stimucoeur 12, 181
22. Shellock FG, Rubin SA, Ellrodt G, et al (1983) Unusual core temperature decrease in exercising heart-failure patients. J Appl Physiol: Respirat Environ Exercise Physiol 54 (2), 544
23. Seger JJ, Edelman SK, Driscoll PO (1987) Comparison of the Nova MR Temperature-Sensing Pacemaker and Activity Rate Responsive Pacing. PACE 10, 1227
24. Smedgard P, Kristensson BE, Kurse I, et al (1987) Rate-responsive Pacing by Means of Activity Sensing Versus Single Rate Ventricular Pacing: A Double-Blind Cross-Over-Study. PACE 10, 902
25. Stangl K, Wirtzfeld A, Lochschmidt O, et al (1987) Möglichkeiten und Grenzen eines „aktivitätsgesteuerten“ Schrittmachersystems. Herz/Kreislauf 19, 351
26. Wirtzfeld AL, Goedel-Meinen, Th. Bock et al (1982) Central venous oxygen saturation for the control of automatic rate-responsive pacing. PACE 5, 829

Authors' address:
PD Dr. med. Eckhard Alt
I. Medizinische Klinik der TU München
Ismaninger Straße 22
8000 München 80, FRG

4. Clinical Value in Pulmonary Diseases

Effects of Inhaled Salbutamol and Oxitropium Bromide on Cardiopulmonary Exercise Capacity in Patients with Chronic Obstructive Pulmonary Disease and Coronary Artery Disease

F. van Erckelens, Th. Hürter, Th. Eitelberg, U. Krobok, Ch. Reupcke, E. Schmitz, M. Sigmund, P. Hanrath

Medical Clinic I, RWTH Aachen

Introduction

In patients with chronic obstructive pulmonary disease (COPD), exercise performance is limited due to reduced ventilatory capacity [6, 9, 15, 23]. Airflow obstruction and its quantitative impact on exercise tolerance is still the subject of investigation [6, 9, 20, 25, 31, 34, 36]. Inhalative therapy of COPD with sympathomimetic and anticholinergic bronchodilators is established [1, 31]. The effects of these agents on exercise performance, however, are controversially discussed [9, 10, 19]. Tachycardia and increase of myocardial oxygen consumption are well-known side-effects of these substances [13, 35].

Relevant narrowing of the main coronary arterial branches with a compromised myocardial oxygen supply causes a limitation of exercise tolerance in coronary artery disease (CAD) [7, 38, 39]. Thus patients suffering from both chronic obstructive pulmonary disease and coronary artery disease are subject to a twofold limitation. The exercise performance of this group has not yet been analyzed.

The present study was designed to quantify the effect of an inhaled sympathomimetic agent: salbutamol and an anticholinergic bronchodilator: oxitropium bromide on cardiopulmonary exercise capacity in patients with COPD and CAD. In addition, special regard was given to cardiac side-effects, e.g. aggravation of ECG-changes suggesting ischemia or arrhythmias caused by an increase of myocardial oxygen demand. We used a combined spiroergometry with continuous ECG monitoring and the none-invasive assessment of key respiratory gas exchange parameters [28, 38, 39] such as oxygen uptake, carbon dioxide outflow, and minute ventilation. As a derived parameter, the anaerobic threshold was determined, characterizing the limit of submaximal work endurance [5, 28, 38, 39].

Methods

Fifteen patients with COPD (mean FEV_1 56 $\pm$ 9% of the predicted value) were recruited from the outpatient department of our hospital. They were clinically stable without symptoms at rest and with a sufficient work tolerance in every-day life. In addition all of them suffered from relevant coronary artery disease that had been angiographically confirmed during the past 6 months (for details see Table 1). Three patients were included with previous anterior myocardial infarction and six with previous inferior infarction. Those with a severely compromised left ventricular performance were excluded so that in all patients ejection fraction was within normal ranges. No one was subject to a symptomatic limitation of work tolerance due to either peripheral arterial occlusive disease or degenerative or rheumatic disorders of the skeletal system.

Each patient's individual therapeutic regimen with regard to cardiac (nitrates, Ca-channel blockers) and pulmonary medication (theophylline, β-agonists, and parasympatholytics, mucolytics) was continued; β_2-agonists and vagolytic agents were withheld for at least 12 h.

The patients underwent spirometry and exercise testing before and after the administration of salbutamol and oxitropium bromide with a dose of 0.2 mg each and placebo with a dose-metered inhaler according to a double-blind protocol in random sequence. Each study period was separated from the next by at least 24 h. Tests were performed at 10 a.m. Baseline spirometry and spiroergometry were repeated 10 resp. 30 minutes after the administration of the aerosol.

The spirogram was recorded using a Jaeger spirometer (Würzburg, FRG) to measure vital capacity (VC) and forced exspiratory volume in one second (FEV_1).

Standardized symptom-limited spiroergometry started at a workload of 25 watts (W) with graded increments of 15 W every minute. The effects of exercise on cardiopulmonary variables were quantified with a computerized breath-by-breath technique employing an infrared CO_2-analyzer, a zirkonium cell O_2-analyzer, and a pneumotachometer (Medical Graphics Corp., St. Paul, USA). Minute ventilation ($\dot{V}E$), oxygen uptake ($\dot{V}O_2$), and carbon dioxide output ($\dot{V}CO_2$) were determined for each breath by direct analysis of expired air. Anaerobic threshold (AT) was calculated from the relation between $\dot{V}CO_2$ and $\dot{V}O_2$, with AT being defined as the point

Table 1. Clinical features and findings in pulmonary function and coronary arteriography of the 15 patients.
Abbrevations: VC = vital capacity (percent of the predicted value); FEV_1 = forced exspiratory ventilation in 1 s (percent of the predicted value). Coronary status: LAD = left anterior descending artery; RCX = circumflex artery; RCA = right coronary artery, (numbers denote percent of stenosis, i.e. = stenosis < 50%; occ. = occlusion); EF = ejection fraction.

No.	Gender/age	FEV 1(%)	VC (%)	Coronary Status			EF (%)
				LAD	RCX	RCA	
1	m/58	46	54	60	—	70	57
2	m/50	64	79	occ.	—	occ.	53
3	m/67	42	78	—	occ.	occ.	61
4	m/72	49	94	60	50	50	61
5	m/62	28	60	50	50	—	71
6	m/67	37	54	50	—	occ.	57
7	m/61	32	69	60	70	50	66
8	m/59	71	77	50	—	occ.	68
9	m/54	75	91	60	60	occ.	75
10	f/56	70	78	90	—	occ.	53
11	m/50	74	93	50	60	occ.	25
12	m/67	33	59	occ.	—	70	45
13	m/58	72	87	50	—	70	50
14	m/59	78	97	—	occ.	60	47
15	m/61	48	92	70	50	occ.	61

of departure from linearity [5, 37]. Throughout exercise, arterial blood pressure was recorded every minute; the ECG was monitored continuously. The study was performed after informed consent.

Data analysis

The results of pulmonary function analysis were expressed as percent change of the predicted normal values.

The effect of inhaled bronchodilator on spiroergometric parameters was quantified as the percent change compared to the baseline examination before the administration of the aerosol.

Analysis of drug-induced changes was performed using Wilcoxon's paired sample rank test [41]. P-values < 0.05 were considered significant.

Results

All of the 15 patients included in the study underwent pulmonary function analysis and sequential cardiopulmonary exercise testing before and after the administration of inhaled salbutamol (S), oxitropium bromide (O), and placebo (P).

The following results were obtained (Fig. 1)

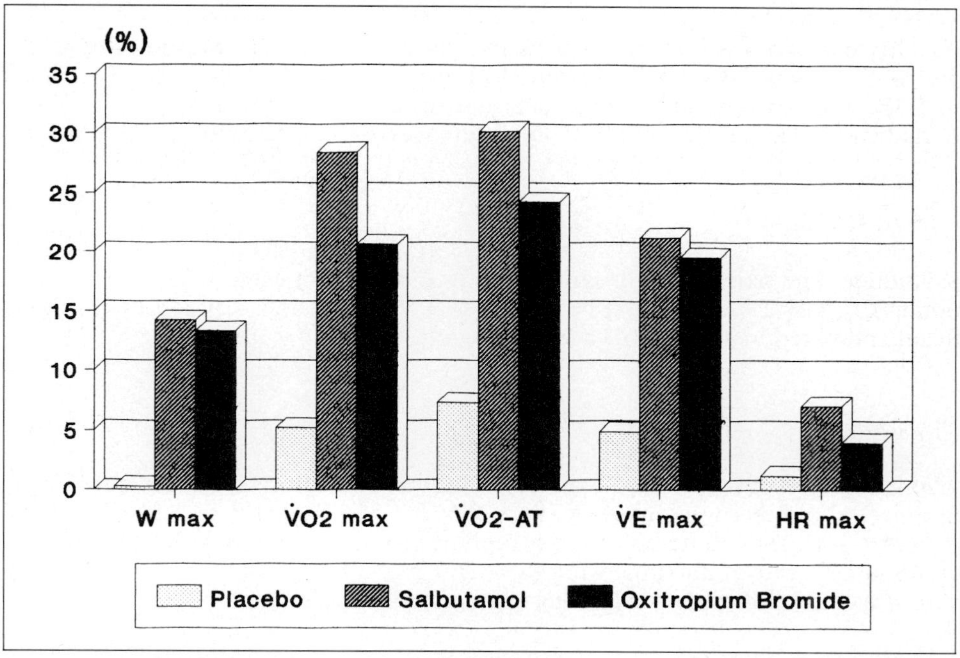

Fig. 1. Effect of inhalation with placebo, salbutamol, and oxitropium bromide on exercise capacity: Increase of cardiopulmonary variables in patients with COPD and CAD expressed in percent of baseline (pre-inhalation test). Abbr.: W_{max} = maximal work load; $\dot{V}O_{2max}$ = maximal oxygen uptake; $\dot{V}O_2$-AT = oxygen uptake at the anaerobic threshold; $\dot{V}E_{max}$ = maximal minute ventilation; HR_{max} = maximal heart rate.

Pulmonary function at rest

FEV_1 increased from baseline after the inhalation: placebo: + 1.2 ± 3.6% (ns); salbutamol: + 11.4 ± 2.1% ($p < 0.05$); oxitropium bromide: + 9.7 ± 1.6% ($p < 0.05$).

Maximal workload

Salbutamol and oxitropium bromide caused a significant ($p < 0.05$) overall increase of W_{max} (S: + 14.2 ± 2.9%, O: + 13.3 ± 6.0%) compared to the effect of placebo: + 0.3 ± 3.4%.

Oxygen uptake

The $\dot{V}O_2$ attained at the peak work rate ($\dot{V}O_{2max}$) was significantly ($p < 0.05$) influenced by salbutamol (+ 28.4 ± 4.4%) and oxitropium bromide (+ 20.6 ± 4.6%) in comparison to placebo (+ 5.2 ± 5.5%).

Anaerobic threshold

For the complete sequence of six tests the anaerobic threshold was detected in 13 out of 15 patients (86.6%). Salbutamol averaged an increase of $\dot{V}O_2$-AT of 30.2 ± 5.3%, and oxitropium bromide caused a mean improvement by 24.2 ± 3.0%. Both displayed a significant ($p < 0.05$) difference from the placebo (+ 7.3 ± 4.7%).

Minute Ventilation

Salbutamol and oxitropium bromide increased maximum exercise minute ventilation ($\dot{V}E_{max}$) by 21.2 ± 3.0% (S) and 19.5 ± 3.1% (O). These differences are significant compared to 4.9 ± 3.6% achieved by placebo.

Heart rate

After inhalation of salbutamol, oxitropium bromide and placebo no relevant change in pulse rate at rest was observed (P: + 0.6 ± 1.8%, S: + 1.3 ± 2.1%, O: + 0.5 ± 3.2%). Neither salbutamol nor oxitropium bromide had a significant influence on peak heart rate at maximal work (S: + 7.0 ± 2.1%, O: + 4.0 ± 1.2%, P: + 1.2 ± 1.4%) compared to the preceeding test before inhalation.

Electrocardiogram

Stress ECG revealed no additional ischemic ST-T-segment changes after salbutamol and oxitropium bromide compared to the test before the administration. An aggra-

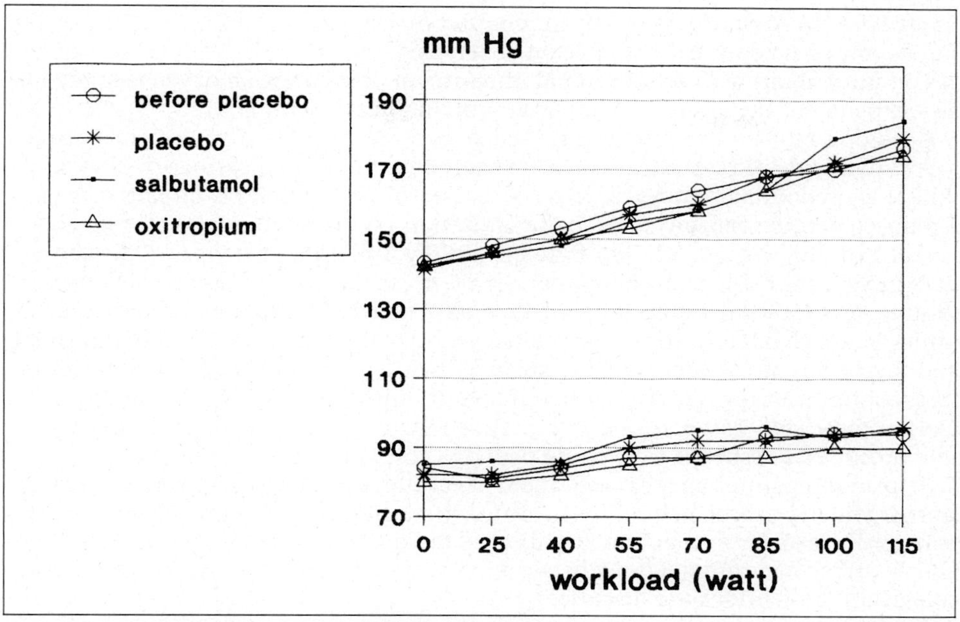

Fig. 2. Blood pressure profile with stepwise work load increase before and after the inhalative administration of placebo, salbutamol, and oxitropium bromide.

vation of preexisting arrhythmias after inhalation at rest and during exercise could not be detected.

Blood Pressure

No significant differences of blood pressure at rest, at each stage of exercise, and at maximal work load between pre- and postinhalation measurements were registered (Fig. 2).

Discussion

Pharmacologic agents used in the management of obstructive airways disease comprise among others β-adrenergic agonists and anticholinergics [1, 13, 31]. Both groups of bronchodilators exert a direct effect on the level of bronchomotor tone by the modulation of sympathetic and parasympathetic activity [1]. β-adrenergic agents are believed to cause bronchodilation mainly in small airways, whereas the site of action of anticholinergic drugs is still under discussion [3, 15, 18]. Due to their immediate onset of action, inhalation therapy with both agents has found a widespread application in respiratory care [1, 11, 33, 35].

The effect of bronchodilation on exercise capacity in patients with respiratory impairment due to chronic obstructive pulmonary disease is a point of special interest with no general agreement among the investigators [9, 10, 17, 19, 22, 27]. Furthermore, no data are available on beneficial or adverse effects of these substances on individuals with an additional impairment of myocardial oxygen supply due to narrowing of the main coronary artery branches.

Cardiopulmonary exercise testing is an appropriate tool to discriminate between a cardiovascular or respiratory cause for exercise limitation. If cardiac or circulatory failure is predominant, oxygen delivery to the working muscles is impaired causing a reduced aerobic capacity. Metabolic limitation occurs when the breathing reserve is still high [28, 29, 36, 37, 38]. Patients mainly limited by respiratory disease underlie exhaustion far from the borders of their cardiovascular capacity. Maximum minute ventilation is reduced by air flow obstruction. Patients with ventilatory limitation are characterized by low peak oxygen uptake, normal anaerobic threshold, and high respiratory rates whereas low maximal oxygen uptake and low anaerobic threshold are suggestive of a cardio-circulatory disorder [28, 29, 37, 38, 39]. Peak oxygen pulse may serve as as crude proportionate of stroke volume and the heart rate profile as a response to exercise demasks chronotropic incompetence.

By providing simultaneous assessment of cardiovascular and respiratory function, spiroergometry can be helpful in the differential diagnosis. In patients with coexistent cardiovascular and pulmonary disease the dominant factor can be identified. On the other hand interactions between both systems and side effects of pharmacological interventions are disclosed.

Thus, the present study was designed to assess the influence of a beta-adrenergic drug, salbutamol, and an anticholinergic agent, oxitropium bromide — on cardiopulmonary exercise capacity of patients with both COPD and CAD. Additional regard was given to adverse cardiac effects, which are of special interest in patients with imbalanced myocardial oxygen supply.

According to our findings, maximal oxygen uptake as well as maximum minute ventilation were significantly increased by salbutamol and oxitropium bromide. Maximum O_2 uptake is generally considered to be the best available index of exercise capacity and can be used for precise objective determination of cardiopulmonary fitness or disability [28, 29, 37, 38, 39]. Other indices, e.g. exercise duration or the stage achieved in a certain protocol have been used to estimate exercise capacity, but they are less reproducible than $\dot{V}O_{2max}$ [28, 39]. Variables influencing the value of these parameters are the patient's effort and motivation [28]. Based on these less objective parameters other authors have tested the influence of bronchodilation on exercise tolerance in COPD. Connolly and coworkers [10] found a significant clinical improvement achieved in a 6-minute walk test after the inhalation of salbutamol and ipratropium bromide in 36 patients with obstructive airways disease. According to Guyatt [17], salbutamol produces an increase in exercise capacity in a 12-minute walk test.

Additionally, bronchodilation with salbutamol and oxitropium bromide was associated with achieving the anaerobic threshold at an increased oxygen comsumption. The anaerobic threshold allows an accurate assessment of the work rate that a patient can sustain for a prolonged period of time without exhibiting an increase in lactate [5, 37, 38—40]. When the metabolic demands of exercise begin to exceed O_2 delivery to working muscles, anaerobic metabolism ensues, limiting the duration of constant work rate exercise [28, 40]. The delayed achievement of the anaerobic threshold at higher levels of oxygen uptake demonstrates improvement of work tolerance at a submaximal level by salbutamol and oxitropium bromide in the patient group studied. The increases achieved with regard to the anaerobic threshold correspond to the patients' daily activities.

Antiobstructive pharmacotherapy of COPD in patients with a concurrent relevant CAD implies the risk of an increase in myocardial oxygen demand potentially provoking ischemic episodes or arrhythmias [13, 26, 35]. To circumvent cardiac side-effects, the older sympathomimetic agents (e.g. epinephrine and isoproterenol) have mostly been replaced by the newer more β_2-specific bronchodilators, such as salbutamol, fenoterol, terbutaline [35]. Anticholinergic drugs applied in the management of COPD are synthetic quarternary ammonium congeners of atropine [2, 11, 15, 26]. Unlike the mother-substance, its derivatives ipratropium bromide and oxitropium bromide exert less adverse cardiac effects [4, 12, 13, 24, 26, 30). Locally administered as an aqueous aerosol, β_2-agonists as well as anticholinergic drugs are unlikely to produce marked side-effects in patients with a healthy cardiovascular system [21, 30, 33].

In our patients with both COPD and CAD neither salbutamol nor oxitropium bromide caused an aggravation of exercise-induced ST-T-segment changes or preexistent arrhythmias. The heart-rate profile at rest, exercise, and during recovery was not significantly influenced; neither was blood pressure affected at rest and during exercise.

The minimal cardiovascular effects of inhaled salbutamol and oxitropium bromide and the significant improvement in oxygen uptake and minute ventilation make us believe that the increase in submaximal and maximal work capacity is mainly due to local bronchodilation.

Conclusion

In patients with COPD and concurrent CAD, inhaled salbutamol as well as oxitropium bromide can markedly increase cardiopulmonary exercise tolerance. Relevant cardiac side-effects seem to be of minor importance.

Summary

In patients with both chronic obstructive pulmonary disease (COPD) and coronary artery disease (CAD) cardiopulmonary exercise testing (CPX) was performed to assess the benefits and adverse cardiac effects of inhaled salbutamol and oxitropium bromide. Fifteen patients suffering from COPD (mean FEV_1 56% of the predicted value) and CAD (10 with two-vessel-, 5 with three-vessel disease, mean ejection fraction 61%) underwent spirometry and standardized spiroergometry. Exercise tests were performed before and after the administration of inhaled salbutamol (S) and oxitropium bromide (O) with a dose of 0.2 mg each and placebo (P). The study was carried out double-blind; the effects were compared intraindividually. P improved FEV_1 by 1.2%, S by 11.4%, and O by 9.7%. Maximum workload was increased significantly ($p < 0.05$) following the administration of S (+ 14.2%) and O (+ 13.3%) compared to P (+ 0.3%). As for maximum minute ventilation the same effect ($p < 0.05$) was shown (S: + 21.1%, O: + 19.5%, P: + 4.9%). S and O caused a significant increase ($p < 0.05$) of maximum oxygen uptake (S: + 28.4%, O: + 20.6%, P: + 5.2%) and of the anaerobic threshold (S: + 30.2%, O: + 24.2%, P:

+ 7.3%) versus the effects of P. For the aforementioned parameters no significant difference between S and O was found. Heart rate response to maximal work load was not significantly influenced by S (+ 7.0%), O (+ 4.0%), and P (+ 1.2%). Stress ECG revealed neither additional exertional ST-T-wave changes nor aggravation of preexisting arrhythmias after bronchodilation by S or O.

Thus, in patients with both COPD and CAD, inhaled salbutamol and oxitropium bromide markedly improved aerobic and anaerobic cardiopulmonary work capacity without adverse cardiac effects.

References

1. American Thoracic Society: Standards for the diagnosis and care of patients with chronic obstructive pulmonary disease (COPD) and asthma. Am Rev Respir Dis (1987); 136: 225
2. Andersen G (1983) Anticholinergic drugs in airways obstruction. Postgrad Med J 59: 64
3. Anthonisen NR, Wright EC, IPPB Trial Group (1986) Bronchodilator response in chronic obstructive pulmonary disease. Am Rev Respir Dis 133: 814
4. Bauer R (1985) Zur Pharmakologie des Bronchospasmolytikums Oxitropiumbromid. Arzneim Forsch 35: 435
5. Beaver WL, Wasserman K, Whipp BJ (1986) A new method for detecting anaerobic threshold by gas exchange. J Appl Phyiol 60: 2020
6. Belman MJ (1986) Exercise in chronic obstructive pulmonary disease. Clinics Chest Med 7: 585
7. Braunwald E (ed) (1988) Heart disease 3rd edition Philadelphia WB Saunders
8. Choo-Kang YFJ, Simpson WT, Grant IWB (1969) Controlled comparison of the bronchodilator effect of three β-adrenergic stimulant drugs administered by inhalation to patients with asthma. Br Med J 2: 287
9. Clark JC, Cochrane LM (1988) Assessment of work performance in asthma for determination of cardiorespiratory fitness and training capacity. Thorax 43: 745
10. Conolly CK, Chan NS (1987) Salbutamol and ipratropium in partially reversible airway obstruction. Br J Dis Chest 81: 55
11. Firstrater E, Mizrachi E, Topilski M (1981) The effect of vagolytic drugs on airway obstruction in patients with bronchial asthma. Ann Allergy 46: 332
12. Floher E, Bischoff KO (1989) Oxitropium bromide, a new anticholinergic drug in a dose-response and placebo comparison in obstructive airway disease. Respiration 38: 98
13. Goodman LS, Gilman A (1989) The pharmacological basis of therapeutics (7th ed.) New York, Mc Millan
14. Gross NJ, Skorodin MS (1984) Anticholinergic, antimuscarinic bronchodilators. Am Rev Respir Dis 129: 856
15. Gross NJ (1986) COPD: a disease of reversible airflow obstruction. Am Rev Respir Dis 113: 725
16. Gross NJ, Bankwala Z: Effects of an anticholinergic bronchodilator on arterial blood gases of hypoxemic patients with chronic obstructive pulmonary disease (1987) comparison with a beta-adrenergic agent. Am Rev Respir Dis 136: 1091
17. Guyatt GH, Towsend M, Keller J, Singer J, Nogradi S (1989) Measuring functional status in chronic lung disease: conclusions from a randomized control trial. Respir Med 83: 293
18. Hensley MJ, O'Cain CF, McFadden ER jr, Ingram RH jr (1978) Distribution of bronchodilatation in normal subjects: beta agonist versus atropine. J Appl Physiol 45: 778
19. Ingeman-Hansen T, Bundgaard A, Halkjer-Kristensen J, Siggard-Andersen J, Weeke B (1980) Maximal oxygen consumption rate in patients with bronchial asthma — the effect of β_2-adrenoceptor stimulation. Scand J Clin Lab Invest 40: 99
20. Jones NL, Jones G, Edwards RHT (1971) Exercise tolerance in chronic airway obstruction. Am Rev Respir Dis 103: 477
21. Kennedy MCS, Simpson WT (1969) Human pharmacological and clinical studies on salbutamol: A specific β-adrenergic bronchodilator. Br J Dis Chest 2: 165

22. Leitch AG, Hopkin JM, Ellis DA, Merchant S, McHardy GJR (1978) The effect of aerosol ipratropium bromide and salbutamol on exercise tolerance in chronic bronchitis. Thorax 33: 711)
23. Loke J, Mahler D, Man SFP, Wiedeman HP, Matthay RA (1984) Exercise impairment in chronic obstructive pulmonary disease. Clin Chest Med 5: 121
24. Lulling J, Delwiche JP, Prignot J (1981) Early bronchodilating effect of oxitropium bromide in comparison with ipratropium bromide. Respiration 42: 188
25. McGavin CR, Artvinly M, Naoe H, McHardy GJR (1978) Dyspnoea, disability, and distance walked: comparison of estimates of exercise performance in respiratory disease. Br Med J 2: 241
26. Minette A, Marcq M (1979) Oxitropium bromide, an advance in the field of anticholinergic bronchodilating treatments. Preliminary results. Rev Inst Hyg Mines 34: 115
27. Mols P, Ham H, Naeije N, Dechamps P, Huyn Ch, Vandenbosch L, Sergysels R (1988) How does salbutamol improve the ventricular performance in patients with chronic obstructive pulmonary disease? Cardiovasc Pharmacol 12: 127
28. Neuberg GW, Friedman SH, Weiss MB, Herman MV (1988) Cardiopulmonary exercise testing. The clinical value of gas exchange data. Arch Intern Med 148: 2221
29. Neuberg GW (1990) Cardiopulmonary exercise testing. 97: 257
30. Pakes GE (1984) Anticholinergic drugs. In: Buckle DR, Smith H (eds.): Development of antiasthmatic drugs. London: Butterworths
31. Paterson JW, Woolcock AJ, Shenfield GM (1979) Bronchodilator drugs. Am Rev Resp Dis 120: 1149
32. Petrie GR, Palmer KNV (1975) Comparison of aerosol ipratropium bromide and salbutamol in chronic bronchitis and asthma. Br Med J 1: 430
33. Riding WD, Dinda P, Catterjee SS (1970) The bronchodilator and cardiac effects of five pressure-packed aerosols in asthma. Br J Dis Chest 64: 37
34. Spiro SG, Hahn HL, Edwards RHT, Pride NB (1975) An analysis of the physiological strain of exercise in patients with chronic obstructive bronchitis. Thorax 30: 415
35. Svedmyr N (1977) Treatment with beta-adrenostimulants. Scand J Resp Dis 58: 5
36. Swinburn CR, Wakefield JM, Jones PW (1985) Performance, ventilation and oxygen consumption in three different types of exercise tests in patients with chronic obstructive lung disease. Thorax 40: 581
37. Wasserman K (1987) Determinants and detection of anaerobic threshold and consequences of exercise above it. Circulation 76 (suppl VI): 29
38. Wasserman K, Hansen JE, Sue DY, Whipp BJ (1987) Principles of exercise testing and interpretation. Philadelphia: Lea & Febiger,
39. Weber KT, Janicki JS (1986) Cardiopulmonary exercise testing. Philadelphia: WB Saunders,
40. Whipp BJ (1987) Dynamics of pulmonary gas exchange. Circulation (1987) 76 (suppl VI): 18
41. Zar JH (1984) Biostatistical analysis (2nd ed.), Prentice-Hall, Inc., Englewood Cliffs, New Jersey

Author's address:
Franz von Erckelens, M.D.
Medical Clinic I
RWTH Aachen
Pauwelsstr. 30
5100 Aachen FRG

Cardiopulmonary Exercise Testing in the Diagnosis of HIV-Infected Patients

G. Pothoff, K. Wassermann, A. Gitt, H. Ostmann, U. J. Winter, H. W. Höpp, H. H. Hilger

Medical Clinic III, University of Cologne, FRG

Introduction

Pulmonary complications are a major cause of morbidity and mortality in patients with acquired immunodeficiency syndrome (AIDS). Full-blown pneumocystis carinii pneumonia (PCP) with fever, cough, dyspnea, interstitial infiltrates in the x-ray, and low oxygen tension in the arterial blood gas analysis is easy to diagnose. In contrast, early diagnosis of PCP is difficult, because x-ray of the chest and arterial oxygen tension are often normal and respiratory symptoms are unspecific. Early treatment of pulmonary complications improves prognosis of the HIV-infected patients, therefore functional screening tests for early recognition are needed. Exercise blood gas analysis (Ex.-BGA) has been proven to be a highly sensitive marker of approaching interstitial pneumonia [1]. Cardiopulmonary exercise testing (CPX) measures pulmonary gas exchange and is a modern computerized version of spiroergometry, used to test cardiopulmonary limitations to exercise. Little is known about CPX in the diagnosis of HIV-associated pulmonary complications. It was therefore the aim of our study to investigate the diagnostic value of CPX for early diagnosis of pulmonary complications in HIV-infected patients.

Patients

Thirty HIV-infected patients with unspecific respiratory symptoms such as cough, mild dyspnea, and fever were included into the study. Twenty-nine patients were male, one female. Mean age was 38 ± 7 years. One patient had mild chronic obstructive airway disease, 13 patients had recovered from a first episode of PCP, and 14 patients were smokers. Eighteen patients were treated with daily application of azido-thymidine; 25 patients took part in a monthly pentamidine inhalation protocol. According to the Walter Reed classification, one patient (pts.) was graded to WR 2, three pts. to WR 4, 11 pts. to WR 5, and 15 pts to WR 6.

To detect approaching pulmonary complications all patients underwent spirometry, CPX-testing, and Ex.-BGA. Due to increasing respiratory symptoms in the days after testing, 16/30 patients underwent flexible-fiber bronchoscopy with bronchoalveolar lavage and transbronchial biopsy. In all 16 patients (group I) bronchoscopy revealed pulmonary complications as listed in Table 1. In the remaining 14 patients (group II) no progress of respiratory symptoms appeared within a follow-up period of 8 weeks. Exercise data of group I and group II were compared in order to detect exercise markers indicating early stages of HIV-associated pulmonary complications.

Table 1. Results of diagnostic fiber bronchoscopy in 16 HIV-infected patients with suspected pulmonary complication.

Total	n = 16
Pneumocystis carinii pneumonia	n = 7
Bacterial bronchitis	n = 2
Tuberculosis	n = 2
Interstitial pneumonitis	n = 3
Kaposi's sarcoma	n = 1
Granulomatous pneumonitis	n = 1

Methods

Spirometric parameters were estimated with a commercially available pneumotachograph (Custovit, Custo Corp.). Decreases < 75% of a standard population [2] in vital capacity (VC) and forced expiratory volume (FEV1) were defined as abnormal.

CPX-measurements were assessed with a bicycle spiroergometer-equipment (Medical Graphics Corp.) using breath-by-breath analysis of respiratory gas exchange. After measurement of resting values, an exercise protocol was used with a workload that increased continuously at a rate of 20 watts/min. Patients pedalled at 60 cycles/min until exhaustion. One patient did not reach the anaerobic threshold. Spiroergometric parameters and criteria for grading them abnormal are listed below:

$\dot{V}O_{2max}$: maximal oxygen uptake; judged by Weber's classification [3] A-E:
A: > 20 ml/min/kg (normal O_2-uptake);
B: 16—20 ml/min/kg (mild decrease);
C: 10—16 ml/min/kg (moderate decrease);
D: 6—10 ml/min/kg (severe decrease);
E: < 6 ml/min/kg (very severe decrease).

AT: anaerobic threshold; judged by Weber's classification [3] A-E:
A: > 14 ml/min/kg (normal AT);
B: 11—14 ml/min/kg (mild decrease);
C: 8—11 ml/min/kg (moderate decrease);
D: 5—8 ml/min/kg (severe decrease);
E: < 4 ml/min/kg (very severe decrease).

HR: heart rate: predictive maximum [4]: 220-age.

O_2-pulse: $\dot{V}O_2$/HR; abnormal < 85 % of a standard population [4].

VD/VT: relation of physiologic dead space to tidal volume; characterized by the difference of exercise VD/VT minus resting VD/VT, abnormal > 0.19 [4].

$AaDO_2$: alveolar to arterial difference of O_2; characterized by the difference of exercise $AaDO_2$ minus resting $AaDO_2$, abnormal > 5 mmHg.

AT was calculated using the V-slope method [5]. VD/VT was measured using the Enghoff modification of the Bohr equation: $(PaCO_2\text{-}PeCO_2)/PaCO_2 - VDm/Vt$, where $PaCO_2$ is arterial PCO_2, $PeCO_2$ is mixed exspired PCO_2, VDm is mechanical dead space (valve), and Vt is tidal volume. $AaDO_2$ was calculated with the equation $(FIO_2 \times (Pb\text{-}\ 47)\text{-}PaCO_2/R) - PaO_2$, where FIO_2 is the fraction of inspired O_2, Pb is the barometric pressure, $PaCO_2$ is the arterial PCO_2, R is the gas-exchange ratio, and PaO_2 is the arterial O_2-tension. Ex.-BGA was estimated with a capillary technique [6]. PO_2, PCO_2, and pH were measured at rest and immediately before stopping exercise, using a conventional blood gas analyzer (ECCO 2000, Eschweiler Corp.).

Unpaired t-test was used to perform statistical analysis; p-values < 0.05 were judged as significant.

Results

Mean values, standard deviations, and statistical comparison of spirometric and CPX-measurements in group I and II are listed in Table 2.

There was no statistical difference in $\dot{V}O_2max$, AT, HR, and O_2-pulse.

In contrast, the exercise difference of $AaDO_2$ was significantly different between both groups. In group II the mean $AaDO_2$-difference from rest to exercise was normal (-0.3 ± 7.3); in group I it was considerably pathologic (13.1 ± 17.4).

Statistically significant differences between groups I and II were also found for VD/VT, FEV1, and VC.

While VD/VT in group II decreased regularly, the decrease in group I was abnormally low.

Mean FEV1 in group I was slightly reduced and normal in group II. Mean VC in both groups was normal despite significant statistical differences between the two groups.

$\dot{V}O_2max$, AT, $AaDO_2$, VD/VT, FEV1, and VC were related to the groups of various pulmonary diseases found at bronchoscopy.

For both groups, $\dot{V}O_2max$ and AT (s. Fig. 1, 2) were randomly distributed within the total range of Weber's classification. No differences were seen between the various groups of PCP and non-PCP complications or with group II.

In contrast, the $AaDO_2$-difference (Fig. 3) differed between group I and group II. Thirteen of 14 pts. in group II had a normal $AaDO_2$, but 6/7 pts. with PCP and 5/9 pts. with non-PCP complications had pathologic $AaDO_2$-differences. High $AaDO_2$-differences > 20 mmHg were noted in 5 pts. of the PCP-group, whereas pathologic values in the non-PCP groups were in a lower range of 9—15 mmHg. The two pts. with bacterial bronchitis had normal $AaDO_2$-differences.

Table 2. Comparison of spirometric and CPX-measurements in 16 HIV-infected patients with pulmonary complications (group I) and a control group of 14 patients (group II). (For further details see text.)

	Group I	Group II	
$\dot{V}O_2max$ (ml/min/kg)	16.7 ± 6.2	19.4 ± 4.4	n.s.
AT (ml/min/kg)	11.4 ± 4.9	14.3 ± 4.0	n.s.
HR (beats/min)	139 ± 13	147 ± 14	n.s.
O_2-pulse ($\dot{V}O_2$/HR)	8.0 ± 3.2	8.9 ± 2.6	n.s.
$AaDO_2$ (ex.-diff.)	13.1 ± 17.4	-0.3 ± 7.3	$p < 0.0005$
VD/VT (ex.-diff.)	-0.13 ± 0.06	-0.23 ± 0.09	$p < 0.05$
FEV1 (%)	68.4 ± 9.8	78.0 ± 6.8	$p < 0.05$
VC (%)	88.2 ± 13.9	97.8 ± 11.3	$p < 0.05$

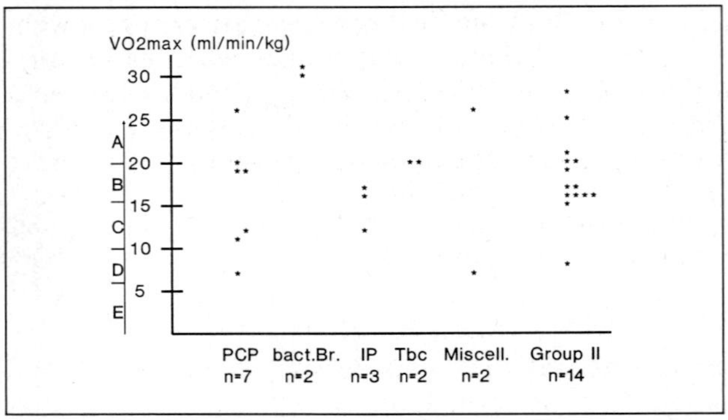

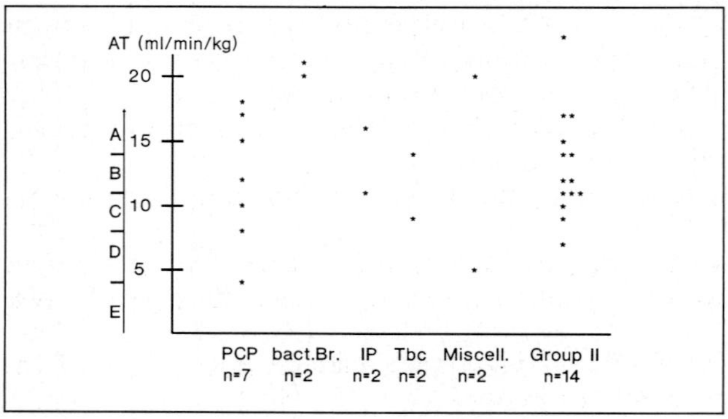

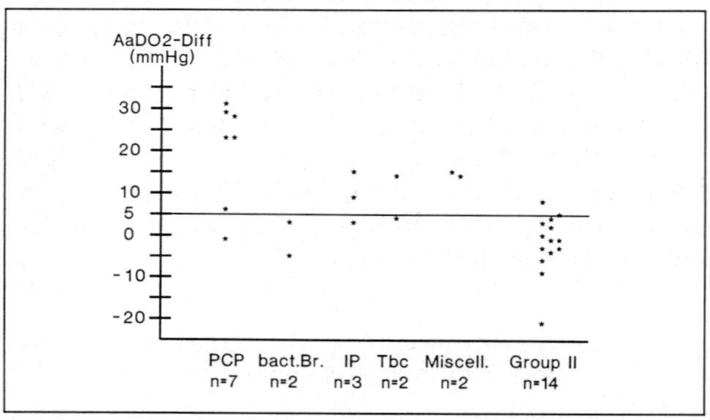

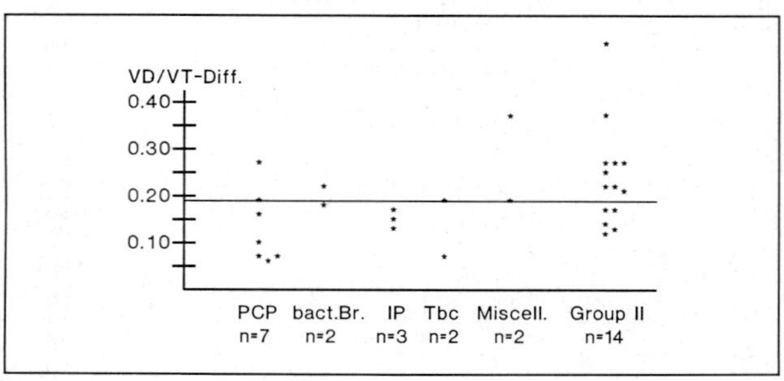

Figs. 1–4. $\dot{V}O_2$max, AT, $AaDO_2$-difference with exercise, and VD/VT-difference with exercise related to groups of various pulmonary diseases assessed by bronchoscopy (PCP = pneumocystis carinii pneumonia; bact. Br. = bacterial bronchitis; IP = interstitial pneumonitis; Tbc = tuberculosis; Miscell. = granulomatous pneumonitis 1 × and Kaposi's sarcoma 1 ×). Group II, as a control-group, is represented by 14 HIV—infected patients without acute pulmonary disease within a period of 8 weeks after CPX-testing. The cross-beam in Figs. 3 and 4 marks the line between normal and pathologic values. Class A-E in Figs. 1 and 2 characterizes Weber's classification. (For interpretation see text.)

VD/VT (Fig. 4) was pathologic in 6/7 pts. of the PCP and 7/9 pts. of the non-PCP subgroups in group I. In contrast to $AaDO_2$, there were more pts. with a pathologic test result in group II. Only 9/14 pts. in group II had a normal VD/VT-difference.

Differences in FEV1 or VC were not observed between the five groups of patients. A reduced FEV1 was measured in 4/7 pts. of the PCP-group, 2/8 of the non-PCP groups, and 2/13 of group II. Normal VC was measured in all but two pts. of the PCP-group. Sensitivity and specificity for the $AaDO_2$-difference were 70% and 94%, and for the VD/VT-difference 86% and 70%, respectively.

Discussion

Functional screening tests for early recognition of pulmonary diseases in HIV-infected patients are needed because early treatment improves prognosis. Ex.-BGA is known to be a reliable parameter with high sensitivity for early diagnosis of PCP [1]. Abnormalities like hyperventilation at rest, however, with changes of PO_2, PCO_2, and the respiratory exchange ratio (RER) are not expressed by Ex.-BGA. This might lead to misjudgement in some cases. The $AaDO_2$ regards PO_2, PCO_2, and RER. Thus, it can be assumed to be a parameter of higher quality than Ex.-BGA. Stover et al. [7] report a 100% sensitivity of the $AaDO_2$-difference with exercise for early diagnosis of PCP, but, inaccurately, they calculated the $AaDO_2$-gradient out of Ex.-BGA, assuming RER at rest and exercise to be 0.8. Yet, they did not measure the true $AaDO_2$- difference.

In our study, $AaDO_2$ was calculated from arterial blood gas analysis and RER measurements with the CPX-equipment. The $AaDO_2$-difference was normal in all but one patient of group II, and abnormal in 11/16 pts. with a bronchoscopy-proven pulmonary disease. PCP was associated with the highest $AaDO_2$-differences in a range of about 20 mmHg, whereas the non-PCP complications had lower, but also definitely pathologic $AaDO_2$-differences. Thus, the $AaDO_2$-difference with exercise is a parameter of high sensitivity (70%) and of even better specificity (94%).

The ratio of VD/VT represents mismatching of ventilation to perfusion. Only 3/16 pts. with pulmonary disease had a normally reduced VD/VT-ratio with exercise. This indicates a high sensitivity (86%) for recognition of beginning pulmonary dysfunction. In contrast, 5/14 patients of group II had a reduced VD/VT with exercise. Thus, specificity of VD/VT (70%) as a marker of disease is lower as compared to the $AaDO_2$-difference.

A relationship of $\dot{V}O_2max$ and AT to early stages of pulmonary diseases could not be found. These findings are most consistent with the idea that $\dot{V}O_2max$ and AT are parameters that especially represent cardiac dysfunction and not ventilatory impairment.

Spirometric data, as well, were not indicators for HIV-associated pulmonary diseases. VC was normal in all but two pts. Likewise, FEV1 was reduced in only a few patients. In conclusion, the differences of $AaDO_2$ and VD/VT with exercise seem to be useful functional screening tests to detect early stages of pulmonary diseases associated with HIV-infection. $\dot{V}O_2max$, AT, and FEV1 seem to be inaccurate in detecting acute pulmonary complications.

References

1. Fätkenheuer G, Salzberger B, Allolio B, Pothoff G, Schrappe-Bächer M (1989) Exercise oximetry for early diagnosis of pneumocystis carinii pneumonia. Lancet 28 (1): 222, letter
2. EKGS (Europäische Gemeinschaft für Kohle und Stahl), Kommission der Europäischen Gemeinschaften: Leitfaden für die praktische Durchführung der Untersuchung der ventilatorischen Funktion durch die Spirographie (1973) Schriftenreihe Arbeitshygiene und Arbeitsmedizin, Luxemburg, Nr. 11
3. Weber KT, Janicki JS (1986) Cardiopulmonary Exercise Testing. WB Sauners, Philadelphia
4. Wasserman K, Hansen JE, Sue DY, Whip BJ (1986) Principles of exercise testing and interpretation, Philadelphia: WB Saunders
5. Hansen JE, Sue DY, Wasserman K (1984) Predicted values for clinical exercise testing. Am Rev Respir Dis 129: 549—55
6. Godfrey S, Wozniak ER, Courtenay RJ, Samuels CS (1971) Ear lobe blood samples for blood gas analysis at rest and during exercise. Brit J Dis Chest 65: 58—64
7. Stover DE, Greeno RA, Gagliardi AJ (1989) The Use of a Simple Exercise Test for the Diagnosis of Pneumocystis carinii Pneumonia in Patients with AIDS. Am Rev Respir Dis 139: 1343—1346

Author's address:

Günter Pothoff, M.D.
Medical Clinic III
University of Cologne
Joseph-Stelzmann-Str. 9
5000 Köln 41, FRG

Respiratory Parameters after Systemic Corticotropin-Releasing Hormone Administration

M. Nink[2], U. Krause[2], M. Coutinho[1], N. Treese[1], E. Salomon[2], H. Lehnert[2], J. Beyer[2]

Second Medical Clinic[1] and Third Medical Clinic[2], Mainz University Hospital, FRG

Introduction

Neuroanatomical studies on the distribution of corticotropin-releasing hormone (CRH) and its receptors (7) as well as physiological data suggest a regulatory function of endogenous CRH in hypothalamic and extrahypothalamic brain areas [1, 4]. Endogenous CRH acts within the endocrine hypothalamo-pituitary-adrenal axis and affects cardiovascular regulation and respiration through extrahypothalamic pathways. CRH also stimulates gluconeogenesis and release of plasma-catecholamines. Our experiments in humans also demonstrate an influence on respiration and on heart rate activity after systemic application of CRH. Respiratory parameters and heart rate were analyzed during steady-state conditions and also under various medications [2, 3] and under CO_2-challenge [6]. In order to evaluate whether the effects observed in experimental animals after central application of CRH were also present after peripheral application in man, we focussed our interest on the intraindividual and interindividual changes of minute volume, tidal volume, and on heart rate after systemic CRH-administration. Our findings should provide a deeper insight into mechanisms of neuronal regulation of respiratory and cardiac function. We also intended to find out whether there is a therapeutic effect on disorders of respiratory regulation in humans by CRH. We used two analogues of CRH, human CRH (hCRH) and ovine CRH (oCRH) (Bissendorf Peptide, Wedemark, FRG) with different biological half-life times. We wanted to specify the therapeutic effect of each analogue and to determine possible side effects.

Findings during conventional spirography

In more than 50 normals and in some patients with respiratory disorders we determined ventilatory flow, minute volume, tidal volume, breathing rate, and ratio of inspiration and expiration time. Partial pressures of CO_2 and O_2 at the mouth were measured with a mass-spectrometer. While performing these experiments, the nose of each subject had to be closed with a clamp and inspiration air was humidified continuously. Heart rate was calculated from ECG-recordings. While rebreathing CO_2, a silicone bag containing a hyperoxic gas mixture (35%O_2) was integrated into

---

This work contains parts of the doctoral thesis by E. Salomon (Mainz, 1991)
This study is supported by Bundesministerium für Forschung und Technologie (BMFT), grant No. 01KE88100

a closed circuit behind the pneumotachograph. Trials lasted for 8—10 minutes and maximal expiratory CO_2-concentration reached 7.5 vol%.

Resulting curves were stored on a continuous paper sheet of an eight-channel recorder. Calibration marks for CO_2 and O_2 and defined volume- and flow-signals were registered. Each parameter was calculated separately by evaluating the curves on the paper sheet. A computer system was used to perform statistical tests for data analysis.

We demonstrated a marked increase (60%—80%, $p < 0.01$) of minute volume in all subjects after systemic application of 33—100 μg hCRH (30s-bolus) [3]. The effects lasted for 5—8 min. Tidal volume also increased significantly ($p < 0.01$). Increases in breathing and heart rate were not significant ($p < 0.05$), although in some individuals marked increases of either parameter were seen. While performing CO_2-rebreathing trials, CRH induced a marked rise of ventilation in all subjects ($n = 12$) [6]. This rise was significant when compared to intraindividual ($p < 0.001$) and interindividual ($p < 0.01$) responses to placebo.

Stimulation of ventilation by CRH was also of therapeutics use in various groups of patients with hypoventilation syndromes.

To economize calculation of experimental data, defined time intervals (e.g. shortly after placebo-application or after CRH-application) were chosen for analysis. Thus, presentation of long-term effects after CRH was limited.

Use of a computerized cardiopulmonary exercise testing-system

In order to elaborate a therapeutic concept for CRH in various groups of hypoventilating patients, we intended to evaluate the effects of ovine CRH in a follow-up study. Since cortisol release after oCRH lasts longer than after hCRH, we wanted to find out whether a oCRH-induced ventilatory stimulation is also longer lasting than after hCRH. Furthermore, we intended to analyze the effects of various application-modes of both analogues (oCRH, hCRH) on resulting patterns of breathing. We further wanted to evaluate whether there are side effects of clinical relevance under specific treatment regimes (e.g. bolus-injection vs. continuous infusion).

We performed steady-state trials with the computerized cardiopulmonary exercise testing system by Medical Graphics Corporation (St. Paul, Minnesota, USA); mode of data display, cf. Fig. 1. The breathing-mask of the system permitted physiological breathing via nasal inspiration, thus preventing desiccation of airways with resulting artifacts induced by coughing. Preliminary tests had shown stable steady state conditions over more than 50 min.

Via a butterfly-cannula a continuous infusion of physiological saline (0.9%) was applied and hCRH or oCRH were injected in random order at alternating doses. Placebo injections (solvent of oCRH or hCRH) were used as control. Drug-induced changes of ventilatory and cardiac parameters were displayed on-line on a monitor. While the trials were still in process, incoming data were very helpful for planning the ongoing procedures of the trial (e.g. additional application of CRH, application of an augmented dose of CRH).

So far, we have performed 19 complex series under hCRH- and oCRH-application. We recognized qualitatively identical effects on ventilation by both analogues, although effects after oCRH were often longer lasting than after hCRH. In a crossover trial we treated 10 healthy volunteers with hCRH and oCRH (bolus of 100 μg

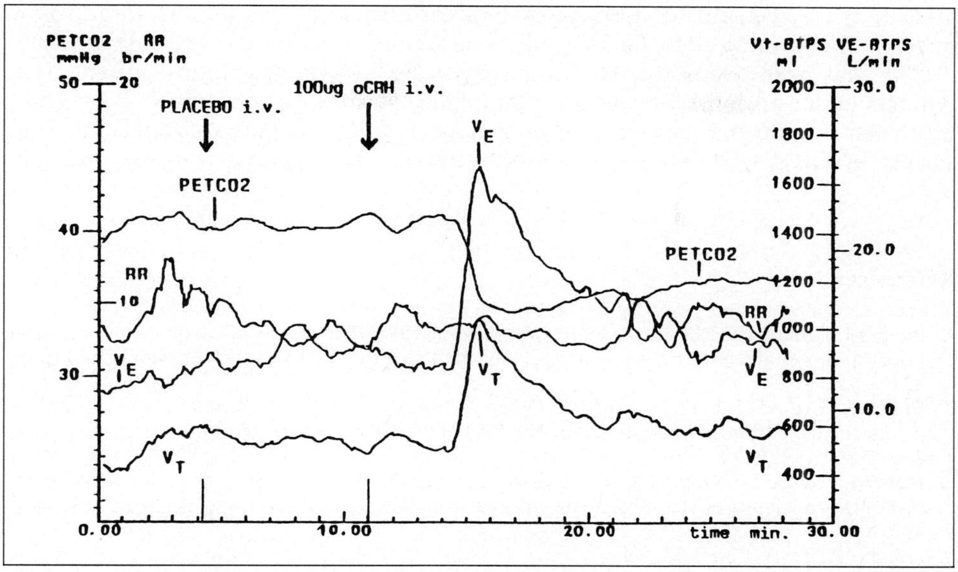

Fig. 1. Ventilatory parameters of a healthy male test subject, 35 years old, height: 1.88 m, body weight: 70 kg, during monitoring with the CPX-system "Medical Graphics 2001". Displayed are endexpiratory partial-pressures of CO_2 ($PETCO_2$), respiration rate (RR), tidal volume (VT), and minute volume ($\dot{V}E$). Initial placebo-application (solvent of CRH, 2 ml i.v.) does not alter steady state conditions. After 100 µg oCRH i.v. a marked stimulation of ventilation is demonstrated. (Original registration with graphical modifications)

each, 30s). Minute volume increased from 8.2 ± 1.7 l (placebo) to 12.0 ± 2.4 l ($p < 0.001$) in the first minute after hCRH and from 8.5 ± 1.2 l (placebo) to 12.6 ± 1.5 l in the first minute after oCRH ($p < 0.001$). Furthermore, an interindividual variety of ventilatory and cardiac drug-response was apparent following the initial peak response after CRH. Although we saw a rapid ventilatory response in all subjects after hCRH- and oCRH-application (see above) with a corresponding increase of heart rate in the majority of this group, cardiac response was little or completely absent in some individuals.

Considering this complex set of data, it is most desirable to install a system-integrated statistical analysis program for rapid data evaluation.

Conclusions

After systemic application of CRH, we showed a strong respiratory stimulation in several studies with human subjects. Only minor side effects were observed. Systemic CRH-application induced similar effects as were demonstrated after topical application at brain sites of experimental animals: both ventilation and heart rate were augmented. According to neuroanatomic findings, exogenous CRH may cross the blood-brain-barrier via defined anatomical structures and thus may reach brain areas that are relevant for respiratory and cardiovascular regulation. In addition, primary effects induced by CRH may be overlapped by secondary (peripheral) ones.

CRH has been tested for its therapeutic value in hypoventilating patients (e.g. patients under prolonged respirator therapy) [5] with positive outcome. There may be further insights in the role of neurohormonal regulation of the autonomic nervous system by CRH when statistically evaluating our data gained from gas exchange tests.

References

1. Bennet L, Gluckman PD, Johnston BM, Vale WW (1990) The effects of corticotropin releasing factor and two antagonists on breathing movements in the fetal sheep. J Physiol (Cambridge) 421: 1—11
2. Brauer A, Krause U, Nink M, Huber I, Velten A, Manz B, Lehnert H, Beyer J (1989) Studies on the mechanism of the respiratory analeptic effect of hCRH: the role of serotonin. Acta Endocrinol 120, Suppl 1: 226
3. Huber I, Krause U, Nink M, Lehnert H, Beyer J (1989) Dexamethasone does not suppress the respiratory analeptic effect of corticotropin-releasing hormone, J Clin Endocrin Metab 69: 440—442
4. Lehnert H, Beyer J, Nink M, Schrezenmeir J, Krause U (1988) Die Bedeutung von Corticotropin-releasing-Faktor für die Regulation autonomer und endokriner Funktionen. Med Klin 83: 763—768
5. Nink M, Lehnert H, Krause U, Brückner R, Welch J, Beyer J (1989) Effects of human corticotropin-releasing hormone (hCRH) on prolonged hypoventilation in patients on postoperative respirator therapy. J Endocrinol Invest 12, Suppl 2 (no. 5): 152
6. Schulz R, Nink M, Krause U, Lehnert H, Schulz V, Beyer J (1989) Einflußnahme von hCRH und TRH auf die CO_2-Atemantwortkurve. Atemwegs- und Lungenkrankheiten 15 (5): 212
7. De Souza EB (1989) Corticotropin-releasing factor receptor in the brain and pituitary: their role in the stress response. In: Tache Y, Morley JE, Brown MR (eds) Neuropeptides and stress. Springer, New York Berlin Heidelberg, pp 1—18

Author's address
Dr. Manfred Nink
III. Medizinische Klinik und Poliklinik-Endokrinologie
Klinikum der Johannes Gutenberg-Universität
Langenbeckstr. 1
6500 Mainz